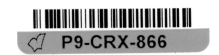
P9-CRX-866

CARDIOVASCULAR DISEASE IN RACIAL AND ETHNIC MINORITIES

CONTEMPORARY CARDIOLOGY

CHRISTOPHER P. CANNON, MD
SERIES EDITOR

For other titles published in this series, go to
www.springer.com/series/7677

CARDIOVASCULAR DISEASE IN RACIAL AND ETHNIC MINORITIES

Edited by

KEITH C. FERDINAND, MD

Cardiology Division,
Emory University,
Atlanta, GA, USA

and

ANNEMARIE ARMANI, MD

Department of Internal Medicine,
New Hanover Regional Medical Center,
Wilmington, NC, USA

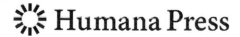 Humana Press

Editors
Keith C. Ferdinand, MD
Emory University
Cardiology Division
5355 Hunter Road
Atlanta GA 30349
USA
kferdinand@abcardio.org

Annemarie Armani, MD
Department of Internal Medicine
New Hanover Regional Medical Center
212 Walnut Street
Wilmington NC 28401 #101
USA
annemarie.armani@gmail.com

ISBN 978-1-58829-981-9   e-ISBN 978-1-59745-410-0
DOI 10.1007/ 978-1-59745-410-0
Springer Dordrecht Heidelberg London New York

Library of Congress Control Number: 2009920398

Printed on acid-free paper

Springer is part of Springer Science+Business Media (www.springer.com)

September 21, 1965

Dear Nar,

If I were Paul I would write an epistle or like Shakespeare I'd put it in drama form or if gifted for writing like Lil Val* I'd give you a vivid account of Hurricane Betsy. Since neither is possible, you must accept this rambling story of our two nights of a dreadful experience which happens only once in an individual's life cycle.........

.........Rescue work by helicopter was slow. That stopped at dark about 7 o'clock & people began to panic. I told Kenneth[†] and Keith and those around me that we may as well make the best of it, for no one knows we are here and help won't come until morning. Let us thank God for the glorious full moon, with which he lit up the sky. God folded all of his handiwork in one massive unit of power that night. The rain fell so hard that I had to take off my glasses & hide my head. The wind blew so hard that had there been one bit of let up everything would have blown dry. The water, still slowly rising, had two more inches to go before it reached the roof top. Our only hope then was the roof of the cafeteria.........

.........The worst part of the storm is going back to clean up. Everything is a total loss. The furniture broke up into splinters. We have not found the chest of drawers which we used to step into the attic. What is not destroyed is so filled with stench & slime that you'll throw it away. The one or two pieces of clothing, after many washings still seem to hold odor. Then too, mildew and other fungi vehemently attack everything.........

We learned: that communication and cooperation are necessary factors for survival in a disaster; that water is the most destructive force in the world; that ice, electricity, and telephone are precious possessions; that people are great.

Yours,

Inola

Excerpts from a letter, written by my mother, the late Inola Copelin Ferdinand, to her sister, Narvalee, after we survived dreadful days on the roof in the aftermath of Hurricane Betsy, which hit New Orleans, Louisiana, September 9, 1965, devastated the Lower Ninth Ward, and killed dozens of citizens, including my paternal grandfather, Vallery Ferdinand, Sr.

This text is dedicated to the people of the Republic of Haiti and New Orleans, Louisiana, United States of America and other victims and survivors of Hurricane Katrina and other natural and un natural disasters, and to the researchers, healers, and all those who have committed themselves to furthering the status and improving the lives of those who have been underserved.

This work is devoted to my wife Daphne, and children Kamau, Rashida, Aminisha, and Jua who are my sources of strength and inspiration.

Keith C. Ferdinand, MD

---

* My eldest brother, Kalamu ya Salaam (Vallery Ferdinand III)

[†] My 2nd eldest brother, Kenneth Ferdinand

I offer this text as a token of my appreciation to Alexander Armani for all his love and patience for his single working mother.

Annemarie Armani, MD

FOREWORD

This textbook, *Cardiovascular Disease in Racial and Ethnic Minorities*, confirms that there is much to be learned about some of the unique aspects of heart and vascular diseases related to various subpopulations. By studying differences in morbidity, mortality, and pathophysiology, the various authors assembled by Keith C. Ferdinand, MD, clearly illustrate areas of concern and much needed further research into health-care disparities, specifically related to race and ethnicity. Before my tenure as director of the Centers for Disease Control and Prevention (CDC), and later 16th Surgeon General and Assistant Secretary for Health, and onward until present time, I am personally committed to defining the best methods to understand health and illness and eliminate disparities related not only to race and ethnicity but also to gender, socioeconomic status, religion, and geography. One of the shared strengths of the American society is the ability to recognize circumstances which are unacceptable and seek means to compassionately address those unfortunate situations.

Prior to the Healthy People 2010 report, health experts including the authors of Healthy People 1990 and 2000, listed decreasing health disparities as a primary goal. However, as clinicians, public health scientists, and others now recognize, our ultimate goal should be and must be the elimination of disparities. As a society, we have effectively increased life expectancy over the last century by greater than 30 years and markedly improved quality of life. Nevertheless, disparities remain and are unacceptable. Therefore, our national goal to eliminate disparities versus short-term objectives related to specific risk factors should have no timeline. Both increasing access to health care and future research into genetics and genomics are essential. Nevertheless, these two areas combined may comprise only 35–40% of overall health determinants. Environmental factors, both physical and social, are paramount and must be addressed in order to eliminate disparities. Health is not just the absence of modern technological interventions. Culture counts; how people manifest diseases and illnesses is directly related to decision making, coping with stressors, life organization, and financial and educational attainment. Social determinants, poverty, and education, including health literacy and cross-culture sensitivity and communication are vital. To eliminate disparities will be a long and arduous task. These unfortunate, adverse situations have developed over centuries and will not be reversed in a few years of enlightened intercession. Dedicated, well-funded approaches to eliminate disparities, specifically related to cardiovascular diseases are essential. Physicians and other clinicians often lack the extensive knowledge base needed to approach cardiovascular disease in various racial and ethnic minorities. As Dr. Martin Luther King, Jr. most eloquently noted, "Of all the forms of inequality, injustice in healthcare is the most shocking and inhumane."

This excellent text, *Cardiovascular Disease in Racial and Ethnic Minorities*, will contribute greatly to our understanding of the present status of multiple cardiovascular conditions and related issues. The various authors and the editor should stimulate clinicians and others to purposeful action.

David Satcher, MD, PHD

PREFACE

This textbook on *Cardiovascular Disease in Racial and Ethnic Minorities* is designed to explore the importance of human genomic variation and the impact of environment on cardiovascular diseases. The Human Genome Project has confirmed that all human populations, regardless of self-identified race or ethnicity, are essentially the same, with widespread variation within self-defined racial groups. In this project, we did not attempt to confirm the validity of race, but to examine to what extent biomedical and scientific literature can clarify the impact of genetic variation versus environment as related to cardiovascular disease.

Specifically, this project was initiated with the encouragement of Annemarie Armani, MD, and is the culmination of our multiple prior collaborations, and our collective efforts to quantify and highlight accurate data and the unique aspects of cardiovascular-related conditions in multiple populations. In choosing varied areas of clinical practice and research, we sought to include experts who have both a history of academic rigor and a thoughtful reflection on these areas of study.

Medical knowledge is more than the simple accumulation of unrelated data. We learn from our patients, and when we delve into these sensitive areas of racial/ethnic disparities, we become better practitioners. In order to keep pace with the shrinking world, medical science must recognize that advances in transportation and communications increase global connectivity. In a 2008 document, the World Health Organization (WHO) confirmed that heart disease remains the top cause of worldwide mortality. Cardiovascular disease, including myocardial infarction, heart failure, and stroke, especially among women, accounts for 29% of deaths worldwide each year. This WHO report on the global burden of disease also confirmed that infectious diseases also contribute to 16.2% of worldwide deaths and thirdly, cancer causes 12.6% of global deaths. Furthermore, the WHO asserted that women die more often from heart disease than men (31.5% versus 26.8%). As noted throughout the text, the primary forces behind the consistent high rates of heart disease in various populations are persistently and increasingly overweight and obesity status, insufficient physical activity, and the excess consumption of fat and salt.

I was nurtured and educated by my parents, Vallery Ferdinand, Jr., and Inola Copelin Ferdinand, to be a force for positive change and contribute to the removal of inequities in our society. My first formal education beyond the shelter of my native Lower 9th Ward and the segregated South occurred as a

Telluride Scholar at Cornell University in Ithaca, New York. As a freshman, initially majoring in history, I was energized by the passion of the youth of the turbulent 1960s to make a difference in other people's lives. Along with several of my fellow student activists, I chose to serve my disadvantaged community through medicine. We considered it essential to use our formal training to impact the welfare of the African-American community and other disadvantaged groups only recently emerging from the shadows of an American experience crippled by racial strife and inequality.

Subsequently, at the historic Howard University, College of Medicine, I became convinced that internal medicine and specifically cardiovascular disease should be my primary area of research and clinical practice since African-Americans were clearly disproportionately affected by hypertension, heart failure, stroke, and end-stage kidney disease. Medical textbooks published before this time considered coronary heart disease to be a rare cause of morbidity/mortality in United States blacks. These earlier concepts were wrong. Cardiovascular heart disease mortality in African-Americans is the highest of all major racial/ethnic subpopulations in the United States.

As recently as 2008, organized medicine, specifically the American Medical Association (AMA), recognized its complicity in propagating racial inequality through an unfortunate history of omission and commission. Apologizing for these past errors, the AMA, along with the National Medical Association and the National Hispanic Medical Association, have created a commission to address healthcare disparities. The coalition's goals are to identify and promulgate means of eliminating health disparities (www.ama-assn.org). In this light, the best means for assessing nuances and significant findings related to cardiovascular disease in various populations is to address a broad range of topics with a diverse group of experts and I have invited submissions from a wide range of geographically and racially/ethnically diverse men and women.

In this book, we explore new findings and implications of genomics and inherence specifically related to single-nucleotide polymorphisms and the concept of ancestry versus the sociopolitical historical category of race. Perhaps in the future, medical research will not use the blunt, inaccurate determination of race as a category but will attempt to define the risk of certain diseases based on genomics, including better understanding and identification of these single-nucleotide polymorphisms. In the interim, the very presence of unacceptable cardiovascular disease disparities, based on race and ethnicity, specifically in the United States, indicates the need for universal access to evidence-based medicine, removal of socioeconomic barriers, and the application of therapeutic lifestyle changes for all individuals at increased risk.

Our understanding of cardiovascular disease in minority populations in the United States and eventually multiple populations worldwide must include the impact of environment. High rates of cardiovascular disease in various racial/ethnic populations will not be curtailed if we do not address obesity, diabetes, and the impact of westernization and urbanization of lifestyle. Describing the essence of Hawaiian culture in the provoking text, *Nā Kua'āina: Living Hawaiian Culture*, Davianna Pōmaika'i McGregor traces the unbroken lineage of native Hawaiians, noting that their very survival is related to their positive relationship to the land and resources where they live and work. Similarly, the various authors in this text recognize the impact of adverse lifestyle, especially urban living conditions on cardiovascular disease, and have weaved new and emerging data related to these findings throughout this work.

Medicine is both art and science. Clinicians who believe that medical knowledge is simply a collection of tangential data cannot fully appreciate the significant interaction between environment, culture, social economic status, and politics that impact the health of each individual in our society. The unique and forward-thinking Ghanaian author, Ayi Kwei Armah, wrote in his groundbreaking fiction/fact-filled novel of the need for Africans to embrace healers. In his 1978 allegorical tale, *The Healers*, he noted that there is greater power in healing than our individual desire for supremacy and accumulation of wealth. This power lies in the ability to help life recreate itself. Although Armah's text refers to African society and the need to overcome the wounds of colonialism, this concept can be applied to any environment where people have been unduly injured and suffer from lack of access to health, unequal application of modern, evidence-based medicine, or live in an environment burdened by poverty and adverse lifestyle.

In 25 years of direct patient care in cardiovascular medicine in my native Ninth Ward, New Orleans, Louisiana, I along with my wife, Daphne Pajeaud Ferdinand, PhD, APRN, maintained an independent, progressive cardiovascular center, Heartbeats Life Center, which served the people of our native Crescent City community. During the development of our clinic, it became increasingly evident that simply prescribing medications, and completing diagnostic testing, and interventional procedures would not successfully curb the disproportionate high levels of cardiovascular morbidity and mortality experienced in the community. On August 29, 2005, the Southern Gulf Coast was devastated by Hurricane Katrina, including the flooding of 80% of New Orleans and the devastated the Lower 9th Ward. Heartbeats Life Center remains at present an empty shell. Nevertheless, the study of cardiovascular medicine and the application of technologically advanced care must continue to respond to the needs of all populations. Working with the Association of Black Cardiologists, the National, Heart, Lung and Blood Institute on its ad-hoc community on minority populations, and the Center for Disease Control and Prevention, and others I have become increasingly aware of the subtle distinctions in how cardiovascular diseases present and are managed in various subgroups.

This compilation hopefully stands as one small effort to define and clarify the nuances of how racial/ethnic groups manifest cardiovascular illnesses and seeks best practices to control risk factors and eliminate unnecessary death and disability. The expert authors will hopefully be recognized for their significant contributions to the medical literature and prompt us to further overcome shortcomings in our understanding of the complex nature of various cardiovascular conditions.

"Wise people are not absorbed in their own needs. They take the needs of all people as their own."

Inspiration from Tao Te Ching

Keith Copelin Ferdinand, MD

ACKNOWLEDGMENT

The editor has been supported during this project and throughout my career by my wife, Daphne P. Ferdinand, RN, MN, PhD. Also, I would like to acknowledge the invaluable contribution of Annemarie Armani, MD in the initial conceptualization and development of this text.

CONTENTS

CONTRIBUTORS

ABRAR AHMED, MD, • *Department of Internal Medicine, Endocrinology and Diabetes Division, University of Missouri Columbia, Harry S Truman VA Hospital, Columbia, MO*

CHERYL A.M. ANDERSON, PhD, • *Johns Hopkins University, Baltimore, MD*

LAWRENCE J. APPEL, MD, MPH, • *Johns Hopkins University, Baltimore, MD*

ANNEMARIE ARMANI, MD, • *Department of Internal Medicine, New Hanover Regional Medical Center, Wilmington, NC*

LAVANYA BELLUMKONDA, MBBS, • *University of Minnesota, Minneapolis, MN*

IVOR J. BENJAMIN, MD, • *Division of Cardiology, University of Utah Health Sciences Center, Salt Lake City, UT*

JADA BENN-TORRES, PhD, • *Department of Anthropology, University of Notre Dame, Notre Dame, IN*

LUTHER T. CLARK, MD, • *State University of New York Downstate Medical Center, Brooklyn, New York*

TONYA L. CORBIN, MD, • *University of Michigan Health System, Department of Internal Medicine, Division of Cardiovascular Medicine, Ann Arbor, MI*

MELVIN R. ECHOLS, MD, • *Duke Clinical Research Institute, Durham, NC*

ERYNNE FAUCETT, BS, • *Michigan State University, School of Medicine, Lansing, MI*

KEITH C. FERDINAND, MD, • *Division of Cardiology, Emory University, Chief Science Officer, Association of Black Cardiologists, Atlanta, GA*

ICILMA V. FERGUS, MD, • *The Columbia University Harlem Hospital Center, Cardiology Division, New York, NY*

JOHN M. FLACK, MD, MPH, • *Division of Clinical Epidemiology and Translational Research and Endocrinology, Metabolism and Hypertension, Department of Internal Medicine, Wayne State University School of Medicine and the Detroit Medical Center, Detroit, MI*

MARY "TONI" FLOWERS, • *St. Joseph Mercy Oakland Hospital, Detroit, MI*

MEGAN E. GAUVEY-KERN, • *Johns Hopkins University, Baltimore, MD*

ROBERT L. GILLESPIE, MD, • *Sharp Rees-Stealy Medical Group, San Diego, CA*

ANUPAM GOEL, MD, • *Division of General Internal Medicine, Department of Medicine, University of California, San Diego School of Medicine, San Diego, CA*

KENNETH A. JAMERSON, MD, • *University of Michigan Health System, Department of Internal Medicine, Division of Cardiovascular Medicine, Ann Arbor, MI*

RICK A. KITTLES, PhD, • *Department of Medicine, Section of Genetic Medicine, The University of Chicago, Chicago, IL*

GUIDO LASTRA, MD, • *Department of Internal Medicine, Endocrinology and Diabetes Division, University of Missouri Columbia, Harry S Truman VA Hospital, Columbia, MO*

AMGAD N. MAKARYUS, MD, • *North Shore University Hospital, Manhasset, NY*

CAMILA MANRIQUE, MD, • *Department of Internal Medicine, Endocrinology and Diabetes Division, University of Missouri Columbia, Harry S Truman VA Hospital, Columbia, MO*

GEORGE A. MENSAH, MD, • *Centers for Disease Control and Prevention (CDC), Atlanta, GA*

JENNIFER H. MIERES, MD, • *New York University School of Medicine, New York, NY*

SAMAR A. NASSER, PA-C, MPH, • *Division of Clinical Epidemiology and Translational Research, Department of Internal Medicine, Wayne State University and the Detroit Medical Center, Detroit, MI*

SHANNON O'CONNOR, • *Michigan State University, School of Medicine, Lansing, MI*

ADE ONI, MD, MPH, • *Cardiovascular Epidemiology, Omni Primary Care Centers, Chattanooga, TN*

THEOPHILUS OWAN, MD, MSc, • *Division of Cardiology, University of Utah Health Sciences Center, Salt Lake City, UT*

LESLEE J. SHAW, PhD, • *Emory University School of Medicine, Atlanta, GA*

SABRINA SHAHEEN, MD • *State University of New York Downstate Medical Center, Brooklyn, NY*

JAMES R. SOWERS, MD, • *Department of Internal Medicine, Endocrinology and Diabetes Division, University of Missouri Columbia, Harry S Truman VA Hospital, Columbia, MO*

ANNE L. TAYLOR, MD, • *Columbia University Medical Center, College of Physicians and Surgeons, New York, NY*

KAROL E. WATSON, MD, • *Division of Cardiology, David Geffen School of Medicine at UCLA, Los Angeles, CA*

PETER W.F. WILSON, MD, • *Emory University School of Medicine, Dept of Medicine, Cardiology Division, Atlanta, GA*

CLYDE W. YANCY, MD, • *Baylor Heart and Vascular Institute, Dallas, TX*

1

Cardiovascular Disease in Racial/Ethnic Minorities: Overview and Perspectives

K.C. Ferdinand, MD
and A. Armani, MD

CONTENTS

Abstract

African-Americans have the highest rate of coronary disease mortality, premature death (including sudden death), stroke (fatal and non-fatal), hypertension, type 2 diabetes, and obesity (especially black females) when compared to whites. Cardiovascular health, life-expectancy, and health care, while improving dramatically for all Americans over the last century, have not been distributed

From: *Contemporary Cardiology: Cardiovascular Disease in Racial and Ethnic Minorities*
Edited by: K.C. Ferdinand and A. Armani, DOI 10.1007/978-1-59745-410-0_1
© Humana Press, a part of Springer Science+Business Media, LLC 2009

equitably. Racial/ethnic-based CVD research may offer the opportunity to clarify vital environmental and inherited aspects in the development of CVD, illustrate the importance of lifestyle, unmask variations in clinical practice, and potentially improve health-care delivery for all Americans. A review of the various chapters of this book is included, specifically highlighting important concepts related to the prevention of cardiovascular conditions in racial/ethnic minorities through the consideration of risk factors, treatment options, and clinical trials.

To combat the distressingly high rates of hypertension morbidity and mortality in African Americans, the International Society on Hypertension in Blacks (ISHIB) promulgated guidelines suggesting combination therapy and more intensive therapy for most black patients. Similarly, the National Cholesterol Education Program Adult Treatment Panel III delineates special considerations in African Americans. Simply identifying racial/ethnic health disparities will not eliminate them. Health-care education in the future should recognize the essential nature of the patient's cultural identity and experiences and understanding social factors and support systems. Clinicians must integrate an understanding of culture, lifestyle, socioeconomic status, the impact of psychological stress, and bias within the health-care system to assist patients with achieving positive outcomes.

Key Words: Cardiovascular disease; Evidence-based therapy; Racial/ethnic health disparities; CVD risk factors.

1. INTRODUCTION

The textbook, *Cardiovascular Disease in Racial and Ethnic Minorities*, is designed to provide clinicians, researchers, public health officials, and others with an advanced, comprehensive portrayal of current and evolving research in this area. The authors, each a leader in his or her respective field of practice and study, provide an evidence-based compilation of current considerations and perspectives. This state-of-the art review of research and clinical practice will hopefully assist with the eventual elimination of racial and ethnic health disparities in cardiovascular disease (CVD).

Despite the apparent continued improvement in cardiovascular (CV) mortality in the United States, CVD persists as the leading cause of death in this country and other industrialized societies. Moreover, the United States is increasingly a more heterogeneous population with larger percentages of racial/ethnic minorities *(1)*. Although race itself is not a biologic or genetic category, documented disparities in certain racial/ethnic subpopulations have been documented and confirm an imperative for public health initiatives to address this situation. Racial/ethnic-based CVD research may, in addition, offer the opportunity to clarify vital environmental and inherited aspects in the development of CVD, illustrate the importance of lifestyle, unmask variations in clinical practice, and potentially improve health-care delivery for all Americans. Alternatively, any proposed race-based, biological differences among subpopulations will become increasingly more difficult to identify as populations continue to merge.

More data are available in regards to African-Americans versus other racial groups because of the larger number and depth of studies involving that subgroup. Unfortunately, African-Americans have the highest rate of coronary disease mortality, premature death (including sudden death), stroke (fatal and non-fatal), hypertension, type 2 diabetes, and obesity (especially black females) when compared to whites *(2)*.

2. CURRENT CONCEPTS OF RACE AND ETHNICITY: FACTS AND FALLACIES

Race is, admittedly, a flawed concept. Furthermore, many social scientists are concerned that utilizing racial/ethnic categories may have the undesired consequence of minimizing important research into the critical areas of socioeconomic status, geography, psychological stress, and lifestyle. Nevertheless, studying CVD in racial/ethnic minorities is necessary to delineate and eventually eliminate unacceptable health disparities in both CV and non-CV conditions. Despite clear degrees of imprecision, specific recommendations of the US Department of Health and Human Services, Food and Drug Administration, Center for Drug Evaluation and Research, Center for Biologic Evaluation and Research, Center for Devices and Radiological Health, and Office of Commissioner were promulgated in September 2005 *(3)*. These guidelines for self-designation of race/ethnicity have become the federal standard, with a two-question approach regarding race and ethnicity, ethnicity preceding race.

Ethnicity, as used in the federal data, is defined as being of either Hispanic or non-Hispanic ancestry *(1)*. Hispanic origin may be considered the heritage, nationality group, lineage, or country of birth of the person or the person's ancestors before their arrival in the United States, regardless of race. For the categories related to race, the various choices include American Indian or Alaska Native, Asian, Black or African American, Native Hawaiian, or Other Pacific Islander, or white *(1)*.

Minorities in the United States continue to increase, with the Hispanic population – the fastest growing subpopulation and largest minority group – numbering 44.3 million in 2006, comprising 14.8% of the total population *(1)*. African-Americans, or blacks, totaled 40.2 million in 2006 and was recognized as the second-largest minority group, followed by Asians (14.9 million), American Indians and Alaskan Natives (4.5 million), and Native Hawaiians and Other Pacific Islanders (1 million). Recently, in 2008, the US Census Bureau estimated that by the year 2042, as much as 50% or more of the United States will be defined as non-white or member of an identified racial/ethnic minority, along with those self-identified as "some other race" or mixed race *(1)*.

The category, "Hispanic," includes Mexican Americans (the largest subgroup), Cuban Americans, Puerto Ricans, and persons with ancestry from South and Central America. The federal guidelines also provide alternative self-identification as Latino or Spanish. However, Hispanics include both individuals with ancestry from the mainly European Iberian Peninsula and darker-skinned persons whose familial ancestry derives from indigenous people from Mexico, Central America, and South America and those of African descent. Nevertheless, in the 2000 census, nine out of ten Hispanics or Latinos self reported as "white" or "some other race" *(1)*.

In the self-selection process, those defined as white may include persons whose immediate ancestry is not only from Europe but also from the Middle East and North Africa. Blacks, or African-Americans, have historically been thought of as descendents of continental Africans brought to the United States during the Atlantic slave trade. Nevertheless, there has been an increasing influx of blacks from Caribbean populations and continental Africa. American Indians and Alaska Natives include the original peoples of North and South America, and also Central America. Asians comprise an extremely heterogeneous category. Some Asian populations have somewhat lower CV risk and others have high degrees of CVD. Asians include persons from the Far East, Southeast Asia, or the Indian subcontinent and also such diverse peoples as those from Cambodia, China, India, Japan, Korea, Malaysia, Pakistan, the Philippine Islands, Thailand, and Vietnam. Native Hawaiian and other Pacific Islanders are also very heterogeneous and include, among others, the people of Hawaii, Guam, Samoa, and other Pacific Islands. Increasingly, Americans have become difficult to categorize at all, and the US Census also permits respondents to select more than one race, reflecting increasing intermixing. "Some other race" is a category available to those who self-identify outside of the five proposed race categories.

Despite the fact that the United States displays increasing diversity and unacceptable imbalances in CV morbidity and mortality, much of the positive evidence on CV medications and interventions has been accumulated essentially to the exclusion of racial and ethnic minorities, who are critically underrepresented in trials. Accordingly, the Agency for Healthcare Research and Quality (AHRQ) and others continue to monitor disparities in quality and access to care *(4)*. Some private and governmental grantors have mandated adequate participation of racial/ethnic groups in clinical research and the full disclosure of race/ethnic cohorts of the population studied. This is reasonable in view of data that in certain instances medications may not have the same efficacy in various racial/ethnic groups, or there may be nuances in terms of bioavailability, dosing, complications, or side effects.

3. OVERVIEW OF CVD IN RACIAL/ETHNIC MINORITIES CHAPTERS

3.1. *Epidemiology of Cardiovascular Diseases and Risk Factors Among Racial and Ethnic Populations in the United States*

The lead chapter of this compilation, by George A. Mensah, MD, *Epidemiology of Cardiovascular Diseases and Risk Factors Among Racial and Ethnic Populations in the United States*, confirms the high importance of epidemiology in defining the burden of CVD and various risk factors among minority populations. He astutely points out that CV epidemiology provides unique tools to assess disease burden and risk factors and leads to specific opportunities to identify increased risk in subpopulations and elucidate the existence of health disparities *(5)*. Mensah maintains that epidemiology plays a fundamental role in promoting and protecting CV health. Nevertheless, clinicians and researchers must recognize inherent weaknesses in the present understanding of racial/ethnic disparities, including a lack of data or different formats in various studies. One striking example of shortcomings in research related to race/ethnicity, he notes, is the prior misclassification of American Indians and Alaskan Natives as having the lowest mortality rates for major CVD, when in fact mortality rates for these populations are among the highest *(6)*.

The paramount importance of epidemiology is further highlighted by Mensah's stimulating discussion on disparities in life expectancy, based on geography and race, heavily impacted by socioeconomic status. He concludes that self-reported behavior and lifestyle risks are strong predictors of CVD rates and makes a powerful call for increasing health care and quality of care to diminish or eliminate disparities. While progress is being made toward multiple Healthy People 2010 CV goals, Mensah notes significant disparities persist by race/ethnicity, gender, educational level, and disability.

3.2. *Unmasking Racial/Ethnic Disparities in Cardiovascular Disease: Nutritional, Socioeconomic, Cultural and Healthcare-Related Contributions*

Building on this detailed review of epidemiology and its relationship to CV disparities, John M. Flack, MD, Samar A. Nasser, PA-C, Anupam Goel, MD, Mary "Toni" Flowers, Shannon O'Connor, and Erynne Faucett describe the *Unmasking Racial/Ethnic Disparities in Cardiovascular Disease: Nutritional, Socioeconomic, Cultural and Healthcare-Related Contributions.* Flack and co-authors point out that the role of genetics in CVD disparities among varied races/ethnicities is complex and difficult to delineate. While they note the potential of genes to influence susceptibility to CVD, common CVD entities have multiple genetic influences and it is very unlikely that genes are primarily responsible for common diseases. While not discounting complex gene–gene and gene–environment interactions, the authors highlight multiple social and environmental factors that affect CVD. For instance, while hypertension has been stated to be higher in African Americans, there is wide variation in blacks from Africa, the West Indies, and the United States and conversely less significant racial disparity in blood pressure based on data from Brazil, Trinidad, and Cuba. They note, therefore, environment and preventable causes of hypertension have a profound effect on prevalence.

One increasing area of research and interest is related to hypovitaminosis D, significantly more prevalent in African-Americans than whites, especially among women. The authors describe a multiplicity of factors which potentially contribute to hypovitaminosis D in African-Americans, including darker skin and more pervasive obesity among women. They propose that low circulating levels of vitamin D are not only associated with elevated blood pressure, but also congestive heart failure, decreased beta-cell function, and insulin sensitivity. In African-Americans, they note the impact of low dietary calcium intake, possibly related to high prevalence ($\sim$80%) of lactose intolerance, interestingly more common in Asian Americans.

Obesity and its relation to CVD is a common thread in many of the chapters of this textbook. As pointed out by Flack and co-authors, the concern falls beyond simple consideration of body image and cosmetics; obesity affects salt sensitivity, which may be complicated by nitric oxide (NO) deficient states, psychosocial stressors, and low intake of dietary potassium (7). The authors also note independent of social class, the high prevalence of physical inactivity in African-Americans versus whites is potentially linked to total and CVD mortality. Finally, the authors suggest that providers implement prevention strategies while actively seeking to understand the patient's culture, including the influence of spirituality or religiosity; cultural competency may be a useful tool to address disparities.

3.3. Race and Genetics

In this section, Rick A. Kittles, PhD, and Jada Benn-Torres, PhD, tackle the controversial area of *Race and Genetics*. Kittles and Benn-Torres note the advent of molecular technology and that, based on genetic research, within group differences far exceed between group differences. In fact, they Human Genome Project confirms all humans, regardless of race/ethnicity, are >99% the same in genetic makeup. The authors describe the benefit of using hundreds of polymorphic loci across the human genome, correlating differences directly with ancestral continent of origin and, hence, continental clustering. Nevertheless, they recognize that genetic variation is a reality and confirm that single-nucleotide polymorphisms (SNPs) are the most common form of DNA variation in the human genome with presently more than 10 million SNPs *(8)*.

Self-identified race and ethnicity remain problematic because race and ethnicity have a multitude of definitions. Indeed, Kittles and Benn-Torres observe that in the United States, no matter how "white" or "black" a person may appear, strikingly, only 34% of African-Americans possess over 90% West African ancestry. Conversely, 98% of European Americans have over 90% European ancestry. Therefore, among persons self-reported as African-American or Hispanic American, there are wide genetic backgrounds. Kittles and Benn-Torres subsequently comment on the emerging popular approach to mapping susceptible genes in admixed populations (admixture mapping) in an attempt to find genes that underlie ethnic differences and disease risk *(9)*. In conclusion, they note that it may be beneficial to use ancestry, instead of race, in biomedical research.

3.4. Race, Genetics, and Cardiovascular Disease

Building on the discussion related to genetics and genomics, Ivor J. Benjamin, MD, and Theophilus Owan, MD, specifically delineate the interaction of various factors in *Race, Genetics and Cardiovascular Disease*. Benjamin and Owan confirm that while ethnic minorities may be afflicted with a higher prevalence of obesity, diabetes, and hypertension compared to whites, multiple factors contribute, including genetics, the environment, and socioeconomics. They specifically point to hypertension as an example of complex gene–environment interactions, especially related to the high prevalence in African-Americans. Interestingly, the authors suggest bioavailability of NO as one possible mechanism to explain difference in vascular function related to racial/ethnic differences in CVD prevalence and outcomes. For instance, Benjamin and Owan comment that alteration of NO production has been linked to polymorphisms in the gene encoding the endothelial nitric oxide synthase (eNOS) and at least one variant is more common in African-Americans than whites, potentially related to a decrease in eNOS expression and NO production. They specifically discuss racial/ethnic-based therapies and propose as an example a possible missed opportunity to explore further understanding of genetic markers in the recent African American Heart Failure Trial (A-HeFT). Although this important trial showed significant morbidity and mortality benefit in African-Americans, Benjamin and Owan highlight important lessons, in areas which need better understanding, and potential pitfalls in A-HeFT construction and interpretation.

Benjamin and Owan comment on future directions that may advance medical understanding of genetics and genomics and specifically acknowledge that an individual's genetic composition will eventually eliminate the utilization of skin color for phenotyping disease susceptibility or resistance.

They point to the International HapMap Project, a scientific collaboration constructed for the purpose of collection and reporting on worldwide genetic variation as a potential source of information to better expose the interactions of genes and CVD in the future.

3.5. Hypertension and Stroke in Racial/Ethnic Groups

One of the most powerful predictors of disparities in CV morbidity and mortality is hypertension and related stroke, especially in African-Americans. Kenneth Jamerson, MD, and Tonya L. Corbin, MD, describe in detail in *Hypertension and Stroke in Racial/Ethnic Groups* that the impact of the widespread burden of hypertension, especially in US blacks, contributing directly to high rates of heart disease, stroke, peripheral vascular disease, and end-stage renal disease. Jamerson and Corbin document the epidemiology of hypertension and pathophysiology, with specific attention to the impact of molecular genetics on salt sensitivity and increased sodium absorption, involving renal sodium transport, specifically in blacks. For instance, they explain the unique aspects of the Liddle syndrome, the mutation in the epithelial sodium channel (ENaC) described in black South Africans with low-renin salt sensitivity hypertension. The authors note this example may suggest continued need for genome-wide studies to identify the potential mechanisms contributing to higher rates of hypertension in blacks versus whites. Furthermore, Jamerson and Corbin elucidate the impact of obesity on the sympathetic nervous system, contributing to hypertension and other risk factors, including glucose intolerance, diabetes, and dyslipidemia. They also note that obesity, especially in black females, is not only a risk factor for hypertension but also may produce sympathetic overreactivity *(10)*.

3.6. Dyslipidemia in Racial and Ethnic Groups

Dyslipidemia in Racial and Ethnic Groups by Luther T. Clark, MD, and Sabrina Shaheen, MD, confirms the key impact of dyslipidemia on coronary heart disease (CHD), especially in African-Americans, who have the highest mortality. Nevertheless, in young to middle-aged adults, low-density lipoprotein (LDL) cholesterol levels were similar in African-Americans and whites *(11)*. Regardless, the relationship between total cholesterol levels and CHD mortality was the same among the 23,490 black and 325,384 white men followed over a decade in the Multiple Risk Factor Intervention Trial (MRFIT) *(12)*. In the Atherosclerosis Risk in Communities (ARIC) study, LDL cholesterol was similarly predictive of CHD events in all races and in both sexes *(13)*. Surprisingly, in some other studies, Clark and Shaheen found the relationship between total or LDL cholesterol, atherosclerotic plaque formation, and CHD events to be somewhat weaker in African-Americans *(14,15)*.

Regardless, the authors document that African-Americans are less likely to achieve treatment goals, more likely to be in the highest risk category, less likely to be using lipid drug therapy, including statins, and less likely to receive care from a subspecialist (16–18). They also highlight the Antihypertensive and Lipid Lowering Treatment to Prevent Heart Attack Trial (ALLHAT-LLT), the only major lipid outcome data in blacks, with a statistically significant 27% reduction in CHD event rates, observed only in black participants, with pravastatin sodium compared to usual care (19). Unfortunately, the apparent benefit in blacks may have resulted from the undertreatment of blacks in the usual care group (20). Along with undertreatment, another major factor in the disease burden in black Americans, as pointed out by Clark and Shaheen, is the presence of multiple risk factor status (1.5 times that of whites) (13, 21–24). Finally, the authors update lipid therapy in blacks with recent studies including the African American Rosuvastatin Investigation of Efficacy and Safety (ARIES) trial (25) and the National Cholesterol Education Program Evaluation Project Utilizing Novel E-Technology (NEPTUNE) II (26).

3.7. Novel and Emerging Risk Factors in Racial/Ethnic Groups

Novel and Emerging Risk Factors in Racial/Ethnic Groups are discussed by Karol E. Watson, MD. She expresses that the relationship between ethnicity and CVD is complicated by a number of variables, such as the effects of migration, generation gaps, and socioeconomic status. While classic CV risk factors undoubtedly explain much of the excess risk faced by certain racial/ethnic minorities, there is increasing interest in a number of newer or "emerging" CV risk markers, specifically homocysteine, lipoprotein(a) [Lp(a)], and inflammatory makers.

Watson points out that elevated plasma homocysteine levels, associated with both an increased risk of atherothrombotic vascular disease and an increased mortality in patients with CVD, differ among racial/ethnic groups, with unknown differential effects on CV morbidity and mortality. Furthermore, she explains that dietary factors impacting these variations in homocysteine levels make defining the role of ethnicity difficult. For instance, a large proportion of Asian Indians have markedly elevated homocysteine, which may be affected by strict vegetarian diets, associated with increased risk of cobalamin deficiency.

She subsequently depicts the significance of Lp(a) and its impact on CVD, including racial/ethnic groups. Lipoprotein(a) is structurally similar to LDL, with an additional disulfide linked glycoprotein termed apolipoprotein(a) [apo(a)],which shares extensive structural homology with plasminogen, but varies in size. Mean Lp(a) levels are more than twice as high in African-Americans versus Caucasians, with questionable association between elevated Lp(a) levels and CHD among African-Americans.

Moreover, Watson notes higher serum Lp(a) concentrations in Asian Indians, possibly associated with carotid atherosclerosis. She further reviews the growing evidence that markers of subclinical inflammation may predict future CHD events, specifically CRP levels, related to obesity and found to be highest among non-Hispanic black men and Mexican American women. Finally, Watson highlights data related to interleukin-6 (IL-6), a proinflammatory cytokine associated with a wide variety of diseases, including CVD, demonstrating higher levels in African-Americans than non-African-Americans *(27)*.

3.8. Therapeutic Lifestyle Interventions in a Multicultural Society

In *Therapeutic Lifestyle Interventions in a Multicultural Society*, data related to this important area are reviewed by Lawrence J. Appel, MD, Megan Gauvey-Kern, BA, and Cheryl A.M. Anderson, PhD. The authors confirm that lifestyle modification, the bedrock of CVD prevention, is an essential component of population-based strategies to prevent blood pressure-related CVD. They also describe the preeminence of obesity as one of the most important public health problems in the United States and throughout most of the world. Distressingly, the authors note that approximately two-thirds of the United States adult population is overweight or obese, and one-third of all children and adolescents are overweight or at risk *(28)*. Appel and co-authors also note well-documented data that the prevalence of overweight or obesity is higher in some minority populations (Hispanics and African American) versus whites. Interestingly, although overweight and obesity in Asian Americans do not exceed that of the white population, the authors explain that standard BMI weight class definitions may be inappropriate for the average Asian body type. Important evidence-based approaches to this public health crisis are subsequently portrayed, emphasizing behavioral counseling rather than simply supplying information.

Unfortunately, the authors also observe that non-Hispanic Black women tend to lose less weight than members of other racial/ethnic groups *(29)*. They observe that weight loss can prevent hypertension among individuals with pre-hypertension and evidence-based approaches are detailed. Appel and others conclude that the magnitude of the obesity epidemic in combination with the lack of effective interventions in minority populations argues strongly for additional research.

3.9. Obesity and the Cardiometabolic Syndrome: Impact on Chronic Kidney Disease and CVD

Obesity and the Cardiometabolic Syndrome: Impact on Chronic Kidney Disease and CVD by James R. Sowers, MD, Abrar Ahmed, MD, Guido Lastra, MD, and Camila Manrique, MD continues to illustrate the relationship of lifestyle and CVD. The authors specifically address the cardiometabolic syndrome (CMS), a cluster of CVD risk factors, including central obesity, dysglycemia, atherogenic dyslipidemia, hypertension, and microalbuminuria. Sowers and co-authors note that obesity largely drives the dramatic increase in the incidence and prevalence of CMS worldwide and the unique aspects of CMS related to race/ethnicity. They delineate the association between adiponectin, insulin sensitivity, and both visceral and subcutaneous-type adiposity; ethnicity-related variation in the role of adiponectin in the development of the CMS is confirmed. Furthermore, they highlight the association between CMS, obesity, and chronic kidney disease and then describe dysfunctional adipose tissue and proinflammatory adipokines including tumor necrosis factor-alpha, IL-1, IL-6, leptin, and resistin, all implicated in the development of insulin resistance. Similar to the other chapters, Sowers and colleagues communicate the need for additional research inclusive of minorities, where data are sparse, including Mexican Americans, other Hispanic Americans, Native Americans, and Asian/Pacific Islanders.

3.10. Risk Calculation and Clustering within Racial/Ethnic Groups

Peter W. F. Wilson, MD discusses *Risk Calculation & Clustering within Racial/Ethnic Groups.* He notes prior to modern computer methods, risk estimation in usual clinical practice was historically difficult and imprecise. Age, sex, blood pressure, cholesterol, cigarette smoking, and diabetes mellitus history were identified as related to risk for initial CHD events, and in 1999, the CHD Prediction Workshop from the National Heart, Lung, and Blood Institute (NHLBI) addressed the use of Framingham CHD risk functions for multiple ethnic groups *(30)*. Wilson notes an important aspect of this analysis, including studies not only in whites but also with various minorities: the ARIC (whites and blacks), the Physicians Health Study, the Honolulu Heart Program (Japanese American men), the Puerto Rican Heart Study (Puerto Rican residents), the Strong Heart Study (Native Americans), and the CV Health Study. He also points out that in regions where CHD risk was low, such as in the Honolulu Heart Program, the Framingham risk algorithms appear to overestimate CHD. In addition, Wilson provocatively suggests that left ventricular hypertrophy (LVH) by electrocardiogram is a CHD risk equivalent and LVH should be assessed in population groups where it is reasonably common, so that aggressive therapy can be instituted and maintained.

3.11. Cardiovascular Imaging in Racial/Ethnic Populations: Implications for the Adequate Application of Cardiovascular Imaging Techniques Guided by Racial and Ethnic Risk

Modern CV care increasingly utilizes novel approaches to cardiac imaging. In *Cardiovascular Imaging in Racial/Ethnic Populations: Implications for the Adequate Application of Cardiovascular Imaging Techniques Guided by Racial and Ethnic Risk Factor Variations,* Jennifer H Mieres, MD, Amgad N. Makaryus, MD, and Leslee J. Shaw, PhD, summarize this growing field. They point out that CV imaging has added to clinicians' awareness and ability to properly risk stratify and categorize patients. Furthermore, increasingly, imaging is used for the identification of patients with subclinical coronary artery disease who are at risk. A recent, large, landmark study, The Multi-Ethnic Study of Atherosclerosis (MESA) of 6,800 patients, supported by the NHLBI, is a major step forward in quantifying risk factors for subclinical atherosclerosis; MESA consisted of racial/ethnic categories, 40% whites, 30% blacks, 20% Hispanic, and 10% Chinese. The authors describe from MESA that African-Americans tend to have higher CVD rates than whites, particularly among women, and Pacific Asians, particularly Chinese Americans, Japanese Americans, and immigrants from Southeast Asia, have lower morbidity mortality rates than whites.

In their forward-looking review, Mieres and co-authors propose that the emerging technologies supporting these techniques vary widely and are in constant evolution. Various diagnostic techniques including electron beam computed tomography (EBCT), multislice cardiac computed tomography scanning and ultra sonography for carotid intima–media thickness are especially important in high-risk racial/ethnic populations. Also, single photon emission computed tomography (SPECT) myocardial perfusion imaging (MPI), a powerful indicator of future cardiac events and may have significant nuances related to race and ethnicity. For instances, they note all-cause mortality for African-Americans with normal SPECT MPI was significantly greater than that in Caucasians.

Moreover, the authors tackle the important area of coronary calcification and the observed ethnic differences in the presence and quantity. In conclusion, the authors call for research and insight into the latest in imaging technology to better delineate the ideal imaging modality for patients of different racial/ethnic backgrounds.

3.12. Unique Aspects of Vascular and Cardiac Ultrasound in Racial/Ethnic Groups

In conjunction with this excellent review of imaging, *Unique Aspects of Vascular and Cardiac Ultrasound in Racial and Ethnic Groups* by Robert L. Gillespie, MD, and Icilma V. Fergus, MD, further describe the unique aspects of CVD presentation in subpopulations and the important contribution of cardiac ultrasound in present and evolving understanding. Gillespie and Fergus first elucidate data on the emerging area of diastolic dysfunction *(31,32)*, defined as impaired left ventricular mechanics with a preserved ejection fraction, and the use echocardiography as the most useful tool for examining its presence and effects. The authors discuss the utility of multiple parameters to measure diastolic abnormalities and grade its severity, including left atrial size and volume, flow velocity across the mitral valve, and increased isovolumic relaxation time.

Sarcoidosis is also highlighted, more common in African-Americans, and manifesting in the heart as nodules, composed of fibrin and other proteins, which potentially lead to multiple arrhythmias, specifically heart block. The authors also highlight amyloidosis, including an autosomal dominant type, formerly described as pre-albumin amyloidosis, now referred to as transthyretin protein amyloid, and potentially treatable *(33)*, seen in African-Americans among others, and amyloidosis secondary to long-standing renal disease. Systemic lupus erythematosus (SLE) also occurring somewhat disproportionately in African-Americans is discussed; SLE may result in a cardiomyopathy or pericardial disease process. Gillespie and Fergus describe left ventricular non-compaction, a distinct form of cardiomyopathy with possible poor prognosis and unique echocardiographic findings *(34)*. Continuing the theme of recognition of obesity and extreme obesity as more prevalent in African-American females, the authors describe the impact of cardiac ultrasound in risk assessment in this population. Finally, they portray Kawasaki Disease, a unique condition specifically of Asian children – including clinical and echocardiographic aspects *(35)*.

3.13. Heart Failure in Racial/Ethnic Populations

Heart Failure in Racial/Ethnic Populations is contributed by Clyde W. Yancy, MD, and Melvin Echols, MD. They note heart failure disproportionately affects certain minorities, often with significantly different phenotypical profile, and they call for appreciation of population-specific research in heart failure as opportunities for reduction of CVD disparities. Prevalence of heart failure in African-Americans is higher than in any other racial/ethnic group, with worrisome prognosis and death rates. Yancy and Echols describe African-American patients with congestive heart failure at younger ages and higher prevalence of hypertension etiology and lower atherosclerotic burden. They also describe the unfortunate reality of potential preference toward Caucasian patients as a factor in disparities in therapeutic and diagnostic approaches. Also, they describe language barriers as contributors to disparities in Hispanics and other non-English-speaking populations. Also, while they note limited studies have evaluated genetic polymorphisms for heart failure in the Hispanic community, Yancy and Echols explain that while trial participation by minorities overall is limited, with Hispanics, data are essentially absent. As noted in prior chapters, they illustrate developing research efforts related to genetic variations between racial/ethnic groups and plausible explanations for the differences seen in therapy between these groups. For example, the authors detail the Genetic Risk Assessment in Heart Failure (GRAHF) subset of the A-HeFT, providing new insight into genetic variants and outcomes of an African-American population with heart failure. They conclude with a review of the responses of beta blockers and angiotensin-converting enzyme inhibitors in African-American with heart failure, along with benefits of the fixed dose combination of isosorbide dinitrate and hydralazine (ISDN/Hyd) *(36,37)*.

3.14. Minority Women and CVD

Anne L. Taylor, MD and Lavanya Bellumkonda, MBBS in the final and vital chapter address *Minority Women and CVD*. Data from multiple studies are reviewed, including the Women's Health Initiative, in which the major correlates of hypertension among postmenopausal women were black race, CVD, physical inactivity, and excess alcohol consumption. Additionally considered is the Dallas Heart Study, which demonstrated that LVH is two- to three-fold more common in black women than white women *(38)*. Tyler and Bellumkonda also depict the impact of diabetes, particularly its severe CV consequences in women, with impaired endothelium-dependent vasodilation when compared to non-diabetic women. A critical component of the authors chapter is a comprehensive description of major CVD risks in women and their harmful effects, including smoking as few as 1–4 cigarettes a day associated with a two-fold increase in risk of fatal *(39)* CHD or non-fatal infarction and the impact of the lack of leisure time physical activity *(40)*.

The authors illustrate the unique aspects of the effects of estrogen, with its vasodilator properties, on stress testing and the greater symptom burden. This occurs despite a lower prevalence of obstructive coronary artery disease by coronary angiography as compared to men. Finally, they highlight a stimulating review of the etiology and presentation of heart failure in women, who are generally more likely to have a history of hypertension compared to men. To confirm the critical need to support and expand evidence-based therapeutic approaches in women, Tyler and Bellumkonda analyze published data for different treatments, including angiotensin-converting enzyme inhibitors, beta-blockers, and fixed dose ISDN/Hyd in A-HeFT *(41)*. In this large clinical trial of 1040 patients, with a cohort of 40% women, the fixed ISDN/Hyd, specifically including subgroup calculations by gender, was highly effective.

4. PERSPECTIVES ON CV MORBIDITY/MORTALITY IN RACIAL/ETHNIC MINORITIES

Cardiovascular health, life-expectancy, and health care, while improving dramatically for all Americans over the last century, have not been distributed equitably. The African-American population has the highest morbidity and mortality for various CVDs and other minorities are at higher risk for hypertension, diabetes, obesity, myocardial infarction, stroke, and kidney disease. Heart disease remains the leading cause of death, and along with cancer – the second leading cause of death – they together account for almost half of all deaths. Certain trends in mortality have become apparent. Life expectancy for white males, white females, and black males remain at the 2004 levels, while life expectancy for black females increased by 0.2 years. Despite the slight increase in black female life expectancy, differences in mortality between black and white populations persist and age-adjusted death rates were 1.3 times greater

Hispanic origin mortality rate is perhaps somewhat understated because of the under-reporting of Hispanic origin on death certificates. There is also the hypothesis of the healthy migrant effect, which argues that Hispanics, especially Mexican Americans, have a large, newly immigrant population which came to the United States with certain baseline good health and robustness. Additionally, there may be a so-called "salmon bias," where US residents of Hispanic origin may actually return to their countries of origin when severely ill or near death. The death rates for certain Hispanic subgroups appear to differ in magnitude.

Significantly, type 2 diabetes mellitus is more than simply a powerful risk factor, but also a CHD equivalent, clearly contributing to the increase in CV mortality in certain racial/ethnic groups, with blacks and Hispanics with a high rate of physician-diagnosed diabetes and undiagnosed diabetes *(2)*.

5. PRACTICAL APPROACHES TO ELIMINATING DISPARITIES

One of the best techniques to eliminating disparities is to implement evidence-based therapies. To combat the distressingly high rates of hypertension morbidity and mortality in African-Americans, the International Society on Hypertension in Blacks (ISHIB) promulgated guidelines suggesting combination therapy and more intensive therapy for most black patients *(43)*. Similarly, the National Cholesterol Education Program Adult Treatment Panel III delineates special considerations in African-Americans. Despite similar LDL cholesterol levels, versus whites, African-Americans noted to have higher levels of uncontrolled dyslipidemia and multiple risk factor status *(44)*. More recently, the International Diabetes Federation recognized abdominal obesity in Asians at lower waist cut-points and promulgated new racial/ethnic-specific waist circumference criteria for patients with metabolic syndrome *(45)*.

Health-care education in the future should recognize the essential nature of the patient's cultural identity and experiences and understanding social factors and support systems. Unfortunately, health-care practitioners, including physicians, nurses, and others, do not proportionately represent an increasingly diverse patient population. Unrepresented minorities including African-Americans, Mexican Americans, Native Americans, and mainland Puerto Ricans comprise approximate 25% of the population, but only 12% of US medical school graduates *(46)*. In addition, medical school faculties are 75% white, with only 5.8% African-American, and 3% Hispanics *(47)*. Moreover, in 2004, African-Americans, Hispanics, Asians, and Native Americans comprised only approximately 12% of the nursing population, with 4.2% Black or African-American, 3.1% Asian, Native Hawaiian, or other Pacific Islander, and 1.7% Hispanic or Latino. In 2006, the number of doctor of pharmacy degrees conferred as first professional degree was 7.4% Black, 4.2% Hispanic, and 0.4% Native American *(48,49)*.

Cultural competency is variously described as the ability of an individual to understand and respect values, attitudes, and beliefs that differ across cultures. Increasingly, health education and interventions must respect cultural differences and utilizing learning models may assist practitioners with understanding cultural competency. For instance, LEARN: Listen to your patient and his or her cultural perspective, Explain your reasons for asking personal information, Acknowledge your patient's concerns, Recommend a course of action, Negotiate a plan that takes into consideration the patient's culture and personal lifestyles *(50)*.

A significant proportion of Americans speaks a language other than English at home, or has limited English proficiency, which limits quality of care and ability to communicate with practitioners, leading to decreased satisfaction and follow-up, and increased medical and non-medical costs *(51)*. Accordingly, hospital translators may improve patient–doctor communication *(52)*. For example, a clinic serving Somali patients in Minneapolis utilizes former Somali health-care professionals and patient advocates *(53)*. Multilingual patient tools also may be valuable, specifically in risk factor control for diabetes, hypertension, and dyslipidemia.

In the future, electronic medical records may assist clinicians with clarifying and eliminating health disparities by accurately reporting race/ethnicity data and uncovering disparities. Certain health plans assist with the identification of disparities, and the Kaiser Foundation and Robert Wood Johnson have launched a major initiative in major medical publications to review evidence on racial/ethnic disparities and care, engaging physicians and other clinicians in the dialogue *(54)*. Moreover, in its research efforts, the NHLBI seeks to alleviate disparities and places a strong emphasis on minority-impacting populations with culturally sensitive and innovative approaches, such as church-based interventions in the black community *(55)*. Similarly, the Centers for Disease Control and Prevention and its various offices support training opportunities for community outreach programs and initiatives in communication and research *(56)*.

6. SOCIOECONOMIC-DISADVANTAGED STATUS AND CVD

To a large extent, CVD and risk factors are affected by not only a person's race or ethnicity but also the socioeconomic status *(57)*. In approaching patients with CVD and limited income, clinicians must first identify barriers to control – including health literacy, beliefs, and adherence – and integrate and understand socioeconomic distress as a risk factor. Therefore, language and cultural barriers in conjunction with low socioeconomic status and decreased literacy are important determinants affecting healthcare outcomes.

Additionally, clinicians must recognize adverse dietary patterns and other lifestyles. Integrated, multidisciplinary teams are beneficial in the elimination of disparities; these partnerships may include nurse practitioners, physician assistants, and community health advocates, along with physicians. One multidisciplinary approach in an inner city African American male cohort effectively controlled blood pressure and improved LVH *(27)*. Additional funding for lifestyle modifications and multilayered interventions is needed to make non-pharmacological interventions available in usual clinical settings *(57)*.

To overcome disparities, disadvantaged minorities and all patients with limited income need medications that are not only effective but also affordable. Beneficial approaches include the use of generics from large department and pharmacy chains, along with easy to access patients-in-need programs to make appropriate medicines available. Nevertheless, generic substitution should avoid under dosing, inappropriate substitution, or utilizing medicines which do not fulfill compelling indications.

Lower socioeconomic status and lower levels of education, found disproportionately in African-American and Hispanics, are powerful predictors of CVD risk factors and mortality. A majority of non-high school graduates have multiple CV risk factors; education and income are negatively correlated to CVD. The recent provocative report, the Eight Americas study, demonstrated that the lowest socioeconomic demographic group with the lowest average income per capita and the highest risk of mortality was southern, low income rural blacks, followed by high-risk urban blacks *(58)*. Disproportionate stress in disadvantaged neighborhoods is a factor. Adequate funding for health insurance, access to care, and reimbursement for therapeutic lifestyle interventions is mandatory.

7. FUTURE CONSIDERATIONS

Simply identifying racial/ethnic health disparities will not eliminate them. In any individual patient, the recognition of racial/ethnic status may affect certain nuances of care, but does not address the multiple barriers to controlling risk factors, adverse lifestyle, bias within the health-care system, and low socioeconomic status. The application of life-saving, evidence-based medications should be afforded to all patients. The question is not only who is at increased risk for CVD, but what lifestyle choices and steps can be made to continue the downward trend in CVD by controlling risk factors. It is clearly inappropriate to have an excessive reliance on skin color, language, or ethnicity to make final decisions on an individual patient's care. Nevertheless, clinicians must integrate an understanding of culture, lifestyle, socioeconomic status, the impact of psychological stress, and bias within the health-care system to assist patients with achieving positive outcomes. Regardless of a patient's race or ethnicity, no matter what scientific breakthroughs continue to be reported in evidenced-based literature, the complexities of living a healthy life and receiving the benefits of modern health care must be applied on a one-to-one basis.

REFERENCES

1. U.S. Census Bureau News. U.S. Department of Commerce. An Older and More Diverse Nation by Midcentury. [Internet] Washington, D.C. [Modified 2008 Aug 14; cited 2008 Sept 2] Accessed from: www.census.gov/Press-Release/www/releases/archives/population/012496.html
2. Rosamond W, Flegal K, Furie K, et al. Heart disease and stroke statistics–2008 update: a report from the American Heart Association Statistics Committee and Stroke Statistics Subcommittee. *Circulation* 2008; 117(4):e25–146.
3. U.S. Department of Health and Human Services, Food and Drug Administration, Center for Drug Evaluation and Research (CDER), Center for Biologics Evaluation and Research (CBER), Center for Devices and Radiologic Health (CDRH), Office of the Commissioner (OC). Clinical Medical Guidance for Industry: Collection of Race and Ethnicity Data in Clinical Trials. [Modified 2005 Oct 3; cited 2008 Sept 2] Accessed from: http://www.fda.gov/cder/Guidance/5656fnl.htm
4. Addressing Racial and Ethnic Disparities in Health Care Fact Sheet. AHRQ Publication No. 00-PO41. [Internet] Agency for Healthcare Research and Quality, Rockville, MD. [Modified 2000 Feb; cited 2008 Sept 2] Accessed from: http://www.ahrq.gov/research/disparit.htm
5. Anderson GM, Bronskill SE, Mustard CA, Culyer A, Alter DA, Manuel DG. Both clinical epidemiology and population health perspectives can define the role of health care in reducing health disparities. *J Clin Epidemiol* 2005; 58(8):757–762.
6. Rhoades DA. Racial misclassification and disparities in cardiovascular disease among American Indians and Alaska Natives. *Circulation* 2005; 111(10):1250–1256.
7. Flack JM, Wiist WH. Epidemiology of hypertension and hypertensive target-organ damage in the United States. *J Assoc Acad Minor Phys* 1991; 2(4):143–150.
8. Crawford DC, Akey DT, Nickerson DA. The patterns of natural variation in human genes. *Annu Rev Genomics Hum Genet* 2005; 6:287–312.
9. McKeigue PM. Prospects for admixture mapping of complex traits. *Am J Hum Genet* 2005; 76(1):1–7.
10. Abate NI, Mansour YH, Meryem T, et al. Overweight and sympathetic overactivity in Black Americans. *Hypertension* 2001; 38:379–383.
11. Gidding SS, Liu K, Bild DE, et al. Prevalence and identification of abnormal lipoprotein levels in a biracial population aged 23 to 35 years (the CARDIA study). The Coronary Risk Development in Young Adults study. *Am J Cardiol* 1996; 78:304–308.

12. Watkins LO, Neaton JD, Kuller LH. Racial differences in high-density lipoprotein cholesterol and coronary heart disease incidence in the usual care group of the Multiple Risk Factor Intervention Trial. *Am J Cardiol* 1986; 57:538–545.

13. Hutchinson RG, Watson RL, Davis CE, et al. Racial differences in risk factors for atherosclerosis. The ARIC study. *Angiology* 1997; 48:279–290.

14. Clark LT, Ferdinand KC, Flack JM, et al. Coronary heart disease in African Americans. *Heart Dis* 2001; 3:97–108.

15. Keil JE, Sutherland SE, Hames CG, et al. Coronary disease mortality and risk factors in black and white men. Results from the combined Charleston, SC, and Evans County, Georgia, heart studies. *Arch Intern Med* 1995; 155(14):1521–1527.

16. Clark LT, Maki KC, Galant R, Maron DJ, Pearson TA, Davidson MH. Ethnic differences in achievement of cholesterol treatment goals: results from the National Cholesterol Education Program Evaluation Project Utilizing Novel E-Technology (NEPTUNE) II. *J Gen Intern Med* 2006; 21(4):320–6.

17. Pearson TA, Laurora I, Chu H, Kafonek S. The lipid treatment assessment project (L-TAP): a multicenter survey to evaluate the percentages of dyslipidemic patients receiving lipid-lowering therapy and achieving low density lipoprotein cholesterol goals. *Arch Intern Med* 2000; 28:459–67.

18. Williams ML, Morris MT, Ahmad U, Yousseff M, Li W, Ertel N. Racial differences in compliance with NCEP II recommendations for secondary prevention at a veterans affairs medical center. *Ethn Dis* 2002; 12:S1-58–62.

19. ALLHAT Officers and Coordinators of the ALLHAT Collaborative Research Group. Major outcomes in moderately hypercholesterolemic, hypertensive patients randomized to pravastatin versus usual care. The Antihypertensive and Lipid-Lowering Treatment to Prevent Heart Attack Trial (ALLHAT-LLT). *JAMA* 2002; 288:2988–3007.

20. Vega GL, Clark LT, Tang A, Marcovina S, Grundy SM, Cohen JC. Hepatic lipase activity is lower in African American men than in white American men: effects of 5' flanking polymorphism in the hepatic lipase gene (LIPC). *J Lipid Res* 1998; 39(1): 228–232.

21. Hall WD, Clark LT, Wenger NK, et al. The metabolic syndrome in African Americans: a review. *Ethn Dis* 2003; 13:414–428.

22. Ford ES, Giles WH, Dietz WH. Prevalence of the metabolic syndrome among US adults: Findings from the Third National Health and Nutritional Examination Survey. *JAMA* 2002; 287(3):356–359.

23. Rowland ML, Fulwood R. Coronary heart disease risk factor trends in blacks between the first and second National Health and Nutrition Examination Surveys, United States, 1971-1980. *Am Heart J* 1984; 108:771–779.

24. Cutter GR, Burke GL, Dyer AR, et al. Cardiovascular risk factors in young adults. The CARDIA baseline monograph. *Control Clin Trials* 1991; 12:1S–25S, 51S–77S.

25. Ferdinand KC, Clark LT, Watson KE, et al. Comparison of efficacy and safety of rosuvastatin versus atorvastatin in African-American patients in a six-week trial. *Am J Cardiol* 2006; 97(2):229–35.

26. Davidson MH, Maki KC, Pearson TA, et al. Results of the National Cholesterol Education (NCEP) Program Evaluation ProjecT Utilizing Novel E-Technology (NEPTUNE) II survey and implications for treatment under the recent NCEP Writing Group recommendations. *Am J Cardiol* 2005; 96(4):556–563.

27. Hassan MI, Aschner Y, Manning CH, et al. Racial differences in selected cytokine allelic and genotypic frequencies among healthy, pregnant women in North Carolina. *Cytokine* 2003; 21:10–16.

28. Ogden CL, Carroll MD, Curtin LR, McDowell MA, Tabak CJ, Flegal KM. Prevalence of overweight and obesity in the united states, 1999-2004. *JAMA* 2006; 295: 1549–1555.

29. Kumanyika S. Obesity treatment in minorities. In: Wadden TA, Stunkard AJ, eds. Handbook of obesity treatment. New York: The Guilford Press; 2002:416–446.
30. D'Agostino RB Sr, Grundy S, Sullivan LM, Wilson P. Validation of the Framingham Coronary Heart Disease Prediction Scores: results of a multiple ethnic groups investigation. *JAMA* 2001; 286(2):180–187.
31. Fox ER, Taylor J, Taylor H, et al. Left ventricular geometric patterns in the Jackson cohort of the Atherosclerotic Risk in Communities (ARIC) Study: clinical correlates and influences on systolic and diastolic dysfunction. *Am Heart J* 2007; 153(2):238–244.
32. Rovner A, de las Fuentes L, Waggoner AD, et al. Characterization of left ventricular diastolic function in hypertension by use of Doppler tissue imaging and color M-mode techniques. *J Am Soc Echocardiogr* 2006; 19(7):872–879.
33. Jacobson DR, Pastore RD, Yaghoubian R, et al. Variant-sequence transthyretin (isoleucine 122) in late-onset cardiac amyloidosis in black Americans. *N Engl J Med* 1997; 336(7):466–473.
34. Kohli SK, Pantazis AA, Shah JS, et al. Diagnosis of left-ventricular non-compaction in patients with left-ventricular systolic dysfunction: time for a reappraisal of diagnostic criteria? *Eur Heart J* 2008; 29(1):89–95.
35. Joffe A, Kabani A, Jadavji T. Atypical and complicated Kawasaki disease in infants. Do we need criteria? *West J Med* 1995 Apr; 162(4):322–327.
36. Dries DL, Exner DV, Gersh BJ, et al. Racial differences in the outcome of left ventricular dysfunction. *N Engl J Med* 1999; 340:609–616.
37. Exner DV, Dries DL, Domanski MJ, Cohn JN. Lesser response to angiotensin-converting-enzyme inhibitor therapy in black as compared with white patients with left ventricular dysfunction. *N Engl J Med* 2001; 344:1351–1357.
38. Drazner MH, Dries DL, Peshock RM, Cooper RS, Klassen C, Kazi F, Willett D, Victor RG. Left ventricular hypertrophy is more prevalent in blacks than whites in the general population: the Dallas Heart Study. *Hypertension* 2005 Jul; 46(1):124–129.
39. Steinberg HO, Paradisi G, Cronin J Type II diabetes abrogates sex differences in endothelial function in premenopausal women. *Circulation* 2000; 101(17):2040–2046.
40. Koh KK, Kang MH, Jin DK, et al. Vascular effects of estrogen in type II diabetic postmenopausal women. *J Am Coll Cardiol* 2001; 38(5):1409–1415.
41. Shekelle PG, Rich MW, Morton SC, et al. Efficacy of angiotensin-converting enzyme inhibitors and beta-blockers in the management of left ventricular systolic dysfunction according to race, gender, and diabetic status: a meta-analysis of major clinical trials. *J Am Coll Cardiol* 2003; 41(9):1529–1538.
42. Taylor AL, Lindenfeld J, Ziesche S, et al. Outcomes by gender in the African-American Heart Failure Trial. *J Am Coll Cardiol* 2006; 48(11):2263–2267.
43. Douglas JG, Bakris GL, Epstein M, et al. Management of high blood pressure in African Americans: consensus statement of the Hypertension in African Americans Working Group of the International Society on Hypertension in Blacks. *Arch Intern Med* 2003; 163(5):525–541.
44. National Cholesterol Education Program (NCEP) Expert Panel on Detection, Evaluation, and Treatment of High Blood Cholesterol in Adults (Adult Treatment Panel III). Third Report of the National Cholesterol Education Program (NCEP) Expert Panel on Detection, Evaluation, and Treatment of High Blood Cholesterol in Adults (Adult Treatment Panel III) final report. *Circulation* 2002; 106(25):3143–3421.
45. Alberti KG, Zimmet P, Shaw J The metabolic syndrome—a new worldwide definition. *Lancet* 2005; 366(9491):1059–1062
46. Cohen JJ. The consequences of premature abandonment of affirmative action in medical school admissions. *JAMA* 2003; 289(9):1143–1149.
47. Barzansky B, Etzel SI. Educational programs in U.S. medical schools, 2002-2003. *JAMA* 2003; 290(9):1190–1196.

48. U.S. Department of Health and Human Services, Health Resources and Services Administration, Bureau of Health Professions. [Internet] The Registered Nurse Population: Findings from the March 2004 National Sample Survey of Registered Nurses [Modified 2006 June; cited 2008 Sept 2]. Accessed from: http://bhpr.hrsa.gov/healthworkforce/rnsurvey04/3.htm

49. Hayes, B. Increasing the representation of underrepresented minority groups in US colleges and schools of pharmacy. *Am J Pharm Educ* 2008; 72(1):14.

50. Berlin EA, Fowkes WC. A teaching framework for cross-cultural health care: application in family practice. *West J Med* 1983; 139(6):934–938.

51. Carrasquillo O, Orav EJ, Brennan TA, Burstin HR. Impact of language barriers on patient satisfaction in an emergency department. *J Gen Intern Med* 1999; 14(2):82–87.

52. Baker DW, Hayes R, Fortier JP. Interpreter use and satisfaction with interpersonal aspects of care for Spanish-speaking patients. *Med Care* 1998; 36(10):1461–1470.

53. Cole PM. Cultural competence now mainstream medicine. Responding to increasing diversity and changing demographics. *Postgrad Med* 2004; 116(6):51–53.

54. Henry J Kaiser Family Foundation, American College of Cardiology Foundation (ACCF). Racial/Ethnic Differences in Cardiac Care: The Weight of the Evidence [Internet] [modified 2002 Oct 8; cited 2008 Sept 2]. Available from: http://www.kff.org/whythedifference/6040fullreport.pdf

55. Department of Health and Human Services, National Institutes of Health, National Heart, Lung, and Blood Institute. Strategy for Addressing Health Disparities FY 2002 — 2006 [Internet] [cited 2008 Sept 2]. Available from: http://www.nhlbi.nih.gov/resources/docs/plandisp.htm

56. Department of Health and Human Services, Centers for Disease Control and Prevention. Racial and Ethnic Approaches to Community Health (REACH). [Internet] Atlanta, GA. [Modified 2008 May 1; cited 2008 Sept 2]. Available from: http://www.cdc.gov/reach

57. Ferdinand KC. Lessons learned from the Healthy Heart Community Prevention Project in reaching the African American population. *J Health Care Poor Underserved* 1997; 8:366–371.

58. Murray CJL, Kulkarni SC, Michaud C, et al. Eight Americas: investigating mortality disparities across races, counties, and race-counties in the United States. *PLoS Med* 2006; 3(9): e260.

2

Epidemiology of Cardiovascular Diseases and Risk Factors Among Racial/Ethnic Populations in the United States

G.A. Mensah, MD

CONTENTS

The findings and conclusions in this chapter are those of the author and do not necessarily represent the views of the Centers for Disease Control and Prevention.

From: *Contemporary Cardiology: Cardiovascular Disease in Racial and Ethnic Minorities*
Edited by: K.C. Ferdinand and A. Armani, DOI 10.1007/978-1-59745-410-0_2
© Humana Press, a part of Springer Science+Business Media, LLC 2009

1. SUMMARY

Cardiovascular epidemiology plays a fundamental role in the assessment of disease burden and evaluation of health disparities. Although current epidemiologic data have important limitations, they nevertheless provide compelling evidence that racial and ethnic disparities in cardiovascular health are pervasive and that they contribute to a lower life expectancy, excess morbidity, and reduced quality of life in several racial and ethnic minority populations. The largest of these disparities is found in race–county comparisons of mortality and summary measures of morbidity. The causes of these disparities are complex. However, established racial and ethnic differences in traditional risk factors and socioeconomic, educational, and environmental determinants contribute to these health disparities. Although stroke and coronary heart disease mortality rates have declined for men and women in all racial and ethnic groups, they remain significantly higher than the national Healthy People 2010 targets in African-Americans. In particular, racial and ethnic disparities associated with these mortality rates have increased, and disparities in access to care and quality of health care persist. Elimination of these disparities, in addition to increasing years and quality of life for all Americans, must remain the overarching national health objectives in the years ahead.

2. INTRODUCTION

Contemporary and future considerations of cardiovascular diseases (CVD) in racial and ethnic minority populations must take into account the burden of cardiovascular events, risk factors, mortality, disabling sequelae, and secular trends by race and ethnicity (1). Cardiovascular epidemiology provides unique tools for assessing all of these and the opportunity to identify population subgroups at increased risk for CVD and outcomes (2). Through this exercise, cardiovascular epidemiology also provides the data for identifying the existence of health disparities. Additionally, the monitoring and surveillance components of cardiovascular epidemiology provide clues to new and emerging cardiovascular threats and permit assessment of the effectiveness of current measures to prevent and control established CVD. Taken together, these properties summarize the fundamental role that epidemiology plays in promoting and protecting cardiovascular health and informing program and policy development for the prevention and control of CVD (2–4).

This chapter begins with the strengths and limitations of the existing epidemiological data on CVD and risk factors by race and ethnicity in the United States. It then presents the most recently available data and trends for summary measures of overall health. Data on state-specific self-reported lifestyle and behavioral risk factors are then discussed. National prevalence of measured risk factors and their recent trends are also presented. Racial and ethnic differences in the recent epidemiological data on total CVD burden and measures of quality care and outcomes are then presented and discussed. Finally, epidemiological data from the mid-course review of the Healthy People 2010 national health objectives for heart disease and stroke by race and ethnicity are then discussed to show the progress made and persisting challenges in the endeavor to eliminate health disparities.

3. STRENGTHS AND LIMITATIONS OF THE EXISTING EPIDEMIOLOGIC DATA

Although the advantages of CVD epidemiology are well recognized, epidemiologic data are typically not available for all racial and ethnic groups. Often, data on specific racial and ethnic populations are not collected or collected in formats that differ from federal standards (5). The accuracy and quality of data on race and ethnicity may also vary by factors such as the type of data collected and the source of information (6,7). When high-quality data are appropriately collected, the data may be insufficient to generate reliable estimates for specific racial and ethnic groups where sample sizes are small (5). Additionally, even in settings where stable estimates can be generated, the miscoding or misclassification of race, which disproportionately affects American Indians and Alaska Natives (8–10) can lead to flawed data in these comparisons.

For example, Rhoades et al. (8) showed that vital events data unadjusted for racial misclassification show American Indians and Alaska Natives as having the lowest mortality rates from major CVD. However, after appropriate adjustment, American Indians and Alaska Natives had the highest mortality rates that demonstrated a rapidly growing disparity when compared with rates in the US all-races and white populations (8). These limitations and challenges in the existing epidemiologic data by race and ethnicity must be recognized.

In interpreting and using the epidemiological data presented in this chapter, the racial and ethnic categories should be viewed as social, not biological constructs (11–13). Although genetics, gene–gene, and the gene–environment interactions are important influences on the data presented (14), racial and ethnic differences seen should not be assumed to be necessarily caused by genetic or biological differences (11–15). Other key determinants of disparities such as access to care, quality of care delivered, systems of care, geographic and environmental influences, income and educational levels, prejudice, discrimination, provider bias, psychosocial stressors, and personal behaviors and lifestyle choices all play important roles in causing disparities (16). Appropriate recognition of these limitations, challenges, and caveats in the use of these data are important in the contemporary and future considerations in the prevention and control of CVD in racial and ethnic minority populations.

4. LIFE EXPECTANCY AND SUMMARY MEASURES OF POPULATION HEALTH

A summary measure of population health is an epidemiological index that combines mortality and non-fatal health outcomes with functional and quality of life dimensions into a single indicator to measure a population's overall state of health *(17–19)*. Together with life expectancy, these measures provide an important assessment of the first overarching goal of the Healthy People 2010 national health agenda (to increase the years and quality of healthy life), as well as the second overarching goal (to eliminate health disparities) when these measures are examined by race and ethnicity *(18–21)*.

Life expectancy at birth and at age 65 years are two of the most commonly used summary measures of mortality. In 2005, life expectancy at birth for the total US population reached a record high of 77.9 years and was higher in whites by 5.1 years compared with that in blacks *(22)*. Compared with black men and women, life expectancy at birth was higher in white men and women by 6.1 and 4.3 years, respectively (Fig. 1) *(22)*. Although

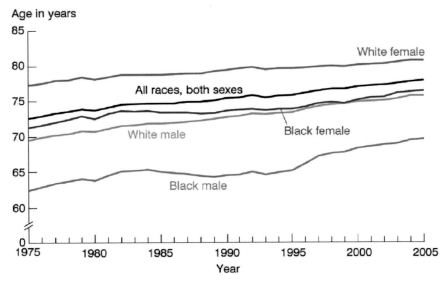

Fig. 1. Life expectancy at birth, by race, and sex: United States, 1975–2004 final and 2005 preliminary.
Source: CDC/NCHS, National Vital Statistics System. From Kung HC, Hoyert DL, Xu J, Murphy SL. Deaths: Preliminary data for 2005. Health E-Stats. Sept 2007. www.cdc.gov/nchs/products/pubs/pubd/hestats/prelimdeaths05/prelimdeaths05.htm *(22)*.

the National Center for Health Statistics does not report life expectancy data for other race or ethnic groups, other sources show marked disparities in life expectancy between Asian Americans who have the highest life expectancy and poor whites living in Appalachia and the Mississippi Valley, Native Americans living on reservations in the West, poor blacks living in the rural South, and other race–county subgroups (Fig. 2) *(23)*. Examination of life expectancy across race-county groups shows even greater disparities (Figs. 3 and 4). For example, Murray et al. showed that Native American males in a cluster of Bennet, Jackson, Mellette, Shannon, Todd, and Washabaugh Counties in South Dakota had a life expectancy of 58 years in 1997–2001, compared to Asian females in Bergen County, New Jersey, with a life expectancy of 91 years, a gap of 33 years. The Eight Americas study confirmed that the largest measurable disparities observed in the United States to-date are those revealed by examining the disparities across race–county groups *(23)*.

Cardiovascular diseases, the leading cause of death in the United States plays an important role in these disparities. In one study of the disparities in life expectancy stratified by race and educational level, Wong et al. showed that cardiovascular diseases account for 35.3% of the black–white difference in potential life-years lost, in large part because of the impact of hypertension *(24)*. African-Americans and American Indians also suffer disproportionate shares of total burden relative to their population size when assessed by the disability adjusted life years as a measure of premature death and disability (Figs. 5 and 6) *(25)*. The marked disparities in burden experienced

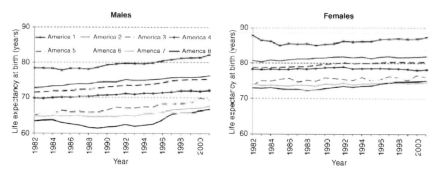

Fig. 2. Life expectancy at birth in the Eight Americas (1982–2001). The "Eight Americas" as used in this study, represent distinct subgroups of the US population where 1 = Asian; 2 = Northland low-income rural white; 3 = Middle America; 4 = low-income whites in Appalachia and the Mississippi valley; 5 = Western Native American; 6 = Black Middle America; 7 = Southern low-income rural black; and 8 = high-risk urban black.
Reproduced with permission from PLoS.
Source: Murray CJ, Kulkarni S, Ezzati M. Eight Americas: new perspectives on U.S. health disparities. *Am J Prev Med* 2005 December; 29(5 Suppl. 1):4–10 *(23)*.

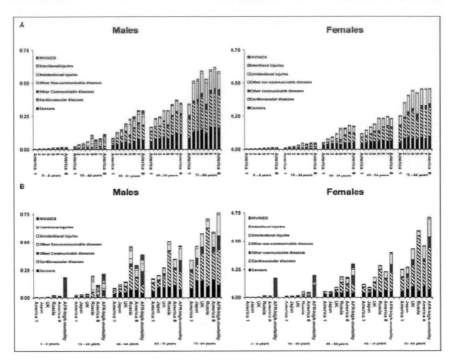

Fig. 3. Probability of dying in specific age ranges in the Eight Americas as defined in Fig. 2. (**A**) Probability of death by sex, age, and disease for the Eight Americas in 2001. (**B**) Probability of death by sex, age, and disease for Americas 1 and 8 compared to Japan, United Kingdom, the Russian Federation, and high-mortality countries in sub-Saharan Africa (AFR-high-mortality; made up largely of countries in West Africa and excluding countries with very high mortality due to HIV/AIDS) in 2001. Results are not shown for ages 5–14 year because there are few deaths in this age range in the United States.
Reproduced with permission from PLoS.
Source: Murray CJ, Kulkarni S, Ezzati M. Eight Americas: new perspectives on U.S. health disparities. *Am J Prev Med* 2005 December; 29(5 Suppl. 1):4–10 *(23)*.

by African-Americans is most evident for cerebrovascular diseases as shown in Fig. 6.

5. CARDIOVASCULAR RISK FACTORS AND BIOMARKERS

An important contributor to population differences in cardiovascular disease events and outcomes is the magnitude of the population-level differences in traditional risk factor levels and emerging biomarkers. For example, in the INTERHEART standardized case–control study of acute myocardial infarction in 52 countries, representing 15,152 cases and 14,820 controls, Yusuf et al. *(26)* found that collectively, nine risk factors accounted for

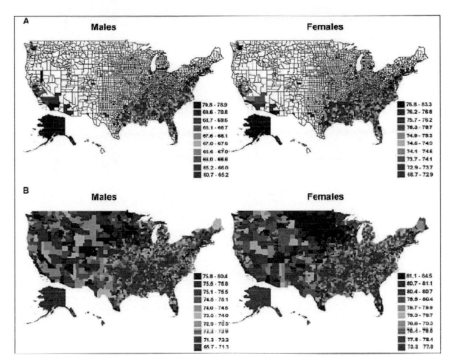

Fig. 4. County life expectancies by race (Fig. 1). Deaths were averaged for 1997–2001 to reduce sensitivity to small numbers and outliers. (**A**) Life expectancy at birth for black males and females. Only counties with more than five deaths for any 5-year age group (0–85) were mapped, to avoid unstable results. (**B**) Life expectancy at birth for white males and females.
Reproduced with permission from PLoS.
Source: Murray CJ, Kulkarni S, Ezzati M. Eight Americas: new perspectives on U.S. health disparities. *Am J Prev Med* 2005 December; 29(5 Suppl. 1):4–10 *(23).*

90% of the population attributable fraction of acute myocardial infarction in men and 94% in women. These nine risk factors included cigarette smoking, raised ApoB/ApoA1 ratio, history of hypertension, diabetes, abdominal obesity, psychosocial factors, daily consumption of fruits and vegetables, regular alcohol consumption, and regular physical activity. Their significant associations with acute myocardial infarction were noted in men and women, old and young, and in all regions of the world *(26).* As discussed in the sections below, racial and ethnic differences in these traditional risk factors contribute to the established racial and ethnic disparities in cardiovascular health. In addition to differences in traditional risk factors, differences in cardiovascular biomarkers such as high sensitivity C-reactive protein (CRP), soluble intercellular adhesion molecule, homocysteine, and fibrinogen may contribute to or serve as markers for differences in disease burden and outcomes *(27–32).*

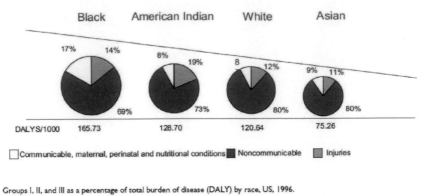

Groups I, II, and III as a percentage of total burden of disease (DALY) by race, US, 1996.

Fig. 5. The main categories of diseases and conditions expressed as a percentage of total burden of disease (DALY) by race, United States, 1996.
Reproduced with permission from PLoS.
Source: Michaud CM, McKenna MT, Begg S, et al. The burden of disease and injury in the United States 1996. *Popul Health Metr* 2006 October 18;4:11 *(25)*.

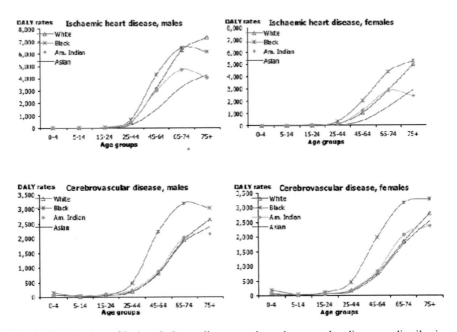

Fig. 6. The burden of ischemic heart disease and cerebrovascular diseases: distribution of DALY rates/100,000 by age, race, and sex, United States, 1996.
Reproduced with permission from PLoS.
Source: Michaud CM, McKenna MT, Begg S, et al. The burden of disease and injury in the United States 1996. *Popul Health Metr* 2006 October 18;4:11 *(25)*.

5.1. Self-Reported Behavioral and Lifestyle Risks

Self-reported behavioral and lifestyle risk factors for CVD vary by sex, race, ethnicity, and education level and contribute to the established disparities in cardiovascular health *(33)*. In the United States, several national and state-based surveillance systems provide crucial information on self-reported personal behaviors and lifestyle risks such as tobacco use, alcohol intake, consumption of fruits and vegetables, lack of participation in leisure-time physical activity, acceptance of seasonal influenza vaccination, and measures of overweight and obesity *(34–37)*.

In one comprehensive review of the state of disparities in these behavioral and lifestyle risk factors, the prevalence of "no physical activity" was common in all racial and ethnic groups, especially in women with less than high school education (Table 1) *(33)*. Daily intake of five or more servings of fruits and vegetables was low in all groups and lowest in African-American and white men with less than a high school education *(33)*. African-American men and women had the highest self-reported prevalence of diagnosed diabetes and high blood pressure, and African-American men had the highest rate of smoking *(33)*. Importantly, the prevalence of two or more risk factors (among six risk factors for heart disease and stroke: high blood pressure, high cholesterol, diabetes, current smoking, physical inactivity, and obesity) in adults aged 18 years and older was highest among blacks (48.7%) and American Indians/Alaska Natives (46.7%) and lowest among Asians (25.9%) *(38)*.

As shown in Fig. 7, the most recent data on the percentages of adults with selected unhealthy behavior characteristics from the National Health Interview Survey varied by race during 2002—2004, with usually high prevalence in African-Americans, American Indians and Alaska Natives, and Native Hawaiian or other Pacific Islanders *(39)*. Increasingly, the important contextual influences that social networks, social support, social norms, and policy and environmental changes have as modifying factors on these lifestyles and behaviors are increasingly being recognized *(40,41)*

5.2. Prevalence and Trends in Measured Risk Factors

Since the early 1960s, the National Health and Nutrition Examination Survey (NHANES) has periodically provided health data on the noninstitutionalized civilian US population and designated subgroups, including race and ethnicity *(35,42)*. Among the measured traditional risk factors, the most important in the pathogenesis of CVD include systolic blood pressure; total blood cholesterol, low-density and high-density lipoprotein cholesterol; body mass index; hemoglobin A1c; and the calculated prevalences of persons diagnosed, treated, and controlled for hypertension, diabetes, and dyslipidemia. Important racial and ethnic variations in all of these risks are well

Table 1

Unadjusted Prevalence of Risk Factors for Cardiovascular Diseases Among US Adults ≥18 Years of Age, The Behavioral Risk Factor Surveillance System, 2003

	Whites				Blacks				Mexican-Americans			
	<High School		≥High School		<High School		≥High School		<High School		≥High School	
	%	SE	%	SE	%	SE	%	SE	%	SE	%	SE
Current smoker												
Men	40.6	1.1	22.9	0.3	41.8	2.7	27.4	1.0	27.3	1.7	22.6	1.1
Women	34.6	0.9	19.9	0.2	25.6	1.6	17.8	0.7	10.6	1.0	12.9	0.7
Total	37.5	0.7	21.4	0.2	33.0	1.5	22.0	0.6	18.6	1.0	17.7	0.7
No physical activity												
Men	40.1	1.0	17.7	0.2	42.1	2.7	24.7	1.0	46.5	1.9	24.9	1.1
Women	45.3	0.9	21.5	0.2	50.7	1.9	32.2	0.8	52.2	1.7	33.3	1.0
Total	42.8	0.7	19.7	0.2	46.8	1.6	28.9	0.6	49.4	1.3	29.1	0.8
≥5 Servings of fruits and vegetables												
Men	13.3	0.7	18.6	0.3	14.6	2.0	18.9	0.9	18.2	1.6	17.4	1.1
Women	20.6	0.7	29.5	0.2	22.5	1.8	25.8	0.8	24.1	1.5	25.3	1.0
Total	17.1	0.5	24.3	0.2	18.9	1.3	22.8	0.6	21.3	1.1	21.4	0.7
Told to have diabetes												
Men	11.9	0.7	7.0	0.2	14.6	1.7	10.1	0.7	9.0	1.0	5.6	0.6
Women	13.3	0.5	5.9	0.1	19.2	1.3	10.6	0.5	11.5	1.0	6.4	0.5
Total	12.6	0.4	6.4	0.1	17.1	1.1	10.4	0.4	10.3	0.7	6.0	0.4

Reproduced with permission from Elsevier.
Source: Mensah GA, Mokdad AH, Ford ES, Greenlund KJ, Croft JB. State of disparities in cardiovascular health in the United States. *Circulation* 2005 March 15; 111(10):1233–1241 (*33*).

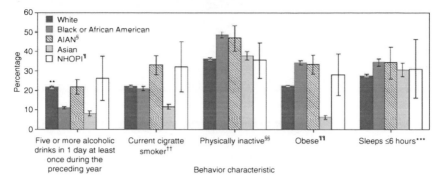

Fig. 7. The percentage of adults with selected unhealthy behavior characteristics varied by race during 2002–2004.

Source: Centers for Disease Control and Prevention. QuickStats: Prevalence of Selected Unhealthy Behavior Characteristics Among Adults Aged 18 Years, by Race* — National Health Interview Survey, United States, 2002–2004. *MMWR Morb Mort Wkly Rep* 2007 February 2;56(04):79 *(39)*.

*Racial categories include persons who indicated a single race only and are consistent with the 1997 Office of Management and Budget federal guidelines for race reporting. [†]Estimates are age adjusted using the 2000 projected US population as the standard population and using three age groups: 18–44, 45–64, and >65 years. Estimates are based on household interviews of a sample of the civilian, noninstitutionalized US adult population. Denominators for each percentage exclude persons with unknown health-behavior characteristics. [§] American Indian or Alaska Native;
[¶] Native Hawaiian or other Pacific Islander;
[**] 95% confidence interval;
[††] smoked at least 100 cigarettes in lifetime and currently smoked;
[§§] Never engaged in any light, moderate, or vigorous leisure-time physical activity;
[¶¶] Defined as a body mass index (weight [kg]/height [m^2]) of >30.

known and so contribute to the well-recognized disparities in CVD burden and outcomes *(33)*.

Generally, the prevalence of hypertension is highest among African Americans regardless of sex or educational status. The prevalence of hypercholesterolemia is usually highest among white and Mexican American men and white women in both education level groups. The prevalence of low concentrations of high-density lipoprotein cholesterol and hypertriglyceridemia is most favorable among African-Americans, although among the most educated women, whites and African-Americans have a similar prevalence of low concentration of high-density lipoprotein cholesterol. The prevalence of measured levels of hemoglobin A1c ≥7% is highest in African-American men and women (Table 2).

These racial and ethnic differences have also held up in more recent surveillance data. For example, in 2005–2006, the NHANES data showed that non-Hispanic blacks had a significantly higher prevalence of hypertension than the non-Hispanic white and Mexican American populations

Table 2

Prevalence of Measured Traditional Risk Factors for Cardiovascular Diseases Among US Adults ≥18 Years of Age, NHANES, 1999–2002

	Whites				Blacks				Mexican Americans			
	<High School		≥High School		<High School		≥High School		<High School		≥High School	
	%	SE	%	SE	%	SE	%	SE	%	SE	%	SE
Obesity (BMI ≥30 kg/m²)												
Men	28.4	2.0	27.2	1.1	25.1	1.8	26.9	2.2	22.3	1.7	29.2	2.5
Women	36.8	2.6	29.6	1.5	47.7	3.2	47.1	2.3	37.8	3.0	32.8	2.8
Men and women	32.8	1.7	28.5	1.1	37.2	1.8	38.4	1.6	29.5	1.7	31.0	1.9
Large waist												
(men >102 cm; women >88 cm)												
Men	44.9	2.6	39.6	1.2	29.4	1.8	27.2	1.7	25.2	1.7	34.2	2.0
Women	68.0	3.3	52.9	1.8	71.9	2.3	67.0	1.6	62.2	2.6	53.9	2.9
Men and women	56.8	2.2	46.4	1.4	51.9	1.6	49.8	1.4	42.3	1.2	43.9	1.6
Hypertension												
Men	39.3	2.5	29.8	1.2	45.9	2.8	31.8	1.7	21.1	2.2	16.5	2.1
Women	47.4	2.6	31.3	1.3	51.2	2.8	37.0	1.9	24.2	2.4	15.5	1.8
Men and women	43.5	1.9	30.6	1.0	48.7	2.4	34.7	1.3	22.6	1.8	16.0	1.3
Total cholesterol ≥200 mg/dl												
Men	45.5	3.0	49.2	1.5	37.7	2.8	41.7	2.3	49.2	2.7	45.5	2.8
Women	56.9	2.5	52.4	1.2	45.8	3.0	42.6	2.2	38.7	2.2	37.9	2.2
Men and women	51.4	2.0	50.8	1.0	41.9	2.0	42.2	1.8	44.4	2.0	41.7	1.6

Table 2
(Continued)

Glycosylated hemoglobin ≥7%												
Men	7.5	1.3	3.8	0.4	10.1	1.4	3.7	0.7	4.9	0.8	4.3	0.9
Women	6.2	1.2	2.2	0.3	10.9	1.9	6.7	0.9	7.8	1.2	3.6	0.7
Men and women	6.8	0.9	3.0	0.3	10.5	1.5	5.4	0.6	6.3	0.7	4.0	0.6
NHANES 1999–2000												
Low HDL cholesterol												
(men <40 mg/dl; women <50 mg/dl)												
Men	41.2	3.1	35.9	2.2	27.0	4.3	23.8	3.4	35.6	3.5	25.6	4.6
Women	54.8	4.3	38.8	2.4	33.8	3.9	39.7	3.4	47.4	2.5	45.7	3.6
Men and women	48.0	3.1	37.4	1.9	30.4	2.9	33.0	2.4	41.1	2.4	36.2	3.0
LDL-cholesterol ≥130 mg/dl												
Men	49.5	7.0	46.7	2.9	27.2	5.4	31.0	5.8	46.7	4.6	54.3	7.0
Women	33.6	7.5	42.3	2.8	36.3	7.4	25.1	4.3	30.1	4.8	28.0	4.9
Men and women	41.9	5.8	44.4	2.0	31.9	5.0	27.5	4.1	38.8	2.8	41.0	5.2
Triglycerides ≥150 mg/dl												
Men	38.3	7.7	35.7	3.2	...	...	...	...	40.5	4.2	40.2	9.1
Women	39.2	6.2	33.2	3.3	14.0	4.2	11.5	3.0	40.9	5.2	30.0	5.8
Men and women	38.7	4.6	34.4	2.4	15.4	4.2	10.4	2.6	40.7	3.7	35.2	6.6

Reproduced with permission from Elsevier.

Source: Mensah GA, Mokdad AH, Ford ES, Greenlund KJ, Croft JB. State of disparities in cardiovascular health in the United States. *Circulation* 2005 March 15; 111(10):1233–1241 (33).

(41% vs. 28% and 22%, respectively) *(43)*. No statistically significant differences were noted by race/ethnicity in the prevalence of prehypertension (defined as systolic BP 120–139 mmHg or diastolic BP 80–89 mmHg, and not pharmacologically treated for high BP) *(43)*. Hypertension awareness and treatment were highest in non-Hispanic blacks compared to non-Hispanic whites and Mexican Americans. However, no statistically significant differences were noted in control rates among persons treated for hypertension (64% overall) *(43)*.

Although glycemic control improved between 1999 and 2004 *(44)*, Mexican Americans and non-Hispanic Blacks were less likely to achieve good control (35.4 and 36.9%, respectively) compared with non-Hispanic Whites (48.6%) *(45)*. These racial and ethnic differences persisted even after multivariable adjustment for measures of socioeconomic status, obesity, healthcare access and utilization, and diabetes treatment *(45)*. Similarly, although the awareness, treatment, and control of high LDL-cholesterol among US adults increased significantly in 1999–2004, control rates remain significantly lower in non-Hispanic blacks and Mexican Americans compared with non-Hispanic whites (17.2% and 16.5% vs. 26.9%, respectively; $p = 0.05$ and $p = 0.008$) *(46)*. The 2005–2006 NHANES data again demonstrate the continuing epidemic of obesity in the United States, and especially the marked racial and ethnic disparities in the prevalence of obesity in women but not in men (Fig. 8) *(47)*.

5.3. Emerging Risk Factors and Biomarkers of Cardiovascular Risk

The NHANES also provides data on the prevalence of emerging risk factors for CVD stratified by sex, race/ethnicity, and education level (Table 3) *(33)*. Among men who had not completed a high school education, the prevalence of elevated concentrations of CRP is high among whites. Among men who had completed high school, the prevalence of elevated concentrations of C-reactive protein was high among African-American and Mexican American men. Among women who had not completed high school, the prevalence was variable among the three racial or ethnic groups, whereas among women who had completed high school, African-American, and Mexican American women tended to have a high prevalence of elevated concentrations of C-reactive protein. Similar patterns were observed for the prevalence of elevated concentrations of fibrinogen. Mexican American men and women had low prevalence of elevated concentrations of homocysteine regardless of educational status. Albuminuria was highest in African-Americans and was nearly twice the prevalence observed in Mexican Americans *(33)*.

In one systematic review of 20 studies that were unadjusted or adjusted for demographic variables, 19 found inverse associations between CRP levels and socioeconomic position. Of 15 similar studies, 14 found differences

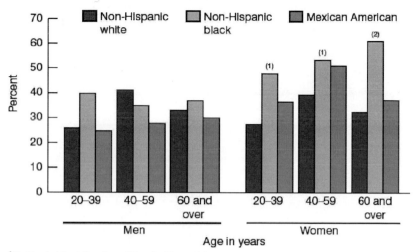

Fig. 8. Prevalence of obesity, by age, race/ethnicity, and sex, adults aged 20 years and older: United States, National Health and Nutrition Examination Survey, 2005–2006. Source: Ogden CL, Carroll MD, McDowell MA, Flegal KM. Obesity among adults in the United States – no change since 2003 2004. NCHS data brief no 1. Hyattsville, MD: National Center for Health Statistics. 2007. Available from:www.cdc.gov/nchs/data/databriefs/db01.pdf *(47)*.

between racial/ethnic groups such that whites had the lowest, while blacks, Hispanics, and South Asians had the highest CRP levels *(30)*. In a large multiethnic cohort study of four American racial/ethnic groups (Caucasian, Black, Hispanic, and Chinese), significant differences in hemostatic and endothelial markers were found *(32)*. Blacks had the highest levels of factor VIII, D-dimer, plasmin–antiplasmin (PAP), and von Willebrand factor, among the highest levels of fibrinogen and E-selectin (women only), but among the lowest levels of intercellular adhesion molecule 1 (ICAM-1), and, in men, the lowest levels of plasminogen activator inhibitor-1 (PAI-1) *(32)*. Whites and Hispanics tended to have intermediate levels of factors and markers, although they had the highest levels of ICAM-1, and Hispanics had the highest mean levels of fibrinogen and E-selectin (women only) *(32)*. Chinese participants had among the highest levels of PAI-1, but the lowest, or among the lowest, of all other factors and markers.

5.4. Markers of Subclinical Cardiovascular Disease

Another established biomarker of atherosclerotic plaque burden or subclinical coronary atherosclerosis is coronary artery calcium score (CACS) *(48)*. In a large, multi-center, ethnically diverse cohort of 14,812 patients,

Table 3
Prevalence of Emerging Risk Factors for CVD Among US Adults ≥18 Years of Age, NHANES, 1999–2002

| | Whites | | | | Blacks | | | | Mexican Americans | | | |
| | <High school | | ≥High school | | <High school | | ≥High school | | <High school | | ≥High school | |
	%	SE	%	SE	%	SE	%	SE	%	SE	%	SE
C-reactive protein >3 mg/L												
Men	37.9	2.9	26.2	1.1	31.7	2.0	32.0	2.2	22.3	2.1	25.6	2.1
Women	53.8	2.6	42.6	1.2	50.1	2.3	50.3	2.5	54.0	2.8	48.9	2.5
Men and women	46.1	1.6	34.6	0.9	41.4	1.5	42.6	1.9	37.0	1.9	37.2	1.8
Fibrinogen >3 g/L												
Men ≥40 year	89.5	2.2	76.2	1.8	84.3	3.6	78.1	2.4	68.8	2.9	73.0	3.5
Women ≥40 year	91.6	1.9	81.7	1.7	95.1	1.7	88.9	2.2	84.5	1.7	87.3	2.5
Men and women ≥40 year	90.6	1.6	79.1	1.5	90.1	2.1	84.3	1.6	76.6	2.1	80.3	2.1
Homocysteine >10 μmol/L												
Men	34.4	2.4	25.2	1.2	31.9	3.4	23.0	1.7	17.7	1.7	15.2	2.2
Women	25.1	2.2	13.7	0.8	22.5	1.9	11.5	1.5	7.9	1.4	4.7	1.4
Men and women	29.6	1.8	19.3	0.8	26.9	1.8	16.4	1.3	13.1	1.2	10.0	1.4
Microalbuminuria ≥30 to <300 mg/g or macroalbuminuria ≥300 mg/g												
Men	12.0	1.6	7.8	0.6	16.5	1.7	9.2	1.3	8.1	0.9	8.9	1.7
Women	16.2	1.5	8.7	0.8	19.6	1.4	10.5	1.0	12.0	1.6	9.6	1.6
Men and women	14.2	1.0	8.2	0.5	18.2	1.0	9.9	0.8	9.9	0.8	9.3	1.0

Reproduced with permission from Elsevier.
Source: Mensah GA, Mokdad AH, Ford ES, Greenlund KJ, Croft JB. State of disparities in cardiovascular health in the United States. *Circulation* 2005 March 15; 111(10):1233–1241 (*33*).

Nasir et al. *(49)* examined the prognostic value of CACS in African-Americans ($n = 637$), Asians ($n = 1,334$), Hispanics ($n = 1,334$), and non-Hispanic whites ($n = 11,776$). The prevalence of CAC scores ≥ 100 was highest in non-Hispanic whites (31%) and lowest for Hispanics (18%) ($p < 0.0001$). However, as also shown in previous studies, lower the CAC score, the better the prognosis, and the higher the CAC score, the worse the prognosis regardless of race or ethnicity. Importantly in this study, the finding of mild or more CAC in African-Americans conferred an all-cause mortality of nearly twice that documented for non-Hispanic whites and Hispanics, with the least all-cause mortality seen in Asians (Fig. 9) *(49)*. In fact, in the 10-year follow-up, the overall survival was 96, 93, and 92% for Asians, non-Hispanic whites, and Hispanics, respectively, as compared with 83% for African-Americans (Fig. 10; $p < 0.0001$) *(49)*. In the accompanying editorial, Rumberger pointed out the importance of underlying traditional risk

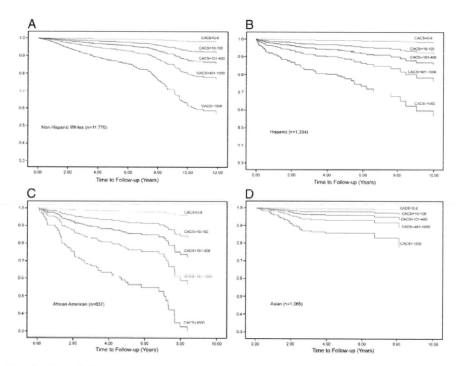

Fig. 9. Cumulative Survival By Coronary Artery Calcium Score (CACS) in ethnic subsets. (**A–D**) Using risk-stratified Cox proportional hazard survival analyses, the survival ranged from 98 to 57% in non-Hispanic whites, 97 to 30% in African-Americans, 99 to 60% in Hispanics, and 100 to 80% in Asians for CACS of 0–10 to 1,000.
Reproduced with permission from Elsevier.
Source: Nasir K, Shaw LJ, Liu ST, et al. Ethnic differences in the prognostic value of coronary artery calcification for all-cause mortality. *J Am Coll Cardiol* 2007 September 4;50(10):953–960 *(49)*.

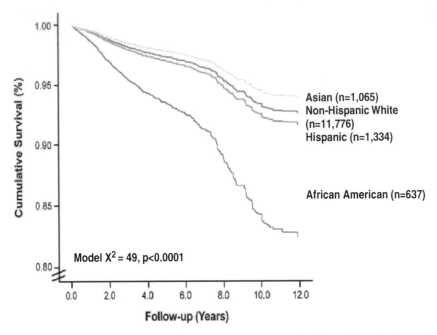

Fig. 10. Long-term survival in ethnic subsets ($n = 14,812$). Overall survival was 96, 93, and 92% for Asians, non-Hispanic whites, and Hispanics as compared with 83% for African-Americans, respectively, ($p = 0.0001$). Among all ethnic groups, the lowest survival was observed in African-Americans (83%, $p < 0.0001$).
Reproduced with permission from Elsevier.
Source: Nasir K, Shaw LJ, Liu ST, et al. Ethnic differences in the prognostic value of coronary artery calcification for all-cause mortality. *J Am Coll Cardiol* 2007 September 4;50 (10):953–960 *(49)*.

factors, with a much higher frequency of "no risk factors" in Asians across ethnic subgroups and greater frequency of 3 or more risk factors in African-Americans *(50)*.

6. CARDIOVASCULAR MORBIDITY

Nearly 81 million Americans, about one in three live with one or more forms of CVD *(51)*. The most common of these include hypertension, coronary heart disease, chronic heart failure, and stroke. Among persons aged 18 years and older in 2005, the age-adjusted percentage of heart disease was highest in American Indians or Alaska Natives (13.0%) and lowest in Asian Americans (6.7%) *(52)*. Stroke was, however, most prevalent in American Indians or Alaska Natives (5.8%) and African-Americans (3.4%) and least prevalent in Asian Americans (2.0%) *(52)*. African-Americans also had the highest age-adjusted percentage of hypertension (31.2%), while the lowest percentages were seen in Hispanics (20.3%) and in whites (21%) *(52)*.

Hospitalizations, especially for chronic heart failure, acute myocardial infarction, and stroke, constitute an important cause of morbidity from cardiovascular diseases. Among Medicare enrollees aged 65 years and older, whites had the highest prevalence of hospitalization for acute myocardial infarction (53,54). In fact, for the period of 1999–2004, the prevalence of acute myocardial infarction was higher in whites than in blacks for persons aged 55 years and older but in younger patients aged 35–54 years, the prevalence was higher in blacks (55). Overall the prevalence of the prevalence of hospitalizations for congestive heart failure was higher in African-Americans, Hispanics, and American Indian/Alaska Natives than among whites (53,54).

The overall prevalence of stroke and stroke hospitalizations Medicare population was highest in African-Americans (53–55).

7. ACCESS TO CARE AND THE QUALITY OF HEALTH CARE DELIVERED

Several publications, including an Institute of Medicine summary of the literature (56–63), and one review, conducted jointly by the American College of Cardiology Foundation and Kaiser Family Foundation (64), concluded (after examining the most rigorous studies investigating racial/ethnic differences in angiography, angioplasty, coronary artery bypass graft surgery, and thrombolytic therapy) that disparities in the quality of medical care are pervasive and they persist even after adjustment for potentially confounding factors. In addition, data from recent national health-care surveys and national health-care reports on disparities and health-care quality provide compelling evidence of the pervasiveness of disparities in quality of health care (65–67).

For example, the third annual *National Healthcare Disparities Report* published by the Agency for Health Research and Quality showed that disparities were observed in almost all aspects of health care and across all dimensions of quality of health care including effectiveness, patient safety, timeliness, and patient centeredness (65). In addition, these disparities were present across many levels and types of care including preventive care, treatment of acute conditions, and management of chronic diseases including cardiovascular diseases (65). Overall in that report, Hispanics received poorer quality of care than whites in 53% of the most important measures; blacks received poorer quality of care in 43% of these measures; and American Indians and Alaska Natives received poorer quality of care in 38% of the key measures (65).

In fact, the subsequent report for 2006 showed that for most core quality measures, Blacks (73%), Hispanics (77%), and poor people (71%) received worse quality care than their respective reference groups (66). Blacks and Asians had worse access to care than Whites for a third of core measures and Hispanics had worse access than non-Hispanic Whites for 83% of core measures *(66)*. Importantly, for most measures in racial and ethnic minorities, significant changes in disparities were not observed, although disparities were increasing for most (80%) measures for Hispanics *(66)*.

The Fifth National Health-Care Report on disparities observed that overall disparities in quality and access for minority groups and poor populations have not been reduced since publication of the first report 5 years earlier *(68)*. In addition, the report concluded that comparing data from 2000 to 2001 with those from 2004 to 2005, the number of measures on which disparities have significantly worsened or have remained unchanged since the first report is higher than the number of measures on which disparities have significantly improved for Blacks, Hispanics, American Indians and Alaska Natives, Asians, and poor populations *(68)*.

8. PROGRESS MADE IN THE ELIMINATION OF HEALTH DISPARITIES

Healthy People 2010 is the US national health promotion and disease prevention framework with the overarching goals of increasing the quality and years of healthy life (Goal-1) and eliminating health disparities (Goal-2) *(69)*. Periodic reviews are conducted to assess progress in achieving objectives for these goals *(69,70)*. Nineteen objectives and subobjectives established for heart disease and stroke were examined at the mid-course review to gauge progress made in addressing the two overarching goals and the 19 objectives and subobjectives *(71)*. This review observed numerous disparities in access to health care for several objectives and subobjectives (specific objective numbers in parentheses) *(71)*.

Overall, significant progress was made during the first half of the decade in improving cardiovascular health. The death rate from coronary heart disease and stroke declined to their lowest levels; hospitalizations due to heart failure declined; the proportion of adults with high blood pressure under control increased; and the target for reducing the proportion of persons with high blood cholesterol levels was met by the 1999–2002 period *(71–73)*. However, hypertension prevalence moved in the wrong direction, away from the 2010 target *(71,72)*. Of the 19 national objectives and subobjectives, 3 have met their respective targets, 7 others have moved toward their target, 1 has moved in the wrong direction away from the target, and 7 others could not be evaluated because the appropriate data were not available at the time of the review or have only recently become available *(72)*.

Most importantly, however, significant disparities persist by race/ethnicity, gender, educational level, and disability. For example, the summary index of disparity (SID) by race/ethnicity was <10% or not statistically significant for 6 objectives; however, it exceeded 10–49% for 7 objectives *(71)*. In particular, racial/ethnic disparities associated with coronary heart disease and stroke mortality increased. Similarly, the SID by education showed statistically significant disparities in seven of eight objectives *(71)*. In persons with less than a high school education, significant disparities were present in seven of eight objectives and in five, disparities exceeded 100% in comparison to persons with at least some college education *(71)*. As shown in Fig. 11, the Healthy People 2010 targets for coronary heart disease (Fig. 11) and stroke (Fig. 11) mortality rates were met by 2004 for whites, Hispanics, American Indians, and Asian Americans but not for blacks *(72)*.

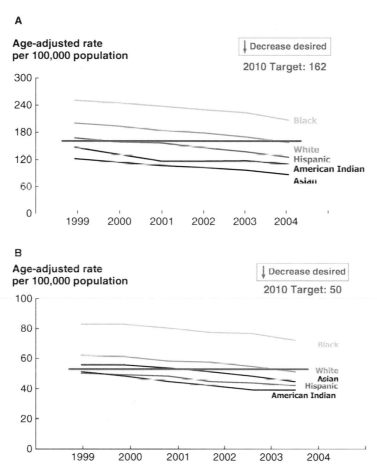

Fig. 11. Age-adjusted death rates for coronary heart disease (**A**) and stroke, by race and ethnicity, United States, 1999 – 2004. Note: Coronary heart disease deaths (**A**) are defined by ICD-10 codes I11, I20–I25 and stroke deaths (**B**) are defined by ICD-10 codes I60–I69. Data are age adjusted to the 2000 standard population. Asian includes Pacific Islander. The black and white categories exclude persons of Hispanic origin. Persons of Hispanic origin may be of any race.
Source: National Vital Statistics System—Mortality (NVSS-M), NCHS, CDC.

Additionally, among racial and ethnic groups, the white non-Hispanic population had the best group rate for the following specific Healthy People 2010 objectives: health insurance (1–1), counseled about smoking cessation (1–3c), a source of ongoing care (1–4a, b, and c), usual primary-care provider (1–5), difficulties or delays in obtaining needed health care (1–6), and delay or difficulty in getting emergency care (1–10) *(71)*. The black non-Hispanic population had the best rate for only two of the sub-objectives: persons counseled about physical activity (1–3a) and diet and nutrition (1–3b). The percentages of the American Indian or Alaska Native population and the Hispanic population that did not have health insurance (1–1) in 2003 were more than twice that of the white non-Hispanic population *(71)*. Similarly, despite a decline in disparity between the poor and the middle/high-income populations, lack of health insurance coverage among the poor and near-poor populations was more than three times that of the middle/high-income population.

Disparities were also noted in the percentage of persons who had a source of ongoing care (1–4). The disparity between the Hispanic population and the white non-Hispanic population exceeded 100% for all age groups. The review noted that the level of disparity has been increasing for all ages and for persons aged 18 years and older (1–4a and c). A similar level of disparity was observed among the Asian and non-Hispanic black populations for persons under 18 years of age (1–4b). Between 1998 and 2003, the disparity between the black non-Hispanic and the white non-Hispanic populations increased by 65 percentage points. Disparities of over 50% were also observed for objective 1–4 between the best income group (middle/high income) and the poor and near-poor populations *(71)*. Persons of two or more races were three times as likely as white non-Hispanic persons to experience delay or difficulty in getting emergency care *(1–10)*. Similarly, the poor and near-poor populations were about twice as likely as the middle/high-income population to have difficulty in obtaining emergency care. Although these measures are not specific for cardiovascular care, the crucial role that they play in overall cardiovascular health is indisputable.

9. SUMMARY AND CONCLUSIONS

Despite its know limitations, epidemiology provides compelling evidence of the pervasiveness of racial and ethnic disparities in cardiovascular health and outcomes. While the most recent evidence documents some progress, stroke and coronary heart disease mortality rates remain high in African-Americans and disparities associated with these rates have increased Table 4. A higher prevalence of lifestyle and behavioral risks, together with a greater prevalence of multiple traditional cardiovascular risk factors and adverse socioeconomic and environmental conditions especially in African-Americans, American Indians/Alaska Natives, contributes to these health

Table 4

a)

Population-based objectives	American Indian or Alaska Native	Asian	Native Hawaiian or other Pacific Islander	Two or more races	Hispanic or Latino	Black non-Hispanic	White non-Hispanic	Summary index
12-1. Coronary heart disease (CHD) death rate (1999, 2002) *			B[1]					
12-2. Knowledge of heart attack symptoms: 20+ years (2001) *							B	
12-3a. Receipt of artery-opening therapy within 1 hour of heart attack symptoms (2000-04)†	B	1				2	2	
12-3b. Receipt of percutaneous intervention within 90 minutes of heart attack symptoms (2000-04)†		1				2	B[2]	
12-4. Cardiopulmonary resuscitation (CPR) training (2001) *				B				
12-6a. Congestive heart failure hospitalizations: 65-74 years (1997, 1999) *							B[2]	
12-6b. Congestive heart failure hospitalizations: 75-84 years (1997, 1999) *						2	B[2]	
12-6c. Congestive heart failure hospitalizations: 85+ years (1997, 1999) *						2	B[2]	
12-7. Stroke death rate (1999, 2002) *	D	↑[1]				↑	↑	
12-8. Knowledge of stroke symptoms: 20+ years (2001) *							B	
12-9. High blood pressure: 20+ years (1988-94, 1999-2002) *					B[3]			
12-10. Controlled blood pressure: 20+ years with high blood pressure (1988-94, 1999-2002) *					3		B	
12-11. Taking action to help control high blood pressure: 18+ years with high blood pressure (1998, 2003) * [4]								
12-12. Blood pressure monitoring: 18+ years with high blood pressure (1998, 2003) *						B		
12-13. Mean total blood cholesterol levels: 20+ years (1988-94, 1999-2002) *					3	B		
12-14. High blood cholesterol levels: 20+ years (1988-94, 1999-2002) *					3	D		
12-15. Blood cholesterol screening within past 5 years: 18+ years (1988, 2003) * [4]		B	b					

Table 4
(Continued)

b)

The best group rate at the most recent data point.	B	The group with the best rate for specified characteristic.	b	Most favorable group rate for specified characteristic, but reliability criterion not met.		Best group rate reliability criterion not met.
				Percent difference from the best group rate		
Disparity from the best group rate at the most recent data point.		Less than 10 percent or not statistically significant		10-49 percent	50-99 percent	100 percent or more
				Increase in disparity (percentage points)		
Changes in disparity over time are shown when the change is greater than or equal to 10 percentage points and statistically significant, or when the change is greater than or equal to 10 percentage points and estimates of variability were not available.			↑ 10-49	↑↑ 50-99	↑↑ 100 or more
				Decrease in disparity (percentage points)		
			↓ 10-49	↓↓ 50-59	↓↓ 100 or more	
Availability of data.		Data not available.			Characteristic not selected for this objective.	

* The variability of best group rates was assessed, and disparities of ≥ 10% are statistically significant at the 0.05 level. Changes in disparity over time, noted with arrows, are statistically significant at the 0.05 level. See Technical Appendix.
† Measures of variability were not available. Thus, the variability of best group rates was not assessed, and the statistical significance of disparities and changes in disparity over time could not be tested. See Technical Appendix.
¹ Data are for Asians or Pacific Islanders.
² Data include persons of Hispanic origin.
³ Data are for Mexican Americans.
⁴ Baseline data by race and ethnicity are for 2003.

Data for objectives 12–5 and 12–16 are unavailable or not applicable. Years in parentheses represent the baseline data year and the most recent data year (if available). Disparity from the best group rate is defined as the percent difference between the best group rate and each of the other group rates for a characteristic (for example, race and ethnicity). The summary index is the average of these percent differences for a characteristic. Change in disparity is estimated by subtracting the disparity at baseline from the disparity at the most recent data point. Change in the summary index is estimated by subtracting the summary index at baseline from the summary index at the most recent data point. See Technical Appendix for more information.
Source: www.healthypeople.gov/data/midcourse/pdf/fa12.pdf.

disparities. Marked disparities in access to care and quality of health care persist, especially for Hispanics, African-Americans, Asians, and poor people of all races and ethnicity. Continued emphasis on strategies for elimination of these disparities, in addition to increasing the years and quality of life for all Americans, is necessary.

REFERENCES

1. Mensah GA, Brown DW. An overview of cardiovascular disease burden in the United States. *Health Aff (Millwood)* 2007; 26(1):38–48.
2. Anderson GM, Bronskill SE, Mustard CA, Culyer A, Alter DA, Manuel DG. Both clinical epidemiology and population health perspectives can define the role of health care in reducing health disparities. *J Clin Epidemiol* 2005; 58(8):757–762.
3. Gillum RF. The epidemiology of cardiovascular disease in black Americans [editorial; comment] [see comments]. *N Engl J Med* 1996; 335(21):1597–1599.
4. Tyroler HA, Hames CG, Gazes PC, et al. Cardiovascular disease epidemiology of blacks in the Evans County and Charleston heart studies. *Epidemiol Atheroscler* 1988.
5. Moy E, Arispe IE, Holmes JS, Andrews RM. Preparing the national healthcare disparities report: gaps in data for assessing racial, ethnic, and socioeconomic disparities in health care. *Med Care* 2005; 43(3 Suppl.):I9–16.

6. Arispe IE, Holmes JS, Moy E. Measurement challenges in developing the national healthcare quality report and the national healthcare disparities report. *Med Care* 2005; 43(3 Suppl.):I17–I23.
7. Buescher PA, Gizlice Z, Jones-Vessey KA. Discrepancies between published data on racial classification and self-reported race: evidence from the 2002 North Carolina live birth records. *Public Health Rep* 2005; 120(4):393–398.
8. Rhoades DA. Racial misclassification and disparities in cardiovascular disease among American Indians and Alaska Natives. *Circulation* 2005; 111(10):1250–1256.
9. Stehr-Green P, Bettles J, Robertson LD. Effect of racial/ethnic misclassification of American Indians and Alaskan Natives on Washington State death certificates, 1989-1997. *Am J Public Health* 2002; 92(3):443–444.
10. Frost F, Taylor V, Fries E. Racial misclassification of Native Americans in a surveillance, epidemiology, and end results cancer registry. *J Natl Cancer Inst* 1992; 84(12):957–962.
11. Cooper RS, Kaufman JS, Ward R. Race and genomics. *N Engl J Med* 2003; 348(12):1166–1170.
12. Cooper RS, Freeman VL. Limitations in the use of race in the study of disease causation. *J Natl Med Assoc* 1999; 91(7):379–383.
13. Cooper RS. A note on the biological concept of race and its application in epidemiological research. *Am Heart J* 1984; 108:706.
14. Arnett DK, Baird AE, Barkley RA, et al. Relevance of genetics and genomics for prevention and treatment of cardiovascular disease: a scientific statement from the American Heart Association Council on Epidemiology and Prevention, the Stroke Council, and the Functional Genomics and Translational Biology Interdisciplinary Working Group. *Circulation* 2007; 115(22):2878–2901.
15. Torres JB, Kittles RA. The relationship between "race" and genetics in biomedical research. *Curr Hypertens* Rep 2007; 9(3):196–201.
16. Mensah GA. Eliminating disparities in cardiovascular health: six strategic imperatives and a framework for action. *Circulation* 2005; 111(10):1332–1336.
17. Murray CJ, Salomon JA, Mathers C. A critical examination of summary measures of population health. *Bull World Health Organ* 2000; 78(8):981–994.
18. Molla MT, Wagener DK, Madans JH. Summary measures of population health: methods for calculating healthy life expectancy. *Healthy People* 2001; 21:1–11.
19. Wagener DK, Molla MT, Crimmins EM, Pamuk E, Madans JH. Summary measures of population health: addressing the first goal of healthy people 2010, improving health expectancy. *Healthy People* 2001; (22):1–13.
20. Levine RS, Foster JE, Fullilove RE, et al. Black-white inequalities in mortality and life expectancy, 1933-1999: implications for healthy people 2010. *Public Health Rep* 2001; 116(5):474–483.
21. Pamuk ER, Wagener DK, Molla MT. Achieving national health objectives: the impact on life expectancy and on healthy life expectancy. *Am J Public Health* 2004; 94(3):378–383.
22. Kung HC, Hoyert DL, Xu J, Murphy SL. Deaths: Preliminary data for 2005. Health E-Stats. Sept 2007. www.cdc.gov/nchs/products/pubs/pubd/hestats/prelimdeaths05/prelimdeaths05.htm. 1-9-2007. Ref Type: Electronic Citation.
23. Murray CJ, Kulkarni S, Ezzati M. Eight Americas: new perspectives on U.S. health disparities. *Am J Prev Med* 2005; 29(5 Suppl. 1):4–10.
24. Wong MD, Shapiro MF, Boscardin WJ, Ettner SL. Contribution of major diseases to disparities in mortality. *N Engl J Med* 2002; 347(20):1585–1592.
25. Michaud CM, McKenna, MT, Begg S, et al. The burden of disease and injury in the United States 1996. *Popul Health Metr* 2006; 4:11.
26. Yusuf S, Hawken S, Ounpuu S, et al. Effect of potentially modifiable risk factors associated with myocardial infarction in 52 countries (the INTERHEART study): case-control study. *Lancet* 2004; 364:937–952.

27. Albert MA. Inflammatory biomarkers, race/ethnicity and cardiovascular disease. *Nutr Rev* 2007; 65(12 Pt 2):S234–S238.
28. Lee S, Gungor N, Bacha F, Arslanian S. Insulin resistance: link to the components of the metabolic syndrome and biomarkers of endothelial dysfunction in youth. *Diabet Care* 2007; 30(8):2091–2097.
29. Marchesi S, Lupattelli G, Sensini A, et al. Racial difference in endothelial function: role of the infective burden. *Atherosclerosis* 2007; 191(1):227–234.
30. Nazmi A, Victora CG. Socioeconomic and racial/ethnic differentials of C-reactive protein levels: a systematic review of population-based studies. *BMC Public Health* 2007; 7(147):212.
31. Forouhi NG, Sattar N. CVD risk factors and ethnicity–a homogeneous relationship? *Atheroscler Suppl* 2006; 7(1):11–19.
32. Lutsey PL, Cushman M, Steffen LM, et al. Plasma hemostatic factors and endothelial markers in four racial/ethnic groups: the MESA study. *J Thromb Haemost* 2006; 4(12):2629–2635.
33. Mensah GA, Mokdad AH, Ford ES, Greenlund KJ, Croft JB. State of disparities in cardiovascular health in the United States. *Circulation* 2005; 111(10):1233–1241.
34. Mokdad AH, Stroup DF, Giles WH. Public health surveillance for behavioral risk factors in a changing environment. Recommendations from the Behavioral Risk Factor Surveillance Team. *MMWR Recomm Rep* 2003; 52(RR-9):1–12.
35. Centers for Disease Control and Prevention. National Health and Nutrition Examination Survey (NHANES 1999-2004). www.cdc.gov/nchs/about/major/nhanes/nhanes99-02.htm. 10-11-2004. 10-5-2004. Ref Type: Electronic Citation.
36. Adams PF, Schoenborn CA. Health behaviors of adults: United States, 2002-04. *Vital Health Stat* 10 2006; 230:1–140.
37. Mokdad AH, Bales VS, Greenlund KJ, Mensah GA. Public health surveillance for disease prevention: lessons from the behavioral risk factor surveillance system. *Ethn Dis* 2003; 13(2 Suppl. 2):S19–S23.
38. Centers for Disease Control and Prevention. Racial/ethnic and socioeconomic disparities in multiple risk factors for heart disease and stroke: United States, 2003. *MMWR Morb Mortal Wkly Rep* 2005; 54:113–117.
39. Centers for Disease Control and Prevention. QuickStats: Prevalence of Selected Unhealthy Behavior Characteristics Among Adults Aged <18 Years, by Race* — National Health Interview Survey, United States, 2002–2004. *MMWR Morb Mort Wkly Rep* 2007; 56(04):79.
40. Emmons KM, Barbeau EM, Gutheil C, Stryker JE, Stoddard AM. Social influences, social context, and health behaviors among working-class, multi-ethnic adults. *Health Educ Behav* 2007; 34 (2):315–334.
41. Association of State and Territorial Directors of Health Promotion and Public Health Education, CDC. Policy and Environmental Change: New Directions for Public Health: Final Report. www.astdhpphe.org/healthpolicyfinalreport.pdf . 2001. Atlanta: CDC. Ref Type: Electronic Citation.
42. Centers for Disease Control and Prevention. National Health and Nutrition Examination Survey. Laboratory procedures manual. www.cdc.gov/nchs/data/nhanes/LAB7-11.pdf. 2004. 10-5-2004. Ref Type: Electronic Citation.
43. Ostchega Y, Yoon SS, Hughes J, Louis T. Hypertension awareness, treatment, and control – continued disparities in adults: United States, 2005-2006. NCHS data brief no 3. Hyattsville, MD: National Center for Health Statistics; 2008.
44. Hoerger TJ, Segel JE, Gregg EW, Saaddine JB. Is glycemic control improving in U.S. adults? *Diabet Care* 2008; 31(1):81–86.
45. Saydah S, Cowie C, Eberhardt MS, De RN, Narayan KM. Race and ethnic differences in glycemic control among adults with diagnosed diabetes in the United States. *Ethn Dis* 2007; 17(3):529–535.

46. Hyre AD, Muntner P, Menke A, Raggi P, He J. Trends in ATP-III-defined high blood cholesterol prevalence, awareness, treatment and control among U.S. adults. *Ann Epidemiol* 2007; 17(7):548–555.
47. Ogden CL, Carroll MD, McDowell MA, Flegal KM. Obesity among adults in the United States— no change since 2003–2004. NCHS data brief no 1. Hyattsville, MD: National Center for Health Statistics; 2007.
48. Rumberger JA, Simons DB, Fitzpatrick LA, Sheedy PF, Schwartz RS. Coronary artery calcium area by electron-beam computed tomography and coronary atherosclerotic plaque area. A histopathologic correlative study. *Circulation* 1995; 92(8):2157–2162.
49. Nasir K, Shaw LJ, Liu ST, et al. Ethnic differences in the prognostic value of coronary artery calcification for all-cause mortality. *J Am Coll Cardiol* 2007; 50(10):953–960.
50. Rumberger JA. The ethnic Rosetta stone: translating risk factors, plaque scores, and mortality. *J Am Coll Cardiol* 2007; 50(10):961–963.
51. Rosamond W, Flegal K, Furie K, et al. Heart disease and stroke statistics–2008 update: a report from the American Heart Association Statistics Committee and Stroke Statistics Subcommittee. *Circulation* 2008; 117(4):e25–146.
52. Pleis JR, Lethbridge-Cejku M. Summary health statistics for U.S. adults: National Health Interview Survey, 2005. *Vital Health Stat* 10 2006;(232):1–153.
53. National Center for Health Statistics. Health, United States, 2003. With chartbook on trends in the health of Americans. Hyattsville, MD: National Center for Health Statistics; 2003.
54. Lethbridge-Çejku M, Schiller JS, Bernadel L. Summary health statistics for U.S. Adults: National Health Interview Survey, 2002. National Center for Health Statistics. Vital Health Stat 10, 1-160. 2004. Ref Type: Electronic Citation.
55. National Heart LaBI. Morbidity and mortality: 2007 chartbook on cardiovascular, lung, and blood diseases. Bethesda, MD: NIH/National Heart, Lung, and Blood Institute; 2007.
56. Gordon HS, Paterniti DA, Wray NP. Race and patient refusal of invasive cardiac procedures. *J Gen Intern Med* 2004; 19(9):962–966.
57. Martin R, Lemos C, Rothrock N, et al. Gender disparities in common sense models of illness among myocardial infarction victims. *Health Psychol* 2004; 23(4):345–353.
58. Rothenberg BM, Pearson T, Zwanziger J, Mukamel D. Explaining disparities in access to high-quality cardiac surgeons. *Ann Thorac Surg* 2004; 78(1):18–24.
59. Walker DR, Stern PM, Landis DL. Examining healthcare disparities in a disease management population. *Am J Manag Care* 2004; 10(2 Pt 1):81–88.
60. Grace SL, Abbey SE, Bisaillon S, Shnek ZM, Irvine J, Stewart DE. Presentation, delay, and contraindication to thrombolytic treatment in females and males with myocardial infarction. *Women's Health Issues* 2003; 13(6):214–221.
61. O'Connell L, Brown SL. Do nonprofit HMOs eliminate racial disparities in cardiac care? *J Health Care Finance* 2003; 30(2):84–94.
62. Litaker D, Koroukian SM. Racial differences in lipid-lowering agent use in medicaid patients with cardiovascular disease. *Med Care* 2004; 42(10):1009–1018.
63. Institute of Medicine. Unequal treatment: confronting racial and ethnic disparities in health care. Washington DC: National Academies Press; 2003.
64. Lillie-Blanton M, Maddox TM, Rushing O, Mensah GA. Disparities in cardiac care: rising to the challenge of Healthy People 2010. *J Am Coll Cardiol* 2004; 44(3):503–508.
65. U.S. Department of Health and Human Services. 2005 National Healthcare Disparities Report. http://www.qualitytools.ahrq.gov/disparitiesreport/documents/Report 207.pdf. 7-1-2005. Ref Type: Electronic Citation.
66. U.S. Department of Health and Human Services. 2006 National Healthcare Disparities Report. http://www.ahrq.gov/qual/nhdr06/nhdr06report.pdf. 2006. Ref Type: Electronic Citation.

67. U.S. Department of Health and Human Services. 2006 National Healthcare Quality Report. www.ahrq.gov/qual/nhqr06/nhqr06report.pdf. 2006. Ref Type: Electronic Citation.
68. Agency for Healthcare Research and Quality. 2007 National Healthcare Disparities Report. AHRQ Pub. No. 08-0041. Rockville, MD: U.S. Department of Health and Human Services, Agency for Healthcare Research and Quality; 2008.
69. U.S. Department of Health and Human Services. Healthy People 2010. With understanding and improving health and objectives for improving health. 2 ed. Washington, DC: U.S. Government Printing Office; 2000.
70. U.S. Department of Health and Human Services. Tracking Healthy People 2010. Washington, DC: U.S. Government Printing Office; 2000.
71. Department of Health and Human Services. Healthy People 2010 Midcourse Review: Focus Area 12 - Heart Disease and Stroke. www.healthypeople.gov/Data/ midcourse/pdf/FA12.pdf. 2007. 9-8-2007. Ref Type: Electronic Citation.
72. Centers for Disease Control and Prevention. Data 2010: The Healthy People 2010 Database. http://wonder.cdc.gov/data2010/obj.htm. 1-14-2008. 3-10-2008. Ref Type: Electronic Citation.
73. Minino AM, Heron MP, Murphy SL, Kochanek KD. Deaths: final data for 2004. *Natl Vital Stat Rep* 2007; 55(19):1–119.

3

Unmasking Racial/Ethnic Disparities in Cardiovascular Disease: Nutritional, Socioeconomic, Cultural, and Health-Care-Related Contributions

J.M. Flack, MD, MPH, S.A. Nasser, PA-C, MPH, A. Goel, MD, M. "Toni" Flowers, BA, S. O'Connor, BS, and E. Faucett, BS

CONTENTS

From: *Contemporary Cardiology: Cardiovascular Disease in Racial and Ethnic Minorities*
Edited by: K.C. Ferdinand and A. Armani, DOI 10.1007/978-1-59745-410-0_3
© Humana Press, a part of Springer Science+Business Media, LLC 2009

SUMMARY
REFERENCES

Abstract

The cardiovascular disease (CVD) burden and disparities within the general population are largely determined by environmental, dietary, and other lifestyle factors. Minority groups have higher rates of morbidity and mortality than do their white counterparts for many diseases, including CVD. Overall, social and environmental factors seem to be more explanatory and influential than genetic factors in explaining the population disease burden of chronic CVD and racial/ethnic differences in the same. When addressing both the risk factors and the health challenges of CVD, it is critical that health-care providers make efforts to understand how racial and ethnic minorities define health, their health beliefs, and health seeking behaviors, as well as how their attitudes, behaviors, and beliefs influence health outcomes. Effective efforts in improving modifiable, lifestyle factors, and deleterious chronic exposures (e.g., positive energy balance) are perhaps the major venue for improving the population CVD burden; and emphasizing cultural competence and raising quality of medical care will be very effective means for reducing disparities in care provision and clinical outcomes in health systems.

Key Words: Cardiovascular disease; Disparities; Ethnicity; Cultural competency; Socioeconomic status; Health-care systems.

1. POPULATION-BASED CVD BURDEN/RACIAL AND ETHNIC DISPARITIES IN CVD

Heart disease and stroke are ranked first and third among the leading causes of death in the United States (US) *(1)*. Of the 2.4 million deaths in 2003, 34.4% were related to CVD. Approximately one in every three American adults has one or more types of CVD; the prevalence increases with age and varies within racial, ethnic, geographic, and sociodemographic groups *(2)*. Within the realm of CVD, the most prevalent conditions are hypertension (65 million), coronary heart disease (13.2 million), stroke (5.5 million), heart failure (5 million), and congenital heart defects (1 million) *(2)*. The total annual cost for health care and lost productivity due to cardiovascular diseases in the United States is $448 billion dollars. Heart disease ranks at the top costing $296 billion in direct health expenditures, $38 billion in indirect cost of morbidity, and $114 billion in indirect cost of mortality *(3)*.

The CVD burden and disparities in the general population are most plausibly attributable to how we live. That is, population disease burden is largely determined by dietary patterns, exercise, the balance between energy intake and expenditure, cigarette smoking, etc. According to the Behavior Risk

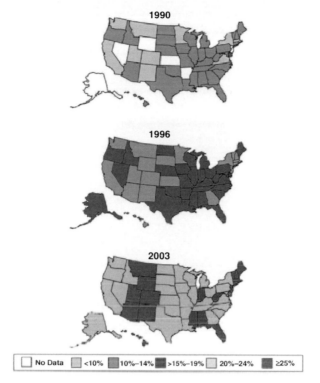

Fig. 1. Trends in obesity (defined as BMI > 30 kg/m^2) among US adults, BRFSS 1990, 1996, and 2003.
Behavioral Risk Factor Surveillance System, CDC.

Factor Surveillance System (BRFSS) run by the Centers for Disease Control (CDC), obesity increased rapidly from 1990 to 2003 (Fig. 1). About 80% of people with hypertension (HTN) in the United States are overweight or obese (body mass index [BMI] $\geq$ 25 kg/m^2). Obesity is related to HTN risk in all racial/ethnic populations. There are many obesity-related physiological effects that contribute to elevated BP, including salt-sensitivity and resistance to antihypertensive drug therapy. Obesity is also a plausible contributor to chronic renal injury. Physical activity among adults has been shown to vary inversely to both income level and educational attainment (in whites and non-whites) and also to be lower in non-white racial/ethnic groups compared to whites (Fig. 2). In 2004, the CDC reported that although physical activity was low in all income/racial groups whites were more active than either Hispanics or blacks at all income levels. Hispanics and blacks had similar activity levels at 16 and 18%, respectively, in those with incomes 100% below poverty levels. Since 1965 cigarette smoking has been on the decline among men and women. In the period between 1965 and

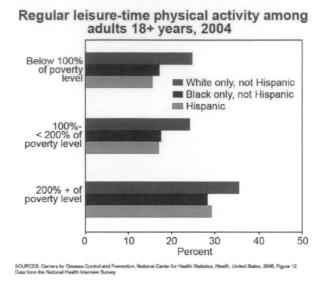

Fig. 2. Physical activity based on ethnic classification and poverty level.

2005, the rates decreased from 51 to 24% for men and from 34% to 20% for women *(2)*. In 2005, about 5.1 million, or 21.5% of, non-Hispanic black adults smoked cigarettes compared to 21.9% of non-Hispanic whites. Blacks accounted for approximately 11% of the 45.1 million adults who were current smokers in the United States during 2005 *(4)*.

Non-Hispanic black women have the highest prevalence of CVD at 49.0%, followed by non-Hispanic black men with 44.6%. Non-Hispanic white men and women as well as Mexican-American women have similar prevalences at 37.2, 35.0, and 34.4%, respectively. Mexican-American men have the lowest prevalence at 31.6% *(5)*. Lower socioeconomic status (SES) in the United States has been linked to increased CVD risk factors in a number of previous studies; the indicators for SES include education, income, and occupational status *(6–9)*.

2. LIKELY CAUSES OF POPULATION-BASED DIFFERENCES IN CVD BURDEN BY RACE/ETHNICITY

In the United States, cardiovascular disease (CVD) is the number one killer of Americans; however, the armamentarium to treat CVD has never been more superior. However, CVD has been widely recognized as being less than optimally treated. Members of minority groups have higher rates of morbidity and mortality than do their white counterparts for many, though not all, diseases including CVD *(10–13)*. Nevertheless, as important as high quality, successful treatment of CVD is among diseased populations, treatment is not an important contributor to racial and ethnic disparities in the population burden of CVD.

2.1. The Role of Genetics in Race/Ethnicity Disparities in CVD

There is little doubt that genes influence susceptibility to CVD. However, a predominant role of genes, per se, in determining the paucity or excess of CVD between racial and ethnic groups, especially for common CVD entities that likely have complex influence from multiple genes, is unlikely. Given the relatively free-flow of genetic loci between racial and ethnic groups because of the continual mixing and migration of human populations throughout history, it is very unlikely that genes responsible for common diseases would be localized to any great differential by race or ethnicity.

Several studies have shown that health-related disparities among racial and ethnic groups disappear or are measurably attenuated once confounding variables such as income and education have been controlled for *(14,15)*. However, even after adjustment for confounding variables, a significant number of studies demonstrate that racial and ethnic disparities remain *(16,17)*. Social and environmental factors seem to be more explanatory and carry more weight than genetic factors in explaining racial/ethnic differences. Nevertheless, this statement does not discount the likely genetic, albeit complex (e.g., gene–gene, gene–environment) interactions and their likely contributions to CVD.

The average proportion of nucleotide differences between a randomly chosen pair of humans is 1 in 1000–1500 *(18)*. Of this 0.1% of DNA that varies among individuals, ~90% of that variability occurs *within* continental racial groups, leaving less than 0.01% (i.e., 1 in 10,000) of genetic variability *between* groups. Thus, humans vary only slightly at the DNA level and only a small proportion of this variation separates continental populations. Studies based on loci have shown that individuals tend to cluster according to their ancestry or geographic origin *(19,20)*. Ancestry also appears to be a more accurate descriptor of individual genetic makeup than race *(21)*. Therefore, although proportions of some important alleles differ between racial/ethnic populations, the hypothesis that this observation accounts for common CVD disease differentials remains unproven.

Consistent with our line of reasoning is a study by Cooper and colleagues that reported the prevalence of hypertension in 85,000 persons. They compared racial groups, sampling white people from eight surveys completed in Europe, the United States, and Canada and contrasted these results with those from three surveys undertaken in black people in Africa, the West Indies, and the United States. Data from Brazil, Trinidad, and Cuba showed a significantly smaller racial disparity in blood pressure than was observed in

North America. In rural Nigeria, the mean blood pressures were low and rose only modestly with age. Accordingly, the authors concluded "These data demonstrate that the consistent emphasis given to the genetic elements of the racial contrasts may be a distraction from the more relevant issue of defining and intervening on the preventable causes of hypertension, which are likely to have a similar impact regardless of ethnic and racial background" *(22)*. Another study which reviewed surveys on hypertension published since 1990 in two North American countries (United States and Canada) and six European nations (England, Finland, Germany, Italy, Spain, and Sweden) found that mean BP measurements and hypertension prevalence were much higher in the six European countries than in Canada and the United States *(23)*.

2.2. Environmental Effects

In a classic 1991 study, Klag and colleagues found that among blacks darker skin color was linked to higher blood pressure levels *(24)*. Klag argued that the correlation between skin color and blood pressure was not biologic or genetic in origin, but sociologic in effect as measured by education, occupation, and ethnicity. This association of skin color with blood pressure was present *only* in the lower levels of socioeconomic strata which may be due to the lesser ability of these groups to deal with psychosocial and environmental stresses associated with darker skin tone; or perhaps attributable to other causes that occur more commonly in persons of lower socioeconomic standing. However, a common misnomer is that non-genetic and/or environmental factors have no measurable impact on biology. As the subsequent example will show, this is a patently untrue assumption.

In the United States, the prevalence of hypovitaminosis D is significantly more prevalent in blacks than whites; this is especially true among women where there is a 10-fold greater prevalence of vitamin $D < 37.5$ nmol/L (42.4% vs. 4.2%). A multiplicity of factors contribute to lower circulating vitamin D in levels in blacks including darker skin and more pervasive obesity, especially among women. Vitamin D deficiency has been associated with congestive heart failure *(25)*, decreased cell function and depressed insulin sensitivity *(26)*, and subsequently, elevated blood pressure/hypertension *(27–29)*. In NHANES III, it was estimated that lower vitamin D levels between blacks might explain ∼one-half of the excess hypertension prevalence in the blacks compared to whites *(28)*. Also, circulating vitamin D level has been inversely linked to the risk of myocardial infarction, even after controlling for known/suspected coronary risk factors *(30)*.

Obesity is clearly correlated with hypovitaminosis D and to reactive rises in parathyroid hormone (PTH) secondary hyperparathyroidism in blacks;

the reactive, and probably deleterious, rise in parathyroid hormone (PTH) metabolic aberrations is probably secondary to both the low levels of vitamin D and the low dietary calcium intake – both of which are highly prevalent among black populations (Fig. 3). Biologically active vitamin D augments intestinal calcium absorption. Additionally, it is very plausible that some of the obesity-related HTN is linked to low dietary calcium intake, hypovitaminosis D, and chronic reactive PTH elevations. Vitamin D production in the skin in response to ultraviolet light is normal in obese persons, however, there is significantly greater sequestration of vitamin D in adipocytes that leads to reduced circulating levels of 25(OH)D. There are also multiple proven physiological pathways through which low vitamin D and/or elevated PTH can cause obesity *(31–33)*. Hypovitaminosis D coupled with low dietary calcium intake, as a consequence of inadequate dairy intakes, plausibly leads to transient reductions in ionized calcium that stimulate the reactive rise in PTH. Figure 3 displays how this occurs and also plausible physiological effects of depressed circulating vitamin D/elevated PTH. The avoidance of dairy products that has been repeatedly identified in

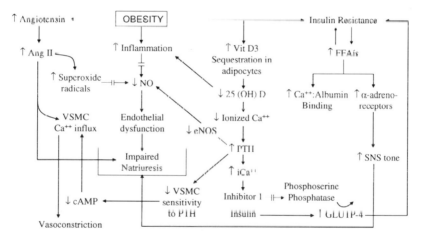

Fig. 3. Obesity-related neurohumoral and endocrine perturbations that raise blood pressure and cause vascular dysfunction.
FFA's, free fatty acids; Ang II, angiotensin II; NO, nitric oxide; Ca++, calcium; eNOS, endothelial nitric oxide; PTH, parathyroid hormone; SNS, sympathetic nervous system; VSMC, vascular smooth muscle cell; GLUTP-4, glucose transporter-4 phosphorylated; cAMP, cyclic adenosine 3′,5′ monophosphate.
This figure provides an integrated schema for how obesity affects the renin–angiotensin system, nitric oxide synthesis, vitamin D, calcium, and PTH metabolism as well as insulin resistance. Persistently high PTH levels raise intracellular calcium concentration. This activates inhibitor 1 leading to diminished phosphoserine phosphatase, an enzyme that dephosphorylates GLUTP-4. Phosphorylated GLUTP-4 is an ineffective transporter of glucose across the cell membrane.

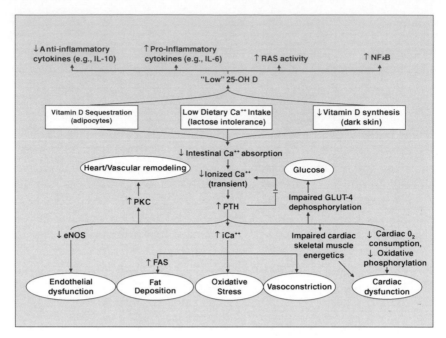

Fig. 4. This figure displays plausible vascular and target-organ effects of vitamin D deficiency and reactive rises in parathyroid hormone, especially in the setting of low dietary calcium intake. This schematic maybe particularly relevant to African-Americans given their high prevalence of lactose intolerance, leading to under-consumption of dairy products and low calcium intake. Left ventricular hypertrophy, obesity, heart failure, high levels of oxidative stress, and excessive/premature vascular remodeling have all been reported as occurring disproportionately.

IL, interleukin; RAS, renin–angiotensin system; NFKB, nuclear factor kappa beta; Ca^{++}, calcium; PKC, proteinkinase C; PTH, parathyroid hormone; eNOS, endothelial nitric oxide; FAS, fatty acid synthase; GLUT-4, glucose transporter-4

blacks probably relates to their relatively high prevalence ($\sim$80%) of lactose intolerance. Asian-Americans are even more lactose intolerant than blacks.

In all likelihood, obesity contributes significantly to HTN risk in all racial/ethnic populations and many racial and ethnic minorities manifest obesity disproportionately. Approximately 80% of people with HTN in the United States are overweight or obese (BMI $\geq$ 25 kg/m^2). In black women, the prevalence of extreme obesity (BMI $>$ 40 kg/m2) is almost one in six, a prevalence that is $\sim$three- to four-fold higher than that of white and Hispanic women. There are marked ethnic and age-based differences in the rates of weight accumulation. Relative to white women (reference group), the onset of obesity occurred sooner for black and Hispanic women. Hispanic men also develop obesity at younger ages than white men. After 28 years of age, black men develop obesity more rapidly than white men.

Anthropometric measures, such as obesity, that correlate inversely with low socioeconomic status (SES), especially in women, can also influence biologic systems involved in BP regulation and the expression of pressure-related target-organ damage (i.e., chronic renal injury). For example, obesity is a major anthropometric correlate of salt sensitivity in blacks and whites and is extremely prevalent among lower SES persons, particularly women.

There is a multiplicity of obesity-related physiological effects that contribute to the intermediate BP phenotype, salt sensitivity *(34,35)*. Dietary sodium-induced attenuation of BP-lowering responsiveness results is also attributable, at least in part, to salt sensitivity. Multiple factors contribute to salt sensitivity including obesity *(36,37)*, NO deficient states *(38,39)*, psychosocial stressors *(40)*, low intake of dietary potassium *(41,42)*, advancing age, and reduced renal mass. Though salt sensitivity has been documented in virtually every ethnic population that has been tested for it, salt sensitivity has often been found to be more prevalent in blacks than whites *(43–45)*. Figure 3 provides an integrated display of how obesity affects vascular function, natriuresis/salt sensitivity, vitamin D/PTH metabolism, and glucose tolerance.

2.3. Low Birth Weight

Maternal obesity increases the risk of preexisting maternal HTN, as well as pregnancy-induced HTN and pre-eclampsia and eclampsia. Obesity is also a risk factor for pre-term delivery. All of these conditions increase the likelihood of preterm delivery and poor intrauterine growth resulting in low birth weight (LBW), which is <2500 g in infants. The risk of delivering a LBW infant is very high among black women. According to the 2003 Centers for Disease Control Pediatric Nutrition Surveillance System, the prevalence of LBW is higher for black infants (12.9%) than for white (8.5%), Asian or Pacific Islander (8.3%), Hispanic (7.3%), and American Indian or Alaska Native (7.1%) infants *(46)*. Low birth weight babies are not found evenly across all geographic locations in the United States, as there is a higher proportion of LBW babies in the southeastern United States compared to other geographic regions. Prematurity and LBW appear to contribute to adult CVD risk in several ways. Low birth weight has been linked to central obesity and higher BMI later in life as well as higher childhood blood pressures. Low birth weight has also been linked to fewer nephrons at birth and to a relatively greater ratio of medullary to cortical glomeruli *(47,46)* – the former being less effective in their ability to autoregulate their glomerular filtration rate and protect against transmission of systemic pressure into the glomerulus. Thus, LBW, an obesity-related conditions, that disproportionately affects non-whites in the United states appears to have an intergenerational effect of augmenting CVD risk.

2.4. Dietary Nutrients and Physiologic Effects upon CVD

Long-term dietary patterns plausibly impact long-term trends in BP. Dietary sodium intake raises BP, at least in susceptible people, in the short-term. There is also evidence that dietary sodium intake augments vascular angiotensin generation *(49)* while, in salt sensitive persons also, reduces urinary nitric oxide (NO) metabolites *(50)*. Dietary sodium downregulates NO, upregulates vascular angiotensin II, and raises oxidative stress via upregulation of NADPH oxidase *(49,51)*. Oxidative stress reflected by release of reactive oxygen species (ROS) such as superoxide anion ($O_2^{\bullet-}$) has several deleterious physiological effects, most importantly a reduction of NO bioactivity. Recently, Fang and colleagues demonstrated that high-salt significantly induces increases in BP as well as plasma asymmetrical dimethylarginine (ADMA), a known inhibitor of NO synthesis, while decreasing plasma NO synthesis and urinary NO excretion in normotensive salt sensitive but not salt-resistant Asians *(52)*. This finding suggests that salt loading may inhibit NO synthesis by increasing the production of ADMA in salt-sensitive subjects. Sodium also enhances urinary calcium excretion and may therefore contribute to reductions in ionized calcium that can upregulate PTH secretion.

Dietary potassium intake has been shown to enhance renal natriuresis as well as to augment NO production. In the setting of ad lib potassium intake, potassium stimulates kallekrein release converting kininogen to bradykinin which increases NO release. Also, recent data documented that dietary potassium intake prevented the sodium-induced rise in circulating ADMA. Moreover, high levels of dietary potassium intake have been shown to modestly lower BP as well as to augment the normal nocturnal fall (10–20% lower than daytime values) in BP. Increasing dietary potassium intake into the range of ~80–120 mmol per day virtually abolished the salt-induced rise in BP during dietary sodium in blacks *(53)*, and, also essentially eliminated the greater salt sensitivity in blacks compared to whites.

Lower dietary intake of calcium has been linked to HTN in blacks. Calcium supplementation has been shown to induce a natriuresis as well as to modestly lower BP, especially in persons with low dietary calcium intake. Thus, in any population, potassium and calcium-rich and low sodium diets should favor lower BP levels. This type of diet would be rich in fresh fruits, vegetables, and low-fat dairy products, while simultaneously being low in sodium. Such a diet is similar, if not identical, to the DASH diet. The adverse physiological impact of low dietary calcium intake is likely greatest in vitamin D-deficient populations given the major influence of vitamin D in augmenting intestinal calcium absorption.

Magnesium is a cofactor in hundreds of enzymatic reactions, thus is important for multiple biochemical reactions involved in the cell cycle, nucleic acid synthesis, mitochondrial integrity, and a modulator of ion transport pumps, carriers, and channels *(54,55)*. Evidence suggests that magnesium deficiency has been shown to have an important role in the pathogenesis of ischemic heart disease, congestive heart failure, sudden cardiac death, cardiac arrhythmias, diabetes mellitus, and hypertension *(56–58)*. Additionally, magnesium affects BP by modifying vascular tone and reactivity and it also acts as a calcium channel antagonist and stimulates production of NO and prostacyclins *(59)*. Cross-sectional studies have shown that magnesium intake correlates significantly with adiposity, insulin resistance, and hypertension *(60,61)*. Higher magnesium intake was associated with lower fasting insulin concentrations among non-diabetics; however, magnesium was inversely associated with systemic inflammation and the prevalence of the metabolic syndrome. Dietary magnesium intake is lower in blacks than whites *(62)*. Dietary magnesium intake is a plausible contributor to the risk for CVD diseases that are more common in blacks and other minority populations than whites.

2.5. Dietary Nutrients, Socioeconomic Status, and Race

Socioeconomic status indicators (e.g., education and income) function as surrogate markers of a constellation of lifestyle characteristics, including diet, physical activity, psychosocial and environmental stressors, social support, coping mechanisms, and health-seeking behaviors, as well as access to health-related information and medical care. During the last three decades, little change in sodium intake has taken place while fat content and alcohol intake have declined, but total intake of calories and obesity prevalence have increased. Moreover, ethnic minority and low-income populations have some of the highest rates of CVD and the highest rates of physical inactivity, especially in lower socioeconomic status women. Blacks are known to have diets deficient/very low in potassium and also to consume sodium in excess of physiological requirements *(63)*. Potassium is found primarily in green leafy vegetables and fruit. Unfortunately, over the last several decades, the cost of fresh fruits and vegetables has risen much more rapidly than energy-dense, high fat foods. Additionally, calcium intake is lower in blacks than whites and is less in lower compared to higher income people. Dairy products account for ~70–75% of total daily calcium intake. Evidence suggests that the daily magnesium intake has declined substantially since the beginning of the century, when it was estimated to be 475–500 mg *(64)*. Recent dietary surveys have shown that the average magnesium intake in western countries is often below the recommended daily allowance *(65)*. Magnesium-rich foods include whole grains, green leafy vegetables, legumes, and nuts. According to a recent study which reviewed both the Continuing Survey of Food Intakes by Individuals 1994–1996, 1998, and the National Health and Nutrition Examination Survey 1999–2000, blacks of all ages did not meet dietary reference intakes for both calcium and magnesium *(66)*. Among blacks 19–30 years of age, approximately 75% of men and 94% of women did not meet the estimated average requirement for magnesium, as compared to 50 and 66% in age-matched whites, respectively. Sub-optimal dietary nutrient intakes over the long term are likely important, modifiable contributors to CVD in populations and, as well, to racial/ethnic disparities in CVD.

2.6. Physical Inactivity

Physical activity levels tend to decrease with advancing age and are also less common in women than men as well as in persons with lower levels of income and education. Black women experience greater age-related decreases in the cross-sectional prevalence of physical activity than white women. Independent of social class, the prevalence of "no leisure-time physical activity" was much higher in non-Hispanic black men (24%) and black women (40%) compared to non-Hispanic white men (13%) and white women (23%) *(67,68)*. Low levels of physical activity have been linked to increased total and CVD mortality. This association can be explained, at least in part, by multiple physiological effects of exercise on the CV system that plausibly explain the beneficial effects of exercise on CVD.

2.7. Geography and Acculturation

Approximately one-half of adult US blacks reside in 13 southeastern states. Thus, race/ethnic contrasts involving US blacks are, to a degree, influenced by geography. Interestingly, the risk of stroke death among blacks varies by geographic region with rates being significantly higher in blacks residing in the Southeast compared to those residing in other regions of the country. Poor BP control, along with dietary factors (e.g., high sodium and low potassium intakes), may be an important factor contributing to the high rate of pressure-related complications among blacks in the southeastern United States.

More recently, Moran and colleagues studied within-ethnic group differences associated with acculturation and the prevalence of hypertension in the United States *(69)*. The association of three measures of acculturation (language spoken at home, place of birth, and years living in the United States) was studied with hypertension in a population sample of whites, blacks, Hispanics, and Chinese participants in the Multiethnic Study of Atherosclerosis (MESA). They found that non-US born individuals who speak a non-English language at home had a lower prevalence of hypertension after adjustment for age, gender, and socioeconomic status than US born individuals who speak a non-English language at home ($P < 0.001$). Furthermore, for those individuals born outside of the United States, each 10-year increment of time in the United States was associated with a higher prevalence of hypertension, after adjustment for other covariates ($P < 0.01$). The associations between acculturation variables and hypertension were weakened after adjustment for race–ethnicity category and risk factors of hypertension. Hypertension prevalence of Hispanics born in Mexico or South America was also lower, while those born in the Caribbean and Central America were higher, compared to US-born Hispanics.

3. SOCIOECONOMIC STATUS AND CARDIOVASCULAR DISEASE

Socioeconomic status affects lifestyle behaviors such as smoking, lack of physical activity, poor dict, and alcohol consumption, all of which are known to be risk factors for CVD. In most developed countries, there is an inverse relationship between CVD and SES (70). For each group in the United States, those with lower income were more obese, had less physical activity, and more often smoked, compared to those with higher income. Figure 5 shows the relationship of income and education with the prevalence of untreated hypertension in the different racial/ethnic groups among women in the United States. In blacks particularly, and to a lesser degree in whites, there was an inverse relationship between SES and prevalence of untreated hypertension.

Morenoff and colleagues suggested that "neighborhoods" in the United States differ in the overall prevalence of hypertension (71). A study from 1971 by Harburg and colleagues found that blacks and whites living in

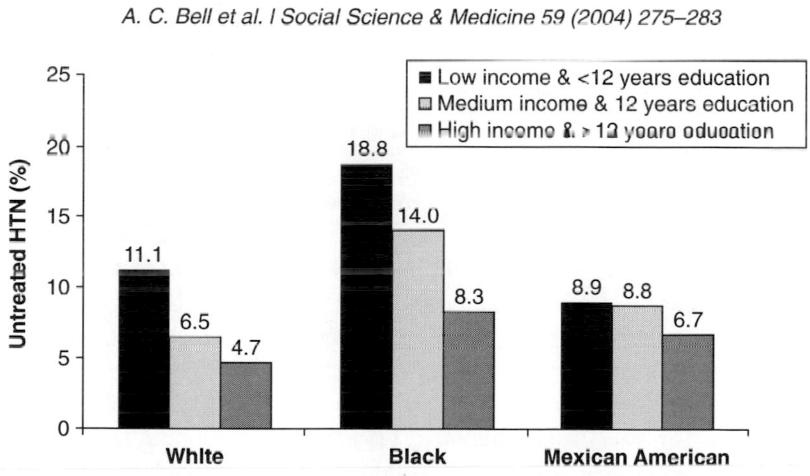

A. C. Bell et al. / Social Science & Medicine 59 (2004) 275–283

Fig. 5. Relationship of income and education to untreated hypertension in the women from the three major race/ethnicity groups in the United States.

lower stress environments had lower levels of blood pressures than their race-matched counterparts living in higher stress areas. The stress of an area was determined by the crime rates, economic stability, and marital instability *(72,73)*. They further examined the impact of neighborhood quality to determine SES and racial/ethnic differences in prevalence, awareness, treatment, and control of hypertension. They found that hypertension risk was lower in more prosperous neighborhoods. In this study, developed neighborhoods were considered to be places with greater numbers of young adults, professionals, and those with higher education/income. Morenoff and colleagues hypothesized that these areas may have a lower prevalence of hypertension due to promoted healthy lifestyles, which included exercising, eating properly, and not smoking, all of which are known to reduce blood pressure levels *(71)*.

Low-income, urban neighborhoods, where more blacks tend to live than whites, are more susceptible to crime and violence than those in affluent areas *(74)*. Violence exposure, which can be defined as "experiencing, witnessing, or hearing about violence in the home, school, or neighborhood" *(75)*, is an environmental and chronic stressor which could be a link to poor cardiovascular health, especially seen in blacks *(71,76)*. Stress experienced on a daily basis can lead to hypertension over time. Anderson and colleagues found that ongoing stressors, such as violence exposure, can increase sympathetic activity, thus releasing neuroendocrine hormones, which over time lead to vascular damage and resultant hypertension *(77)*. This pathophysiologic pathway may explain the relationship between higher stress neighborhoods and elevated blood pressure/hypertension.

4. CARDIOVASCULAR DISEASE DISPARITIES IN HEALTH-CARE SETTINGS

Race-based disparities in cardiovascular conditions can be thought of as differences from the provider (i.e., making the diagnosis or offering appropriate treatment) and differences from the patient (i.e., refusing a treatment option or not adhering to a treatment plan). These differences can be seen across different health-care settings and across different cardiovascular conditions. Given the larger burden of cardiovascular risk factors among non-Hispanic blacks and American Indian/Alaskan natives *(78)*, it is imperative to address disparities within the health-care system to reduce the cardiovascular events and their sequelae for these groups. We will argue that systematic approaches to improving cardiovascular health-care delivery for all patients will address disparities in cardiovascular disease and also should improve the care of all patients with CVD. Though patient preferences do influence the type/intensity of treatment received, and although there are known racial differences in patient preferences (e.g., blacks are less likely to accept procedure-related risk than whites), patient preferences, per se, do not explain the subsequently discussed racial disparities in the intensity of diagnostic testing and invasive interventions for suspected/proven CVD.

4.1. Coronary Ischemia and Myocardial Infarction

Racial disparities within the health-care system may be attributed to providers not offering the most effective treatments. Blacks do not undergo coronary angiography and coronary artery-bypass grafting (CABG) as frequently as their white counterparts (79–84). This disparity could be due to either a lack of providers offering the procedure (85) or a lack of patients accepting the treatment option. One multi-center trial found that whites received newer cardiovascular therapies more often than blacks after a myocardial infraction (86). In one Veteran's Affairs study, removing barriers to access for diagnosis and treatment for coronary ischemia (including CABG) attenuated the racial differences in quality-of-life gains (87), a finding supported by a lack of racial disparities among patients with private insurance (88).

Many treatments for coronary ischemia and myocardial infarction are invasive. In additional to medical therapy, percutaneous transluminal coronary angioplasty, intracoronary stents, and CABG surgery can be offered to patients to treat coronary disease. Although CABG does not prolong life for all patients with coronary ischemia, the procedure can be helpful for patients with diabetes (89).

The outcomes for different ethnic groups vary by intervention. For coronary angioplasty, there appear to be no significant differences in mortality after the procedure (90). However, black patients have higher mortality rates than their white counterparts when undergoing CABG (91).

4.2. Hypertension, Hyperlipidemia, and Other Cardiovascular Risk Factors

Another approach to reduce disparities in cardiovascular care is to focus on risk factors. Unfortunately, disparities exist in this area as well. Blacks are less likely to achieve blood pressure control, even after accounting for medication adherence and literacy (92). Among patients with the same insurance coverage, minorities appear to have a lower likelihood for receiving medications to lower cholesterol and, if those medications are received, a lower likelihood for maintaining those prescriptions over time (93). Even for smoking cessation advice, an intervention that can actually save patients money, disparities have been observed by racial and ethnic group (94).

4.3. Congestive Heart Failure

Heart failure can be considered an end-stage of long-standing hypertension and coronary disease. Medical therapy is the mainstay of treatment for both types of heart failure, but patients with advanced disease can benefit from implantable cardiac defibrillators (ICD), biventricular pacing *(95)*, left ventricular assist devices, and cardiac transplantation. ICD placement rates were initially lower among black patients, but that discrepancy has decreased over time *(96)*. Blacks tend to be admitted to the hospital with congestive heart failure more often than other racial groups. However, this difference does not seem to be due to differences in the care delivered *(97)*. As with coronary artery disease, the disparity between blacks and whites largely disappears in a systems of equal access to cardiovascular treatment (e.g., Veteran's Administration, Medicare) *(98,99)*.

4.4. Health System and Provider Characteristics Linked to CVD Disparities

Health-care system disparities can be categorized as individual beliefs from providers or institutional beliefs from a group of providers or health-care system *(100)*. Health-care provider may recognize that disparities exist in health care, but they are reluctant to attribute these disparities to provider behavior *(101)*. Providers may use mental shortcuts to tailor how they deliver care *(102)*. Based on prior experience with patients of a similar age or race, a provider may alter their treatment recommendation *(103)*.

One theme in studies of medicine and race is the concept of concordance between patient and provider. If the patient and the provider are from the same racial and ethnic background, then the two are *concordant*. Interactions between providers and patients of different racial and ethnic backgrounds are *discordant*. Although some studies have documented a decrease in perceived racism in concordant interactions compared to discordant ones *(104,105)*, the evidence does not consistently show this effect *(106)*. One possible explanation is the patient's perception that racism is a function of the provider (encouraging the patient to look for concordant interactions) or the health-care system in general (making concordance irrelevant) *(107)*. Nevertheless, concordant patient–provider interactions have been shown to be longer and more satisfying to the patient *(104,108–109)*.

Disparities may exist at the level of the health-care system. Not only can patients perceive discrimination from their health-care provider, but they can also sense discrimination from other health-care workers *(110)*. After controlling for patient perceptions of provider racism, some minority groups were still less likely to visit their usual source of care for a health concern compared to non-Hispanic Whites *(111)*.

4.5. Proposed Solutions for Reducing/Eliminating CVD Health Disparities in Health-Care Settings

Efforts to reduce disparities should focus on improved access to the health-care system for all patient groups, providing evidence-based treatments in a timely manner and improve communication between patients and providers to reduce the risk that patients will refuse life-enhancing therapies due to a lack of perceived benefit *(112)*. Improvements in medical quality have been associated with a reduction in cardiovascular treatment disparities *(113)*.

For several cardiovascular risk factors, providers need to monitor risk factor response to treatment and adjust the treatment accordingly. Unfortunately, providers as a group adjust medications less often than they should *(114)*. Clinical inertia is the avoidance of therapy intensification for patients with abnormal risk factor profiles *(115)*. There may be several reasons for providers to avoid intensifying treatment (e.g., medication regimen complexity, costs to the patient, excess faith in patient behavior modification), but the end result is a failure to titrate a patient's medication regimen. At least one group has documented that persistent medications adjustments can eliminate disparities in hypertension control *(116)*.

One potentially attractive strategy is to combat clinical inertia is to provide feedback about all of a provider's patients over a period of time *(117)*. There is also an intuitive appeal for pay for performance schemes. However, clinical trials have not found a strong association between pay-for-performance and better clinical care. In one study in the United Kingdom, pay-for-performance was associated with an increased rate of measuring CVD risk factors, but no corresponding increase in risk factor control among minority populations *(118)*. An additional complication with public reporting of performance measure is the avoidance of treating patients perceived to be at higher risk of complications. In a recent study of CABG rates after public reporting in New York, racial disparities increased *(119)*. A possible remedy to this patient selection is to adjust rates based on racial and socioeconomic characteristics *(120)*. A more proactive approach would be to advise providers to act on elevated risk factors before allowing a patient to leave the clinic. Point-of-care reminders and real-time clinical decision support can serve as independent assessors of a patient's cardiovascular risk and suggest the need to act with a general warning (or even a specific treatment recommendation) to providers. Systematic efforts to improve care quality have eliminated disparities in the inpatient setting as well. One group eliminated survival differences between black and white patients, although a difference in hospitalization rates persisted *(121)*. Such efforts require a conscious decision to identify care disparities and implement interventions that reduce those disparities.

To address the cognitive processes occurring between a patient and a provider during a clinical interaction, it is especially helpful for the provider to recognize the biases they bring to the encounter. This mental check can help identify subtle prejudices that may unduly influence the discussion. Due to the difficulty in monitoring provider and patient cognition, these types of interventions are unlikely to be used systematically. For patients with language barriers that inhibit effective communication with their providers, available translation services may reduce the risk of misunderstanding and

potentially, lower-quality care *(122)*. Another method to address disparities in cardiovascular care is to provide the same written information to
all patients who may be eligible for a medical intervention. This information could be delivered by a medical staff member who is concordant
with the patient. It will be impractical for every medical encounter to be
racially/ethnically concordant *(123)* continued efforts should be made to
train and employ a racially and ethnically diverse workforce in the delivery of health care.

5. CULTURAL COMPETENCY AND CVD HEALTH CARE

5.1. Health-Care Quality and the Underserved

Although cardiovascular disease is the leading cause of death for all
Americans, underserved populations experience higher rates of CVD than
their white counterparts. This coupled with the knowledge that racial and
ethnic demographics of the United States continue to become more diverse
member of these group often experience cross-cultural patient/provider
dyads. For these reason, the topic of cultural competency, as it relates to
cardiovascular disease, is of great and also increasing importance. This
set of circumstances makes the case for the utilization of cultural competency as an intervention tool to reduce health and health-care disparities by
race/ethnicity related to cardiovascular disease.

In March 2001, the Institutes of Medicine published *Crossing the Quality Chasm*; this collection of studies clearly demonstrates the poor level of
quality delivery by the health-care industry. Some of the stark findings were

- 18,000 Americans die each year from heart attacks because they did
  not receive preventive medications, although they were eligible for them
  (124,125)
- Medical errors kill more people per year than breast cancer, AIDS, or motor
  vehicle accidents *(126,127)*
- More than 50% of patients with diabetes, hypertension, tobacco addiction,
  hyperlipidemia, congestive heart failure, asthma, depression, and chronic
  atrial fibrillation are currently managed inadequately *(125,128–134)*

These facts reflect the health-care experience of all Americans. However,
this disproportionate standard of care is especially troubling for ethnically
and racially underserved populations, which are the more vulnerable and
experience poorer health outcomes, specifically those from cardiovascular
diseases.

5.2. Cultural Competency Defined

Culture is define as the set of attitudes, behaviors, and beliefs that are
passed from one generations to the next that assists members to make

meaning of the world around them and give guidance to what it means to be a member of a specific group. Culture provides a wall that helps to contain that meaning which defines each group and their worldviews. It is fluid not static, changing overtime. Culture also influences ideas, thoughts, and behaviors regarding what it means to be both ill and well. It impacts the methods of determining what is appropriate for cure and treatment. Culture will also affect decision making regarding health-seeking behaviors, health practices, and ultimately health outcomes.

Cultural competency is a relatively new term. One definition of culturally competent systems of care is provided by Cross et al. as "a set of congruent behaviors, attitudes, and policies that come together in a system, agency, or amongst professionals and enables that system, agency, or those professionals to work effectively in cross-cultural situations" *(135)*. Betancourt et al. *(136)* describe cultural competency in health care as the "ability of a systems to provide care to patients of diverse backgrounds, including tailoring the delivery of health care to meet patient's social, cultural and linguistic needs". Our use of cultural competency will refers to the active performance of the policies, skills, and abilities acquired by health-care professionals to provide care for the social, cultural, and linguistic needs of patients and their families in cross-cultural situations.

When addressing both the risk factors and the health challenges of cardiovascular disease, it is vital that health-care providers obtain an understanding of the manner in which underserved populations define health, how health beliefs and health-seeking behaviors are demonstrated and ultimately, how factors such as attitudes, behaviors, and beliefs influence health outcomes.

Currently, there is not empirical evidence to support cultural competency as an effaceable tool to eliminate health-care disparities, there is, however, a growing body of literature that sanctions its use to address the problem. Cultural competency is rapidly becoming a more wide spread intervention tool to address the issue of health and health-care disparities. Many national organizations endorse its use and identify it as an emerging efficacious, evidenced based intervention in the work to reduce disparities. A listing of them include are but not limited to the following:

- The Department of Health and Human Services
- The Office of the Surgeon General
- The Office of Minority Health
- The Joint Commission on Accreditation of Health Organizations
- The Centers for Medicaid & Medicare Services
- The Centers for Disease Control
- The American Medical Association
- The Institutes of Medicine.

In the clinical encounter both, patient and provider bring their cultural backgrounds, biases, beliefs, practices with them. These issues can translate into barriers to the provision and acquisition of health-care services. In the case of cardiovascular disease national statistics demonstrate that underserved populations experience significantly greater rates of all preventable causes of death with cardiovascular disease having the highest rates *(137–139)*.

5.3. Cardiovascular Disease and Etiology

What does having CVD or its associated risk factors mean to underserved populations? How do they frame the disease within cultural paradigms? What are the explanatory modules used to bring understanding to signs and symptoms experienced? What methods and strategies will members of various ethnic groups employ to heal themselves? What health beliefs and behaviors do these groups hold and practice regarding cardiovascular disease? Providers should ask these and many other culturally specific questions.

Patients explain their illnesses in many ways. Often citing such reasons as fate, witchcraft, "the evil eye," or spirits. Kleinman recommended that a patient's explanatory models of illness should be elicited using a mini-ethnographic approach that explored their concerns *(140)*. The provider can gain an increased understanding of the subjective experience of illness, and in doing so, partnership and a sharing of power in the provider–patient relationship can occur, with the expected goal of improved health outcomes and increased patient satisfaction.

While there is common ground among underserved populations regarding health attitudes, behaviors, and beliefs, there are vast differences in the ways that these issues are demonstrated daily. A belief that is most common is that of reciprocity or balance. It may be defined in terms of "ying and yang," "what goes around, comes around," or "reaping what you sow." The idea is that balance exists in the world and good behaviors will illicit good results and bad behaviors will illicit bad results.

Hispanic Americans demonstrate this phenomenon in the form of "hot and cold and "wet and dry" illnesses. A "hot" illness requires a "cold" cure, conversely a "cold" illness requires a "hot" cure – balance. Cardiovascular disease is a "hot" illness because it involves "warm" blood. Therefore, its treatment should reflect a "cold" modality. When addressing risk factors associated with CVD such as heart disease, stroke/transient ischemic attack, diabetes, abnormal cholesterol and obesity, understanding the meaning and the framing of these issues are critically important.

5.4. Laizze Faire or Fatalistic Attitudes

Often members of various ethnic and racial groups are labeled as not being concerned or possessing negative/fatalistic attitudes regarding their health and/or treatment plans. Statements such as "insha'Allah (as God wills)," or "this is my lot in life" and "everyone in my family has diabetes it's just my turn now." On the surface these statements may appear laizze faire or fatalistic. However, there are other factors at work. The locus of control of control for many underserved populations is external rather than internal. The concept that "things happen to me" rather than "I make things happen" is what is operationalized. Predetermination is a religious term that refers to the ability of a higher power to choose the future path of an individual. "God is in control" is often the term used to explain this phenomenon. The issue of cardiovascular disease and its risk factors is simply added to the list of things that are beyond their control.

There are strategies that the provider can employ to address this issue, namely

- Engage the patient in conversation regarding their religious beliefs regarding health
- Ask open-ended questions regarding the role of personal responsibility in caring for their bodies
- Inquire about exceptions to the "rules" and if there are other options.

The task of the provider to implement a prevention strategy becomes a daunting one when predetermination is an active element of the patient's culture. The influence of spirituality or religiosity cannot be ignored when providing care to underserved populations. For many, it is a pillar of their culture and without the knowledge of a patient's belief system a provider is void of a tremendous part of the patient history.

The importance of cultural competency as a tool to address disparities in cardiovascular disease has been clearly demonstrated. As cross-cultural patient/provider dyads continue or increase, the need for providers who have educated themselves in the cultural and health practices of the ethnically and racially diverse populations will become vital to their survival in the health-care market place.

6. SUMMARY

Cardiovascular disease is the number one cause of death in the United States and disproportionately affects blacks and other minorities relative to white populations. The population burden of CVD as well as the racial disparities is a reflection of long-term environmental exposures and lifestyle choices. Disparities in process of care measures and CVD outcomes also exist within the health-care system. Focusing on modifiable factors such as dietary quantity and quality, promoting energy expenditure, taking steps to monitor and improve the quality of clinical care, and proactively working to promote cultural competency will likely pay dividends in reducing the population CVD burden and reducing/eliminating CVD disparities within our health system.

REFERENCES

1. National Center for Health Statistics (NCHS), 2005. http://www.statisticstop10. com/Causes of Death in US.html
2. Mensah GA, Brown DW. An overview of cardiovascular disease burden in the United States. *Health Affairs* 2007; 26(1):38–48.
3. National Heart Lung and Blood Institute (NHLBI), 2007. http://www.nhlbi.nih. gov/about/factbook/chapter4.htm
4. Center for Disease Control and Prevention. Morbidity and Mortality Weekly Report. Tobacco Use Among Adults–U.S., 2005. Vol. 42(42); 1145–1145, Oct. 2006. Available at: http://www.cdc.gov/mmwr/preview/mmwrhtml/mm5542a1.htm . Accessed on 9/9/08.
5. Mensah GA, Mokdad AH, Ford ES, Greenlund KJ, Croft JB. State of disparities in cardiovascular health in the United States. *Circulation* 2005; 111:1233–1241.
6. Pierce JP, Fiore MC, Novotny TE, Hatziandreu EJ, Davis RM. Trends in cigarette smoking in the United States. Projections to the year 2000. *JAMA* 1989; 261(1): 61–65.
7. Winkleby MA, Kraemer HC, Ahn DK, Varady AN. Ethnic and socioeconomic differences in cardiovascular disease risk factors. Findings for Women from the Third National Health and Nutrition Examination Survey, 1988-1994. *JAMA* 1998; 280(4):356–362.
8. Luepker RV, Rosamond WD, Murphy R, Sprafka JM, Folsom AR, McGovern PG, et al. Socioeconomic status and coronary heart disease risk factor trends. The Minnesota Heart Survey. *Circulation* 1993; 88(5 Pt 1):2172–2179.
9. Reynes JF, Lasater TM, Feldman H, Assaf AR, Carleton RA. Education and risk factors for coronary heart disease: results from a New England community. *Am J Prev Med* 1993; 9(6):365–371.
10. Sinclair S, Hayes-Reams P, Myers HF, Allen W, Hawes-Dawson J, Kington R. Recruiting African-Americans for health studies: lessons from the Drew-RAND Center on Health and Aging. *J Mental Health Aging* 2002; 6:39–51.
11. Federal Interagency Forum on Aging-Related Statistics. Older American 2004: Key Indicators of Well-Being. Federal Interagency Forum on Aging Related Statistics. 2004.
12. Frist WH. Overcoming disparities in U.S. Health Care. *Health Affairs* 2005; 24: 445–451.
13. Ong KL, Cheung BM, Man YB, Lau CP, Lam KS. Prevalence, awareness, treatment, and control of hypertension among United States adults 1999-2004. *Hypertension* 2007; 49(1):69–75.
14. de Rekeneire N, Rooks RN, Simonsick EM, Shorr RI, Kuller LH, Schwartz AV, Harris TB. Racial differences in glycemic control in a well-functioning older diabetic population: findings from the Health, Aging and Body Composition Study. *Diabet Care* 2003; 26:1986–1992.
15. Bromberger JT, Harlow S, Avis N, Kravitz HM, Cordal A. Racial/ethnic differences in the prevalence of depressive symptoms among middle-aged women: The Study of Women's Health across the Nation. *Am J Public Health* 2004; 94: 1378–1385.
16. Mayberry RM, Mili F, and Ofili E. Racial and ethnic differences in the access of medical care. *MedCare Res Rev* 2000; 57:108–145.

17. Kressin NR, Petersen LA. Racial differences in the use of invasive cardiovascular procedures: review of the literature and prescription for future research. *Ann Intern Med* 2001; 135:352–366.
18. Jorde LB, Wooding SP. Genetic variation, classification and 'race'. *Nat Genet* 2004; 36(Suppl):S28–S33.
19. Shriver MD, Kittles RA. Genetic ancestry and the search for personalized genetic histories. *Nat Rev Genet* 2004; 5(8):611–618.
20. Bamshad MJ, Wooding S, Watkins WS, Ostler CT, Batzer MA, Jorde LB. Human population genetic structure and inference of group membership. *Am J Hum Genet* 2003; 72(3):578–589.
21. Feldman MW, Lewontin RC, King MC. Race: a genetic melting-pot. *Nature* 2003; 424(6947):374.
22. Cooper RS, Wolf-Maier K, Luke A, et al. An international comparison study of blood pressure in populations of European versus African descent. *BMC Med* 2005; 3:22.
23. Wolf-Maier K, Cooper RS, Banegas JR, Giampaoli S, Hense H, Joffres M, et al. Hypertension prevalence and blood pressure levels in 6 European Countries, Canada, and the United States. *JAMA* 2003; 289:2363–2369.
24. Klag MJ, Whelton PK, Coresh J, Grim C, Kuller H. The association of skin color with blood pressure in US blacks with low socioeconomic status. *JAMA* 1991; 265:599–602.
25. Zittermann A, Tenderich G, Berthold HK, Korfer R, Stehle P. Low vitamin D status: a contributing factor in the pathogenesis of congestive heart failure? *J Am Coll Cardiol* 2003; 41:105–112.
26. Chiu KC, Chu A, Go VL, Saad MF. Hypovitaminosis D is associated with insulin resistance and β cell dysfunction. *Am J Clin Nutr* 2004; 79:820–825.
27. Hermann M, Ruschitzka F. Vitamin D and hypertension. *Curr Hypertens Rep* 2008; 10(1):49–51
28. Scragg R, Sowers M, Bell C. Serum 25-hydroxyvitamin D, ethnicity, and blood pressure in the Third National Health and Nutrition Examination Survey. *Am J Hypertens* 2007; 20(7):713–719.
29. Judd SE, Nanes MS, Ziegler TR, Wilson PW, Tangpricha V., Optimal vitamin D status attenuates the age-associated increase in systolic blood pressure in white Americans: results from the third National Health and Nutrition Examination Survey *Am J Clin Nutr* 2008; 87(1):136–141.
30. Giovannucci E, Liu Y, Hollis BW, Rimm EB. 25-hydroxyvitamin D and risk of myocardial infarction in men: a prospective study. *Arch Intern Med* 2008; 168(11):1174–1180.
31. Alemzadeh R, Kichler J, Babar G, Calhoun M. Hypovitaminosis D in obese children and adolescents: relationship with adiposity, insulin sensitivity, ethnicity, and season. *Metabolism* 2008; 57(2):183–91.
32. Ybarra J, Sánchez-Hernández J, Pérez A. Hypovitaminosis D and morbid obesity. *Nurs Clin North Am* 2007; 42(1):19–27.
33. Lips P. Vitamin D physiology. *Prog Biophys Mol Biol* 2006; 92(1):4–8.
34. Rocchini AP. Obesity hypertension, salt sensitivity and insulin resistance. *Nutr Metab Cardiovasc Dis* 2000; 10(5):287.
35. Hall JE, Henegar JR, Dwyer TM, et al. Is obesity a major cause of chronic kidney disease? *Adv Ren Replace Ther* 2004; 11:41.
36. Flack JM, Grimm RH Jr, Staffileno BA, et al. New salt-sensitivity metrics: variability-adjusted blood pressure change and the urinary sodium-to creatinine ratio. *Ethn Dis.* 2002 Winter; 12(1):10.
37. Rocchini AP, Key J, Bondie D, et al. The effect of weight loss on the sensitivity of blood pressure to sodium in obese adolescents. *N Engl J Med* 1989; 321(9):580.
38. Kopkan L, Majid DS. Superoxide contributes to development of salt sensitivity and hypertension induced by nitric oxide deficiency. *Hypertension* 2005; 46(4):1026.

39. Alvarez G, Osuna A, Wangensteen R, Vargas F. Interaction between nitric oxide and mineralocorticoids in the long-term control of blood pressure. *Hypertension* 2000; 35(3):752.

40. Flack JM, Wiist WH. Epidemiology of hypertension and hypertensive target-organ damage in the United States. *J Assoc Acad Minor Phys* 1991; 2(4):143–150.

41. Wilson DK, Sica DA, Miller SB. Effects of potassium on blood pressure in salt-sensitive and salt-resistant black adolescents. *Hypertension* 1999; 34(2):181.

42. Coruzzi P, Brambilla L, Brambilla V, et al. Potassium depletion and salt sensitivity in essential hypertension. *J Clin Endocrinol Metab* 2001; 86(6):2857.

43. Peters RM, Flack JM. Salt sensitivity and hypertension in African Americans: implications for cardiovascular nurses. *Prog Cardiovasc Nurs* 2000; 15(4):138.

44. Wright JT Jr, Rahman M, Scarpa A, et al. Determinants of salt sensitivity in black and white normotensive and hypertensive women. *Hypertension* 2003; 42(6):1087.

45. Sullivan JM, Prewitt RL, Ratts TE. Sodium sensitivity in normotensive and borderline hypertensive humans. *Am J Med Sci* 1988; 295(4):370.

46. Centers for Disease Control and Prevention (National Center for Health Statistics). Births and deaths: preliminary data for 1998. 1999. National Vital Statistics Reports. Washington, DC: Department of Health and Human Services.

47. Douglas-Denton RN, McNamara BJ, Hoy WE, Hughson MD, Bertram JF. Does nephron number matter in the development of kidney disease? *Ethn Dis* 2006 Spring; 16(2 Suppl 2):S2-40-5.

48. Luyckx VA, Brenner BM. Low birth weight, nephron number, and kidney disease. *Kidney Int Suppl.* 2005; (97):S68–77.

49. Boddi M, Poggesi L, Coppo M, et al. Human vascular renin-angiotensin system and its functional changes in relation to different sodium intakes. *Hypertension* 1998; 31(3):836.

50. Cubeddu LX, Alfieri AB, Hoffmann IS, et al. Nitric oxide and salt sensitivity. *Am J Hypertens* 2000; 13:973.

51. Zhou MS, Adam AG, Jaimes EA. In salt-sensitive hypertension, increased superoxide production is linked to functional upregulation of angiotensin II. *Hypertension* 2003; 42(5):945–951.

52. Fang Y, Mu JJ, He LC, Wang SC, Liu ZQ. Salt loading on plasma asymmetrical dimethylarginine and the protective role of potassium supplement in normotensive salt-sensitive Asians. *Hypertension* 2006; 48(4):724–729.

53. Morris RC Jr, Sebastian A, Forman A, Tanaka M, Schmidlin O. Normotensive salt sensitivity: effects of race and dietary potassium. *Hypertension* 1999; 33(1):18–23.

54. Grubbs RD, Maguire ME. Magnesium as a regulatory cation: criteria and evaluation. *Magnesium* 1987; 6:113–127.

55. Beyenbach KW. Transport of magnesium across biological membranes. *Magnes Trace Elem* 1990; 9:233–254.

56. Arsenian M. Magnesium and cardiovascular disease. *Prog Cardiovasc Dis* 1993; 35:271–310.

57. Altura BM, Altura BT. Role of magnesium in the pathogenesis of hypertension updated: relationship to its action on cardiac, vascular smooth muscle, and endothelial cells. In: Larargh J, Brenner BM, editors, Hypertension: pathophysiology, diagnosis, and management. 2nd ed. New York: Raven Press; 1995:1212–1242.

58. van Dam RM, Hu FB, Rosenberg L, Krishnan S, Palmer JR. Dietary calcium and magnesium, major food sources, and risk of type 2 diabetes in U.S. black women. *Diabet Care* 2006; 29: 2238–2243.

59. Sontia B, Touyz RM. Role of magnesium in hypertension. *Arch Biochem Biophys* 2007; 458(1):33–39.

60. Fung TT, Manson JE, Solomon CG, Liu S, Willett WC, Hu FB. The association between magnesium intake and fasting insulin concentration in healthy middle-aged women. *J Am Coll Nutr* 2003; 22:533–538.
61. Song Y, Ridker PM, Manson JE, Cook NR, Buring JE, Liu S. Magnesium intake, C-reactive protein, and the prevalence of metabolic syndrome in middle-aged and older U.S. women. *Diabet Care* 2005; 28:1438–1444.
62. Ford ES, Mokdad AH. Dietary magnesium intake in a national sample of US adults. *J Nutr* 2003; 133(9):2879–2882.
63. Jen KL, Brogan K, Washington OG, Flack JM, Artinian NT. Poor nutrient intake and high obese rate in an urban African American population with hypertension. *J Am Coll Nutr* 2007; 26(1):57–65.
64. Altura BM, Altura BT. Cardiovascular risk factors and magnesium: relationships to atherosclerosis, ischemic heart disease and hypertension. *Magnes Trace Elem* 1991; 10:182–192.
65. USDA. Continuing survey of food intake by individuals. Washington, DC: USDA, 1990.
66. Fulgoni V III, Nicholls J, Reed A, Buckley R, Kafer K, Huth P, Dirienzo D, Miller G. Dairy consumption and related nutrient intake in African-American adults and children in the United States: continuing survey of food intakes by individuals 1994–1996, 1998, and the National Health and Nutrition Examination Survey 1999–2000. *J Am Diet Assoc* 2007; 107(2):256–264
67. Crespo CJ, Keteyian SJ, Heath GW, Sempos CT. Leisure-time physical activity among US adults. Results from the Third National Health and Nutrition Examination Survey. *Arch Intern Med* 1996; 156(1):93.
68. Crespo CJ, Smit E, Andersen RE, et al. Race/ethnicity, social class and their relation to physical inactivity during leisure time: results from the Third National Health and Nutrition Examination Survey, 1988–1994. *Am J Prev Med* 2000; 18(1):46.
69. Moran A, Diez Rouz AV, Jackson SA, Kramer H, Manolio TA, Sharager S, Shea S. Acculturation is associated with hypertension in a multiethnic sample. *Am J Hypertens* 2007; 20: 354–363.
70. Bell AC, Adair LS, Poplin BM. Understanding the role of mediating risk factors and proxy effects in the association between socioeconomic status and untreated hypertension. *Soc Sci Med* 2003; 59:275–283.
71. Morenoff JD, House JS, Hansen BB, Williams DR, Kaplan GA, Hunte HE. Understanding social disparities in hypertension prevalence, awareness, treatment, and control: The role of neighborhood context. *Soc Sci Med* 2007; 65(9):1853–1866.
72. Harburg E, Erfurt JC, Hauenstein L.S, Chape C, Schull WJ, Schork MA. 1973. Socioecological stress, suppressed hostility, skin color, and black-white male blood pressure: Detroit. *Psychosom Med* 1973; 35: 276–296.
73. Harburg E, Erfurt JC, Chape C. Socioecological stress, smoking, skin color, and black-white blood pressure: Detroit. Paper delivered at Michigan Cardiovascular Research Forum, Detroit, Michigan; 1971.
74. Wilson DK, Kirtland KA, Ainsworth BE, Addy CL. Socioeconomic status and perceptions of access and safety for physical activity. *Ann Behav Med* 2004; 28: 20–28.
75. Wilson DK, Kliewer,W, Sica DA. The relationship between exposure to violence and blood pressure mechanisms. *Curr Hypertens Rep* 2004; 6:321–326.
76. Wilson DK, Kliewer W, Teasley N, Plybon L, Sica DA. Violence exposure, catecholamine excretion, and blood pressure nondipping status in African American male versus female adolescents. *Psychosom Med* 2002; 64:906–915.
77. Anderson NB, McNeilly M, Myers HF. Toward understanding race difference in autonomic reactivity: a proposed contextual model. In Individual differences in

cardiovascular response to stress. Turner JR, Sherwood A, Light KC (eds.). New York: Plenum; 1992:125–145.

78. Centers for Disease Control and Prevention (CDC). Racial/ethnic and socioeconomic disparities in multiple risk factors for heart disease and stroke—United States, 2003. *MMWR Morb Mortal Wkly Rep* 2005; 54(5):113–117.

79. Barnhart JM, Fang J, Alderman MH. Differential use of coronary revascularization and hospital mortality following acute myocardial infarction. *J Am Soc Nephrol* 2003; 163(4):461–466.

80. Popescu I, Vaughan-Sarrazin MS, Rosenthal GE. Differences in mortality and use of revascularization in black and white patients with acute MI admitted to hospitals with and without revascularization services. *JAMA* 2007; 297(22):2489–2495.

81. Kressin NR, Petersen LA. Racial differences in the use of invasive cardiovascular procedures: review of the literature and prescription for future research. *Ann Intern Med* 2001; 135(5):352–366.

82. Ibrahim SA, Whittle J, Bean-Mayberry B, Kelley ME, Good C, Conigliaro J. Racial/ethnic variations in physician recommendations for cardiac revascularization. *Am J Public Health* 2003; 93(10):1689–1693.

83. Callier JG, Brown SC, Parsons S, Ardoin PJ, Cruise P. The effect of race and gender on invasive treatment for cardiovascular disease. *J Cult Divers* 2004; 11(3):80–87.

84. Jha AK, Staiger DO, Lucas FL, Chandra A. Do race-specific models explain disparities in treatments after acute myocardial infarction? *Am Heart J* 2007; 153(5): 785–791.

85. Schulman KA, Berlin JA, Harless W, et al. The effect of race and sex on physicians' recommendations for cardiac catheterization. *N Engl J Med* 1999; 340(8): 618–626.

86. Sonel AF, Good CB, Mulgund J, et al. Racial variations in treatment and outcomes of black and white patients with high-risk non-ST-elevation acute coronary syndromes: insights from CRUSADE (Can Rapid Risk Stratification of Unstable Angina Patients Suppress Adverse Outcomes With Early Implementation of the ACC/AHA Guidelines?). *Circulation* 2005; 111(10):1225–1232.

87. Kressin NR, Glickman ME, Peterson ED, Whittle J, Orner MB, Petersen LA. Functional status outcomes among white and African-American cardiac patients in an equal access system. *Am Heart J* 2007; 153(3):418–425.

88. Carlisle DM, Leake BD, Shapiro MF. Racial and ethnic disparities in the use of cardiovascular procedures: associations with type of health insurance. *Am J Public Health* 1997; 87(2):263–267.

89. Bypass Angioplasty Revascularization Investigation (BARI) Investigators. The final 10-year follow-up results from the BARI randomized trial. *J Am Coll Cardiol* 2007; 49(15):1600–1606.

90. Minutello RM, Chou ET, Hong MK, Wong SC. Impact of race and ethnicity on inhospital outcomes after percutaneous coronary intervention (report from the 2000, 2001 New York State Angioplasty Registry). *Am Heart J* 2006; 151(1):164–167.

91. Lucas FL, Stukel TA, Morris AM, Siewers AE, Birkmeyer JD. Race and surgical mortality in the United States. *Ann Surg* 2006; 243(2):281–286.

92. Bosworth HB, Dudley T, Olsen MK, et al. Racial differences in blood pressure control: potential explanatory factors. *Am J Med* 2006; 119(1):70–15.

93. Litaker D, Koroukian S, Frolkis JP, Aron DC. Disparities among the disadvantaged: variation in lipid management in the Ohio Medicaid program. *Prev Med* 2006; 42(4):313–315.

94. Lopez-Quintero C, Crum RM, Neumark YD. Racial/ethnic disparities in report of physician-provided smoking cessation advice: analysis of the 2000 National Health Interview Survey. *Am J Public Health* 2006; 96(12):2235–2239.

95. Shenkman HJ, Pampati V, Khandelwal AK, et al. Congestive heart failure and QRS duration: establishing prognosis study. *Chest* 2002; 122(2):528–534.
96. Stanley A, DeLia D, Cantor JC. Racial disparity and technology diffusion: the case of cardioverter defibrillator implants, 1996–2001. *J Natl Med Assoc* 2007; 99(3): 201–207.
97. Alexander M, Grumbach K, Remy L, Rowell R, Massie BM. Congestive heart failure hospitalizations and survival in California: patterns according to race/ethnicity. *Am Heart J* 1999; 137(5):919–927.
98. Deswal A, Petersen NJ, Urbauer DL, Wright SM, Beyth R. Racial variations in quality of care and outcomes in an ambulatory heart failure cohort. *Am Heart J* 2006; 152(2):348–354.
99. Rathore SS, Foody JM, Wang Y, et al. Race, quality of care, and outcomes of elderly patients hospitalized with heart failure. *JAMA* 2003; 289(19):2517–2524.
100. Fincher C, Williams JE, MacLean V, Allison JJ, Kiefe CI, Canto J. Racial disparities in coronary heart disease: a sociological view of the medical literature on physician bias. 2004; 14(3):360–371.
101. Lurie N, Fremont A, Jain AK, et al. Racial and ethnic disparities in care: the perspectives of cardiologists. *Circulation* 2005; 111(10):1264–1269.
102. Burgess DJ, Fu SS, van RM. Why do providers contribute to disparities and what can be done about it? *J Gen Intern Med* 2004; 19(11):1154–1159.
103. Lutfey KE, Ketcham JD. Patient and provider assessments of adherence and the sources of disparities: evidence from diabetes care. *Health Serv Res* 2005; 40(6 Pt 1): 1803–1817.
104. Saha S, Komaromy M, Koepsell TD, Bindman AB. Patient-physician racial concordance and the perceived quality and use of health care. *J Am Soc Nephrol* 1999; 159(9):997–1004.
105. Gordon HS, Street RL, Jr., Sharf BF, Souchek J. Racial differences in doctors' information-giving and patients' participation. *Cancer* 2006; 107(6):1313–1320.
106. Blanchard J, Nayar S, Lurie N. Patient-provider and patient-staff racial concordance and perceptions of mistreatment in the health care setting. *J Gen Intern Med* 2007; 22(8):1184–1189.
107. Malat J, Hamilton MA. Preference for same-race health care providers and perceptions of interpersonal discrimination in health care. *J Health Soc Behav* 2006; 47(2): 173–187.
108. Cooper-Patrick L, Gallo J, Gonzales J, et al. Race, gender, and partnership in the patient-physician relationship. *JAMA* 1999; 282(6):583–589.
109. Fergusen W, Candib L. Culture, language, and the doctor-patient relationship. *Fam Med* 2002; 34(5):353–361.
110. Johnson RL, Saha S, Arbelaez JJ, Beach MC, Cooper LA. Racial and ethnic differences in patient perceptions of bias and cultural competence in health care. *J Gen Intern Med* 2004; 19(2):101–110.
111. Gaskin DJ, Arbelaez JJ, Brown JR, Petras H, Wagner FA, Cooper LA. Examining racial and ethnic disparities in site of usual source of care. *J Natl Med Assoc* 2007; 99(1):22–30.
112. Clark LT. Issues in minority health: atherosclerosis and coronary heart disease in African Americans. *Med Clin North Am* 2005; 89(5):977–1001, 994.
113. Trivedi AN, Zaslavsky AM, Schneider EC, Ayanian JZ. Trends in the quality of care and racial disparities in Medicare managed care. *N Engl J Med* 2005; 18;353(7): 692–700.
114. Andrade SE, Gurwitz JH, Field TS, et al. Hypertension management: the care gap between clinical guidelines and clinical practice. *Am J Manag Care* 2004; 10(7 Pt 2):481–486.

115. Phillips LS, Branch WT, Cook CB, et al. Clinical inertia. *Ann Intern Med* 2001; 135(9):825–834.
116. Hicks LS, Shaykevich S, Bates DW, Ayanian JZ. Determinants of racial/ethnic differences in blood pressure management among hypertensive patients. *BMC Cardiovasc Disord* 2005; 5(1):16.
117. Hendrix KH, Lackland DT, Egan BM. Cardiovascular risk factor control and treatment patterns in primary care. *Manag Care Interface* 2003; 16(11):21–26.
118. Gray J, Millett C, Saxena S, Netuveli G, Khunti K, Majeed A. Ethnicity and quality of diabetes care in a health system with universal coverage: population-based cross-sectional survey in primary care. *J Gen Intern Med* 2007; 22(9):1317–1320.
119. Werner RM, Asch DA, Polsky D. Racial profiling: the unintended consequences of coronary artery bypass graft report cards. *Circulation* 2005; 111(10):1257–1263.
120. Fiscella K, Franks P, Gold MR, Clancy CM. Inequality in quality: addressing socioeconomic, racial, and ethnic disparities in health care. *JAMA* 2000; 283(19):2579–2584.
121. Pamboukian SV, Costanzo MR, Meyer P, Bartlett L, McLeod M, Heroux A. Influence of race in heart failure and cardiac transplantation: mortality differences are eliminated by specialized, comprehensive care. *J Card Fail* 2003; 9(2):80–86.
122. Clemans-Cope L, Kenney G. Low income parents' reports of communication problems with health care providers: effects of language and insurance. *Public Health Rep* 2007; 122(2):206–216.
123. Chen FM, Fryer GE, Jr, Phillips RL, Jr, Wilson E, Pathman DE. Patients' beliefs about racism, preferences for physician race, and satisfaction with care. *Ann Fam Med* 2005; 3(2):138–143.
124. Chassin MR. Assessing strategies for quality improvement. *Health Aff (Millwood)* 1997; 16(3):151–161.
125. Institute of Medicine. Fostering Rapid Advances in Health Care: Learning from System Demonstrations. JM. Corrigan, A. Greiner, SM. Erickson, eds. Washington, DC: National Academy Press. 2003a.
126. Institute of Medicine. To Err Is Human: building a safer health system. Kohn LT, Corrigan JM, Donaldson MS, eds. Washington, DC: National Academy Press. 2000.
127. Centers for Disease Control and Prevention (National Center for Health Statistics). Births and Deaths: preliminary data for 1998. National Vital Statistics Reports. Washington, DC: Department of Health and Human Services; 1999.
128. Clark CM, Fradkin JE, Hiss RG, Lorenz RA, Vinicor F, Warren-Boulton E. Promoting early diagnosis and treatment of type 2 diabetes: The National Diabetes Education Program. *JAMA* 2000; 284(3):363–365.
129. Legorreta AP, Liu X, Zaher CA, Jatulis DE. Variation in managing asthma: Experience at the medical group level in California. *Am J Manag Care* 2000; 6(4):445–453.
130. McBride P, Schrott HG, Plane MB, Underbakke G, Brown RL. Primary care practice adherence to National Cholesterol Education Program guidelines for patients with coronary heart disease. *Arch Intern Med* 1998; 158(11):1238–1244.
131. Ni H, Nauman DJ, Hershberger RE. Managed care and outcomes of hospitalization among elderly patients with congestive heart failure. *Arch Intern Med* 1998; 158(11):1231–1236.
132. Perez-Stable EJ, Fuentes-Afflick E. Role of clinicians in cigarette smoking prevention. *West J Med* 1998; 169(1):23–29.
133. Samsa GP, Matchar DB, Goldstein LB, Bonito AJ, Lux LJ, Witter DM, Bian J. Quality of anticoagulation management among patients with atrial fibrillation: Results of a review of medical records from 2 communities. *Arch Intern Med* 2000; 160(7): 967–973.
134. Young AS, Klap R, Sherbourne CD, Wells KB. The quality of care for depressive and anxiety disorders in the United States. *Arch Gen Psychiatry* 2001; 58(1):55–61.

135. Cross T, Bazron B, Dennis K, Isaacs M. Towards a culturally competent system of care, volume I. Washington, DC: Georgetown University Child Development Center, CASSP Technical Assistance Center; 1989.
136. Betancourt J, Green A, Carmillo J, Cultural Competence in Health Care: Emerging Frameworks and Practical Approaches. The Commonwealth Fund Field Report. October 2002. http// www.cmwf.org
137. Institutes of Medicine. Guidance for the National Healthcare Disparities Report. Washington DC: National Academies Press; 2004.
138. Lillie-Blanton M, Maddox TM, Rushing O, et al. Disparities in cardiac care: rising to the challenge of healthy people 2010. *J Am Coll Cardiol* 2004; 44:503–508.
139. Institutes of Medicine. Unequal treatment: confronting racial and ethnic disparities in health care. Washington, DC: National Academies Press; 2003.
140. Kleinman A. Culture, illness and cure: Clinical lesions from anthropologic and cross-cultural research. *Annals Int Med* 1978; 88:251–258.

4   Race and Genetics

R.A. Kittles, PhD, and
J. Benn-Torres, PhD

CONTENTS

Abstract

Race is an enigma, exhibiting no clear biological definition yet strong cultural and social meanings, particularly in the United States. However, the advent of molecular technology led to a new realization that within-group differences far exceeded between-group differences. Our knowledge of human genetic variation has grown enormously over the past few decades. Single-nucleotide polymorphisms (SNPs) are the most common form of DNA variation in the human genome. At present, there are more than 10 million SNPs in the human genome. At most genetic loci, African populations harbor some relatively common alleles that are absent in non-African populations; however, most of the alleles that are common in non-African populations are also common in African populations. Given the genetic data now available across diverse human populations, it is becoming increasingly clear that the frequency of most genetic markers do not vary much among the major continental populations. However, a number of studies that examine genetic variation across the genome have found that

From: *Contemporary Cardiology: Cardiovascular Disease in Racial and Ethnic Minorities*
Edited by: K.C. Ferdinand and A. Armani, DOI 10.1007/978-1-59745-410-0_4
© Humana Press, a part of Springer Science+Business Media, LLC 2009

individuals with similar ancestral continental origins tend to cluster together, and in general, these clusters correspond to four continental groups: Sub-Saharan Africa, Europe/Western Asia, Asia, and the Americas.

Not withstanding the large amount of genetic variation shared across human groups there is a small but significant fraction of polymorphisms that are quite informative for estimating biogeographic ancestry. Interestingly, individuals self-report as African-American due to skin color and the historical classification schema referred to as the "one-drop" rule which denotes an individual with an African ancestor as Black. The first striking feature observed is that 98% of the European Americans had over 90% European ancestry, while only 34% of the African-Americans possessed over 90% West African ancestry. Variance in genetic background of study subjects is becoming more of an issue with the increasing number of genetic association studies on complex disease. Differences in genetic background among study individuals may impact the power and reliability of genetic association studies. We suggest that ancestry be used instead of race. Genetic ancestry has several salient features which are useful for biomedical studies.

Key Words: Race; Genetics; AIMs; Population structure; Genetic ancestry; Genetic variation; Admixture.

1. INTRODUCTION

Knowledge from human genetic research continuously challenges the notion that race and genetics are inextricably linked with implications across biomedical and public health disciplines. Race is an enigma, exhibiting no clear biological definition yet strong cultural and social meanings, particularly in the United States. Historically, racial groups have been classified by various physical attributes, such as skull volume and size, skin color, facial features, and other physical attributes. The Swedish naturalist, Carl Linneaus's *Systema Naturae* (1758) defined four racial groups: *Homo sapiens europaeus, Homo sapiens asiaticus, Homo sapiens americanus*, and *Homo sapiens afrer*. Johann Friedrich Blumenbach (1775) then provided a classification of five varieties humans based on skin color. These racial schema predated the modern genomic era yet are still used today when describing populations around the world *(1,2)* and are used in genetic studies to classify individuals *(3)*.

However, the arrival of molecular technology led to a new realization that within-group differences far exceeded between-group differences. In addition, the revelation from the Human Genome Project that all humans, regardless of race/ethnicity, are >99% the same at the DNA sequence level should have nullified the existence of biologically distinct racial groups. Instead, the use of genetics to explain racial and ethnic differences in diseases and other traits intensified. Studies using hundreds of polymorphic loci across the genome have shown that groupings of individuals correlate directly with ancestral continent of origin *(4,5)*. And that the continental clustering appears to correspond to the following division of human beings: sub-Saharan Africans; Europeans, western Asians, and northern Africans; eastern Asians; Polynesians and other inhabitants of Oceania; and Native Americans *(1,4)*. Not surprisingly, human genome research has increasingly projected population comparisons at the genetic level and genetic variation continues to be used to explain racial and ethnic group differences in health *(3,6)*. But what are these racial groupings? Are they continental groups? How accurately do they define bounded homogeneous entities? Are the differences in health outcomes due to biological differences among the so-called "races"? Obviously, there continues to be a paradoxical relationship between race and genetics.

2. HOW IS GENETIC VARIATION STRUCTURED?

Human genetic variation is structured by the history of our species. The pattern of this structure, however, is not bounded or discrete, but continuous, resulting from the demographic history of populations shaped by forces such as natural and social (mate) selection. Our knowledge of human genetic variation has grown enormously over the past few decades. Single-nucleotide polymorphisms (SNPs) are the most common form of DNA variation in the human genome. At present, there are more than 10 million SNPs in the human genome *(7)*. A large fraction of these SNPs are found at a frequency less than 5% and thus are private or common in only a single population *(8)*. SNPs have been used to explore how genetic variation is structured within- and between-human populations. Gabriel et al. *(9)* examined 3738 SNPs across 51 autosomal regions in sampled populations of Africans, African-Americans, Asians, and Europeans. The alleles for consecutive SNPs along a chromosome which are inherited as a unit are called "haplotypes." These haplotypes were then compared between the groups. While 51% of the haplotypes were shared between all groups, on average, Africans (which included African-Americans) possessed the most haplotypes. This finding indicates that the variation observed in European and Asian populations is a subset of African variation and furthermore supports a single African origin for all humans.

Guthery et al. *(10)* arrived at similar conclusions when they examined population structure of common genetic variants in African, European, Asian, and Hispanic American populations. At most genetic loci, African populations harbor some relatively common alleles that are absent in non-African populations; however, most of the alleles that are common in non-African populations are also common in African populations. Thus, the pattern of genetic variation is one of nested subsets, such that the variation in non-African populations is a subset of the variation found in African populations. The recent out of Africa model, which postulates an African origin of modern humans and subsequent migrations out into Eurasia and the Americas best fits with this genetic data *(11)*.

In addition to finding the most variation within the African-American population, Guthery et al. also noted that the genetic structure of common variants within African-American populations was different than the genetic structure of other US populations, meaning that genetic elements involved in disease may differ between African-Americans and other US groups. They attributed this difference in genetic structure to a difference in genetic ancestry between the populations. As a result, they suggest that future genetic association studies consider both genetic ancestry and population structure of the study populations. Furthermore, considering that in the past many of the genetic association studies have included only European populations and that those findings may not be applicable to other populations, in particular African-Americans, they suggest that future studies should either "oversample" African-Americans or focus on understanding how genetic variation within African-American populations contributes to disease.

Given the genetic data now available across diverse human populations, it is becoming increasingly clear that the frequency of most genetic markers do not vary much among the major continental populations. Population geneticists use a statistic called F_{ST} to describe the amount of total variation within subpopulations relative to the total population *(12)*. This index can range from 0 to 1, where 0 indicates that there is no variation between the subpopulations (little genetic differentiation) and 1 indicates that all the variation is between the subpopulations (high genetic differentiation). F_{ST} can also be described as a measurement of genetic distance where as F_{ST} increases, subpopulations become more distant and/or unrelated, from each other *(13)*.

Genetic variation among human groups is typically quoted as having an F_{ST} value of 0.09–0.13 *(14)*. This value is small compared to other species with comparable geographical ranges to humans. The F_{ST} value indicates that between 9% and 13% of the variation is between continental groups while the majority of variation, 87–91%, is within continental groups. This observation that more variation exists within continental groups than between groups blurs boundaries between groups; this has been used to argue against the biological basis to race *(15,16)*. However, a number of studies that examine genetic variation across the genome have found that individuals with similar ancestral continental origins tend to cluster together, and in general, these clusters correspond to four continental groups: Sub-Saharan Africa, Europe/Western Asia, Asia, and the Americas *(4)*. Additionally, Tang et al. *(17)* in 2005 showed that self-identified race/ethnicity can parallel these clusters. In spite of this, the relationship between race/ethnicity and genetics remains uncertain for some. Problems regarding this issue have arisen because the terms race and ethnicity have a multitude of definitions.

In addition, the words race and ethnicity are sometimes ascribed with a negative and prejudiced connotation, often associated with a particular social hierarchy. Finally, despite the continental clustering of those with shared ancestry, there are no discrete genetic boundaries that define any race or ethnicity *(18)*.

While most genetic markers have low F_{ST} levels, a small number ($\sim$5%) have significantly higher F_{ST} than expected *(8)*. These markers with higher than expected F_{ST} values are within regions of the genome that many believe may have been under natural selection sometime during the history of the population. The human genome should not be thought of as a single entity but an assortment of segments which have evolved differently due to diverse environmental pressures. Thus, the human genome is made up of segments with vastly different histories.

3. MEASURE AND USE OF GENETIC ANCESTRY

Not withstanding the large amount of genetic variation shared across human groups there is a small but significant fraction of polymorphisms that are quite informative for estimating biogeographic ancestry. Less than 5% of polymorphisms have large allele frequency difference between continental populations (i.e., West Africans, Europeans, and Asian/Native Americans). We call these markers "ancestry informative markers" because of their high information content for continental or biogeographical ancestry *(19)*.

In the United Stated, variation in genetic background exists within most self-identified racial–ethnic groups (SIRE) groups. For instance, African and Hispanic Americans represent recently admixed populations with diverse ancestries due to social and biological factors. Hispanic Americans are a complex macro-ethnic group who share a common language yet can trace their ancestries to multiple continents *(20)*. Interestingly, individuals self-report as African-American due to skin color and the historical classification schema referred to as the "one-drop" rule which denotes an individual with an African ancestor as Black. No matter how physically "white" or "black" the person looked, he or she would be considered "Black" or African-American. This racial paradigm emerged from the antebellum south and then became the nation's definition accepted by almost everyone *(21)*. Because of this social model of one-way gene flow, the one-drop rule has increased the genetic heterogeneity of the African-American population in the United States.

There lacks consensus on the use of SIRE data in biomedical research but its reliability varies across populations *(2,15)*. In Fig. 1, we show a histogram depicting percentage West African ancestry measured using AIMs in three SIRE populations, European Americans from State College PA; African-Americans from Washington, DC; and Hispanic Americans (Puerto Ricans) living in NYC. The first striking feature observed is that 98% of the

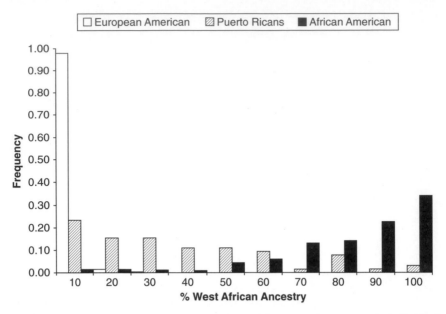

Fig. 1. Frequency histogram of percentage West African genetic ancestry in individuals who self-reported as African-American, European American, and Puerto Rican. Data from *(22,23)*.

European Americans had over 90% European ancestry, while only 34% of the African-Americans possessed over 90% West African ancestry. A broad range of ancestry is observed among the African and Hispanic American populations. The distribution in West African ancestry was inversely related between the two admixed populations with about 20% of the African-Americans had less than 60% West African ancestry compared to over 80% of Puerto Ricans.

Contrary to some published reports self-report for African and Hispanic Americans is not necessarily a strong proxy for genetic background. Our figure highlights that differences related to geographic or continental ancestry deconstruct traditional racial categorization. We also note that this distribution is reflective only of the black/white dichotomy and does not factor in the Native American component in these populations. The Native American component is much higher in Puerto Ricans than in European and African American populations due to the historical experiences of many Hispanic groups *(24)*.

Variance in genetic background of study subjects is becoming more of an issue with the increasing number of genetic association studies on complex disease. Differences in genetic background among study individuals may impact the power and reliability of genetic association studies *(25)*. Methods to detect and control for differences in ancestry in genetic association studies utilize AIMs.

AIMs have high utility in biomedical research since they can be used to accurately measure individual ancestry (IA) of subjects enrolled in studies. Almost all outbred populations show variation in individual ancestry which can introduce population stratification and impact the success of genetic studies *(26)*. Most importantly these IA estimates can be used to control for heterogeneity in genetic studies in recently admixed populations like African-Americans and Hispanic Americans. In fact, the use of AIMs to control for genetic heterogeneity and population stratification in genetics studies is becoming widespread. AIMs were used to control for stratification in studies of risk factors for hypertension *(27)*, myocardial infarction *(28)*, and asthma *(29)*. Controlling for population stratification due to admixture is referred to as "admixture adjustment" since IA is used as a covariate in the regression analyses.

4. FINDING DISEASE SUSCEPTIBILITY GENES IN ADMIXED POPULATIONS

An emerging popular approach to mapping susceptibility genes in recently admixed populations is called admixture mapping. This novel approach attempts to find genes that underlie ethnic differences in disease risk *(30)*. Recent gene flow (admixture) between long separated populations creates linkage disequilibrium (LD) between loci which can extend over large chromosomal regions (exceeding 30 cM). In this approach, we type genome spanning AIMs in the clinical population to infer ancestry at each locus and then test locus ancestry for association with the trait of interest in the population. However, once potential regions are located using admixture mapping, conventional association tests are needed to locate the causative locus. Admixture proportions and dynamics and marker (AIMs) characteristics all influence the power of mapping *(30,31)*. Admixture mapping has been successful for mapping disease and trait loci for multiple sclerosis *(32)*, hypertension *(33)*, and prostate cancer *(34)*. However, not all diseases which exhibit differential risk across populations are amenable to the admixture mapping approach especially when disease alleles are similar in frequency in parental populations and disease risk is due to differences in environmental and social influences. This may be the case for many disease disparities since they are largely influenced by social determinants.

5. HAS NATURAL SELECTION SHAPED GENETIC VARIATION?

The extent and pattern of genetic variation in human populations have been influenced by natural selection. Natural selection is complex and recent studies have produced interesting new data. Natural selection can shape genetic variation in a population by removing harmful variants, spreading favorable ones, or maintaining variation at particular genetic loci. Has historical selection influenced the frequency of many genetic variants that contribute to population differences in disease prevalence and drug response? If so, how much of an effect has natural selection had on shaping variation in genes which affect traits involved in disease pathways such as cardiovascular disease (CVD)? Several recent studies have utilized large genetic datasets to search for signatures of recent selection in the human genome *(35,36)*. These studies indicate that genes involved in inflammatory response to infectious disease show a pattern of variation different from other regions of the genome. Other categories of genes which may have been impacted by selective pressures include pigmentation, fertility, and reproduction genes *(35,36)*. Interestingly, recent work exploring gene expression differences between West Africans and Europeans is consistent with the pattern of SNP variation within many of these genes *(37)*.

Differences in the pattern of genetic variation across human populations can be assessed using different methods. As mentioned earlier, FST summarizes genetic differentiation between populations. Haplotype structure and frequency also provides some clues for potential selective events. Most haplotypes are shared across populations but for a subset of genes, haplotype structure and frequencies vary significantly across populations. Haplotype structure and frequencies for genes influencing physiological pathways involved in fat storage, salt sensitivity *(38)*, and testosterone have been shown to vary significantly across groups. Several reasons for these patterns include bottleneck effects, selection, and genetic hitchhiking events.

There is compelling data emerging that selection has shaped genetic susceptibility for several common diseases *(39)*. Recently, a number of researchers have shown that certain alleles that are involved in causing common diseases, including CVD, may have at one time conferred an evolutionary advantage to ancestral human populations. However, with changes in modern lifestyle, e.g., sedentism, diet, new environmental exposures, these alleles are no longer advantageous but instead increase disease risk.

Selection during the out-of-Africa expansion of human populations may have influenced risk for hypertension (HTN) *(40)*. Data has shown that the effect of ancestral susceptibility alleles on risk for HTN varies across latitude. The hypothesis suggests that the differential susceptibility to HTN may be due to gradients of exposure to selective pressures once human populations migrated out of Africa about 80,000–100,000 years ago *(40)*. There are clear genetic signals of selection in support of this hypothesis for several genes (such as AGT, CYP3A5, and GNB3) which may influence HTN and CVD *(39,40)*.

6. CONCLUSION

Since a large fraction of genetic variation may be localized to particular geographic regions much attention has been focused on whether geographic ancestral origins contributes to the differential distribution of disease and mortality *(41)*. These studies continue to utilize sociopolitical constructs that are inappropriate for investigations on genetic contributions to the etiology of complex disease, drug response, and more importantly, health disparities. While race may be an important determinant to monitor health status and health-care quality *(42)*, it lacks biological integrity. In fact, the use of race to identify groups may confound biomedical studies. This is because race reflects deeply confounded sociocultural as well as biological factors.

We suggest that ancestry be used instead of race. Genetic ancestry has several salient features which are useful for biomedical studies. First, genetic ancestry has strong utility as an index for human biological variation *(19,26)*. Also when ancestry is used to describe genetic background, it allows for more sophisticated investigation of biological risk factors. Additionally, there is no historical baggage associated with genetic ancestry and it has promoted increased discourse between disciplines *(43,44)*. There is an urgent need for biomedical research to develop interdisciplinary research designs and embrace research on social determinants of health and how they influence genetic risk factors. The key features of genetic ancestry also demand that more work be done in order to better assess individual genetic ancestry and most importantly how it may be correlated with social factors such as SES and racism. Most would agree that information on genetic ancestry is potentially more useful for efficient analyses of genetics of complex disease and pharmacogenetics than the traditional racial classifications.

REFERENCES

1. Risch N, Burchard E, Ziv E, Tang H. Categorization of humans in biomedical research: genes, race and disease. *Genome Biol* 2002; 3(7): comment 2007.
2. Burchard EG, Ziv E, Coyle N, et al. The importance of race and ethnic background in biomedical research and clinical practice. *N Engl J Med* 2003; 348(12):1170–1175.
3. Kittles RA, Weiss KM. Race, ancestry, and genes: implications for defining disease risk. *Annu Rev Genomics Hum Genet* 2003; 4:33–67.
4. Rosenberg NA, Pritchard JK, Weber JL, et al. Genetic structure of human populations. *Science* 2002; 298(5602):2381–2385.
5. Serre D, Paabo S. Evidence for gradients of human genetic diversity within and among continents. *Genome Res* 2004; 14(9):1679.
6. Goodman AH. Why genes don't count (for racial differences in health). *Am J Public Health* 2000; 90(11):1699–1702.
7. Crawford DC, Akey DT, Nickerson DA. The patterns of natural variation in human genes. *Annu Rev Genomics Hum Genet* 2005; 6:287–312.
8. Hinds DA, Stuve LL, Nilsen GB, et al. Whole-genome patterns of common DNA variation in three human populations. *Science* 2005; 307(5712):1072–1079.
9. Gabriel SB, Schaffner SF, Nguyen H, et al. The structure of haplotype blocks in the human genome. *Science* 2002; 296(5576):2225–2259.
10. Guthery SL, Salisbury BA, Pungliya MS, Stephens JC, Bamshad M. The structure of common genetic variation in United States populations. *Am J Hum Genet* 2007; 81(6):1221–1231.

11. Cavalli-Sforza LL, Feldman MW. The application of molecular genetic approaches to the study of human evolution. *Nat Genet* 2003; 33(Suppl.):266–75.
12. Cockerham CC, Weir BS. Covariances of relatives stemming from a population undergoing mixed self and random mating. *Biometrics* 1984; 40(1):157–164.
13. Weir BS, Hill WG. Estimating f-statistics. *Annu Rev Genet* 2002; 36:721–50.
14. Jobling MA, Hurles M, Tyler-Smith C. Human evolutionary genetics: origins, peoples & disease. New York: Garland Science; 2004.
15. Cooper RS, Kaufman JS, Ward R. Race and genomics. *N Engl J Med* 2003; 348(12): 1166–1170.
16. Lewontin RC. The apportionment of human diversity. *Evol Biol* 1972; 6:381–398.
17. Tang H, Quertermous T, Rodriguez B, et al. Genetic structure, self-identified race/ethnicity, and confounding in case-control association studies. *Am J Hum Genet* 2005; 76(2):268–275.
18. Collins FS. What we do and don't know about 'race', 'ethnicity', genetics and health at the dawn of the genome era. *Nat Genet* 2004; 36(11 Suppl):S13–15.
19. Shriver MD, Kittles RA. Genetic ancestry and the search for personalized genetic histories. *Nat Rev Genet* 2004; 5(8):611–618.
20. Burchard EG, Borrell LN, Choudhry S, et al. Race, genetics, and health disparities. Latino populations: a unique opportunity for the study of race, genetics, and social environment in epidemiological research. *Am J Pub Health* 2005; 95(12):2161–8.
21. Harris BK. Southern savory. Chapel Hill: University of North Carolina Press; 1964.
22. Bonilla C, Shriver MD, Parra EJ, Jones A, Fernandez JR. Ancestral proportions and their association with skin pigmentation and bone mineral density in Puerto Rican women from New York city. *Hum Genet* 2004; 115(1):57–68.
23. Shriver MD, Parra EJ, Dios S, et al. Skin pigmentation, biogeographical ancestry and admixture mapping. *Hum Genet* 2003; 112(4):387–399.
24. Parra EJ, Kittles RA, Shriver MD. Implications of correlations between skin color and genetic ancestry for biomedical research. *Nat Genet* 2004; 36(11 Suppl):S54–S60.
25. Choudhry S, Coyle NE, Tang H, et al. Population stratification confounds genetic association studies among Latinos. *Hum Genet* 2006; 118(5): 652–664.
26. Halder I, Shriver MD. Measuring and using admixture to study the genetics of complex diseases. *Hum Genomics* 2003; 1(1): 52–62.
27. Tang H, Jorgenson E, Gadde M, et al. Racial admixture and its impact on BMI and blood pressure in African and Mexican Americans. *Hum Genet* 2006; 119(6):624–633.
28. Helgadottir A, Manolescu A, Helgason A, et al. A variant of the gene encoding leukotriene A4 hydrolase confers ethnicity-specific risk of myocardial infarction. *Nat Genet* 2006; 38(1):68–74.
29. Salari K, Choudhry S, Tang H, et al. Genetic admixture and asthma-related phenotypes in Mexican American and Puerto Rican asthmatics. *Genet Epidemiol* 2005; 29(1):76–86.
30. McKeigue PM. Prospects for admixture mapping of complex traits. *Am J Hum Genet* 2005; 76(1):1–7.
31. Reich D, Patterson N. Will admixture mapping work to find disease genes? *Philos Trans R Soc Lond B Biol Sci* 2005; 360(1460):1605–1607.
32. Reich D, Patterson N, De Jager PL, et al. A whole-genome admixture scan finds a candidate locus for multiple sclerosis susceptibility. *Nat Genet* 2005; 37(10):1113–1118.
33. Zhu X, Luke A, Cooper RS, et al. Admixture mapping for hypertension loci with genome-scan markers. *Nat Genet* 2005; 37(2):177–181.
34. Freedman ML, Haiman CA, Patterson N, et al. Admixture mapping identifies 8q24 as a prostate cancer risk locus in African-American men. *Proc Natl Acad Sci U S A* 2006; 103(38):14068–14073.
35. Akey JM, Eberle MA, Rieder MJ, et al. Population history and natural selection shape patterns of genetic variation in 132 genes. *PLoS Biol* 2004; 2(10):e286.

36. Voight BF, Kudaravalli S, Wen X, Pritchard JK. A map of recent positive selection in the human genome. *PLoS Biol* 2006; 4(3):e72.
37. Storey JD, Madeoy J, Strout JL, Wurfel M, Ronald J, Akey JM. Gene-expression variation within and among human populations. *Am J Hum Genet* 2007; 80(3):502–509.
38. Thompson EE, Kuttab-Boulos H, Yang L, Roe BA, Di Rienzo A. Sequence diversity and haplotype structure at the human CYP3A cluster. *Pharmacogenomics J* 2006; 6(2): 105–114.
39. DiRienzo A, Richard RH. An evolutionary framework for common disease: the ancestral-susceptibility model. *Trends Genet* 2005; 21(11):596–601.
40. Young JH, Chang YP, Kim JD, et al. Differential susceptibility to hypertension is due to selection during the out-of-Africa expansion. *PLoS Genet* 2005; 1(6):e82.
41. Keita SO, Kittles RA, Royal CD, et al. Conceptualizing human variation. *Nat Genet* 2004; 36(11 Suppl.):S17–S20.
42. LaVeist TA. Beyond dummy variables and sample selection: what health services researchers ought to know about race as a variable. *Health Serv Res* 1994; 29(1):1–16.
43. Rebbeck TR, Sankar P. Ethnicity, ancestry, and race in molecular epidemiologic research. *Cancer Epidemiol Biomarkers Prev* 2005; 14(11 Pt 1):2467–2471.
44. Shields AE, Fortun M, Hammonds EM, et al. The use of race variables in genetic studies of complex traits and the goal of reducing health disparities: a transdisciplinary perspective. *Am Psychol* 2005; 60(1):77–103.

5

Race, Genetics and Cardiovascular Disease

Ivor J. Benjamin, MD,
and Theophilus Owan, MD, MSc

CONTENTS

Abstract

Significant strides from personalized medicine hold great promise to improve early detection, guide targeted therapies, and enhance disease monitoring while simultaneously incorporating specific contributions from race and ethnicity in disease pathogenesis. Hypertension underscores complex gene–environment interactions related to salt sensitivity. Genetic disorders in which certain candidate genes result in a loss of function and the aberrant expression of an abnormal gene product might give rise to either autosomal dominant or recessive inheritance patters. For example, impaired vascular function has been reported in both healthy and hypertensive African Americans. To account for ethnic differences in cardiovascular disease prevalence and outcome, however, the bioavailability of nitric oxide has been proposed as one mechanism to explain difference in

From: *Contemporary Cardiology: Cardiovascular Disease in Racial and Ethnic Minorities*
Edited by: K.C. Ferdinand and A. Armani, DOI 10.1007/978-1-59745-410-0_5
© Humana Press, a part of Springer Science+Business Media, LLC 2009

vascular function. Alteration of nitric oxide production has been linked to oly-
morphisms in the gene encoding the endothelial nitric oxide synthase (ecNOS)
in African Americans.

Distinctive variations, either by gender or by ethnicity, in the prevalence of
significant CAD and mortality are often attributed to provider bias, in equities
in heath care access or both. In spite of the earlier literature showing gaps by
gender or ethnicity for heath-care access and treatment, direct evidence that disparities might be explained only by biases is lacking. Investigations such as the
African-American Heart Failure Trial (A-HeFT) may now serve as a powerful reminder for us to avoid similar missed opportunities to explore emerging
disciplines such as pharmacogenetics in the genomic era. Future guidelines on
beta-adrenergic blockade for patients with heart failure or cardiac ischemia will
inevitably be revised when the genetic information is available utilizing pharmacogenetics. Specific knowledge of an individual's genetic composition will
eliminate existing proxies using skin color for phenotyping disease susceptibility or resistance while enabling adequate monitoring and surveillance measures
to be instituted.

Key Words: Genetic haplotyping; Single nucleotide polymorphism; Endothelial nitric oxide synthase; Pharmacogenetics; Phenotype.

1. INTRODUCTION

Recent years have witnessed an overall improvement in the clinical prevalence and outcome of cardiovascular diseases in the US population. However, specific ethnic groups such as African-American are burdened with
striking disparities in cardiovascular disease compared with white patients.
What factors might account for an African-American male, between the ages
of 45 and 65, to be four times more likely than his white counterpart to have
a stroke? Ethnic minorities are afflicted with a higher prevalence of obesity,
diabetes, and hypertension compared with whites for which genetics, the
environment, and socioeconomics are contributing factors.

There is growing evidence that the existing clinical model used for generating practice guidelines will be inadequate to cope with the overwhelming
costs for generating "evidence-based" medicine, incremental benefits of new
therapies, and the demographic shifts toward age-related chronic diseases.
Significant strides from personalized medicine, however, hold great promise
to improve early detection, guide-targeted therapies, and enhance disease
monitoring while simultaneously incorporating specific contributions from
race and ethnicity in disease pathogenesis *(1)*. While an exhaustive trea-
tise on race and genetics is beyond the scope of this chapter, we intend
to focus on the predisposing factors, underlying pathophysiologic mechanisms, challenges, and likely opportunities to make transformative progress
on the unfolding complex interplay between race, ethnicity, and cardiovascular genomic medicine.

2. PREDISPOSITION

Traditional cardiovascular risk factors such as hypertension, diabetes, family history, and smoking also are predisposing conditions for ischemic heart disease. Occlusive coronary artery disease and hypertension, however, are examples of polygenic diseases since multiple genes, molecular pathways, and environmental elements have been implicated in disease pathogenesis by incompletely understood mechanisms. Hypertension underscores complex gene–environment interactions related to salt sensitivity but has, with inconclusive evidence, been postulated to centuries old conditions during the slave trade to account for the high prevalence in African-Americans. In contrast, a genetic predisposition for an inheritable disease refers to the increased susceptibility for clinical manifestation arising from one or more gene mutations. Autosomal dominant or recessive inheritance patters arise from factors in which certain candidate genes result in a loss of function, and/or in either a loss or gain or function and aberrant expression of an abnormal gene product.

Single nucleotide polymorphism (SNPs) refers to a genetic variation in a sequence of either a purine or a pyrimidine base, and occuring at a frequency of at least 1% in a given population. Genetic polymorphisms might be linked to several disease conditions. Alleles are alternative forms of a gene at a locus on a chromosome and may occur singly on a locus (heterozygote) or in pairs (homozygote). Haplotypes are combination of alleles on each chromosome, which are closely linked enough to be inherited together. Single gene disorders causing cardiovascular diseases are primarily missense mutations in which a base-pair substitution results in the replacement of a single amino acid. We will examine more broadly the genetic factors that predispose to disease phenotypes with an emphasis on cardiovascular and related diseases in racial and ethnic groups. When the nucleotide adenine is replaced by thymine in the genetic code (A to T), introducing an incorrect amino acid into the protein sequence of the β-globin gene, the gene defect results in glutamate to be substituted by valine at position 6. Autosomal recessive inheritance of the Glu$\Rightarrow$Val substitution in β-globin gene found on chromosome 6 causes sickle cell anemia. In endemic regions with malaria, the sickle cell gene confers a selective advantage for carriers whose red blood cells are inhospitable against the parasites.

Viruses (e.g., Coxsackie's B3, parvovirus) in susceptible individuals can attack the heart and are the major etiologic factors for idiopathic dilated cardiomyopathy (IDCM). Such postviral sequalae include both acute and chronic relapsing inflammation, triggering apoptosis, and ventricular remodeling (2). Chemical mutagenesis is more widely used experimentally to introduce genetic mutations in which the exogenous trigger or mutagen overwhelms the endogenous repair schemes, resulting either in gain or loss of functions in the organism. The alkylating chemotheraputic agent, doxorubicin, is a highly effective anticancer agent but triggers dose-dependent-increased susceptibility for cardiomyopathy in humans.

3. SCREENING

Genetic screening and counseling are now routinely performed at birth for many heritable metabolic disorders (e.g., maple syrup urine disease, Tay–Sacks disease) at birth. More recently attention has focused on molecular genetic testing for closely related regions of DNA, which might give rise to linkage studies for a given trait in linkage disequilibrium for a group of genetic markers. A bit of *caveat emptor* is warranted in this emerging arena as the temptations for profiteering on genetic tests are constantly being fueled by the hype surrounding the potential cures being promoted with each new scientific discovery *(3)*. Notwithstanding, there is growing scientific interest in the field for establishing multigenic effects on disease susceptibility, which must be examined in the context of an individual's genomic and environmental contributions.

Distinctive variations, either by gender or by ethnicity, in the prevalence of significant CAD and mortality are often attributed to provider bias, inequities in heath-care access or both. Substantial differences in the prevalence and severity of atherosclerotic disease witnessed among whites, blacks, Hispanics, and Asians are not simply or easily explained by the levels of traditional risk factors. Unlike gender, for categorical ethnicity is a continuous it remains controversial whether variable whose complex influences in disease pathogenesis are inextricably linked to traditional risk factors of hypertension, hyperlipidemia, diabetes, smoking, exercise, dietary, and environmental factors. Further, present focus on health disparities might be missing the future challenges and opportunities to exploit potential differences in genetic variation for understanding disease pathogenesis and causal mechanisms. Using electron beam tomography for asymptomatic assessment of atherosclerosis, Budoff and colleagues have reported on the relative risks for coronary calcification among African-American, Asian, Caucasian, and Hispanic women and men *(4)*. When adjusted for risk factors multivariate analysis, the relative risk of coronary calcification was least likely for African-American men, whereas the odds ratio was most likely for African-American women compared with other ethnicities *(4)*, illustrating the importance for population-specific nomograms for different genders. Similar results to this physician-referral cohort were shown in the population-based multi-ethnic study of atherosclerosis (MESA), comprising four ethnic groups (12% Chinese, 38% white, 22% Hispanic, and 28% black) of 6814 women and men aged 45–84 years *(5)*. However, the prognostic potential of coronary or extracardiac calcification for predicting subsequent cardiovascular events has not been settled *(6)*.

4. PATHOPHYSIOLOGY

In this section, we will highlight some common polymorphisms associated with cardiovascular disease phenotypes with emphasis on those particularly prevalent in US minority populations. Given ethnic differences in cardiovascular disease prevalence and outcome, bioavailability of nitric oxide has been proposed as one mechanism to explain difference in vascular function *(7)*. Impaired vascular function has been reported in both healthy and hypertensive African-Americans compared with whites *(8,9)*. As a mediator of vascular homeostasis, a deficiency of bioactive endothelial nitric oxide might be predicted to impair multiple actions important for vasodilation, anti-inflammatory function, platelet inhibition, and smooth muscle cell growth inhibition.

Alteration of nitric oxide production has been linked to polymorphisms in the gene encoding the endothelial nitric oxide synthase (ecNOS). Among African-Americans, the 4a variant in the 4a/4b polymorphism is more common among whites and is associated with a decrease in ecNOS expression and nitric oxide production *(10,11)*. Hooper and coworkers have recently reported that homozygosity for the 4a polymorphism substantially increased the risk of myocardial infarction in African-Americans before the age of 45 years *(12)*.

Both enzymatic and non-enzymatic antioxidants are required to counterbalance pro-oxidants such as superoxide and hydroxyl radical generated under pathologic states such as myocardial ischemia and heart failure.

Antioxidant production in the form of reduced glutathione (GSH) and the co-factor, NADPH, is linked to glucose-6-phosphate dehydrogenase (G6PD), the rate-limiting enzyme of the pentose phosphate pathway. G6PD generates NADPH synthesis, a key co-factor of glutathione reductase, which catalyzes the reduction of glutathione disulfide to glutathione. G6PD deficiency is the most common enzymopathy worldwide but is especially common among the African-American population in which the prevalence is ~11 to 15%. Among the first genetic disorders to be described in the twentieth century, G6PD deficiency was discovered in certain African-American soldiers who developed hemolytic anemia after treatment with primaquine *(13,14)*. The mechanism of action of antimalarials is to increase oxidative stress and creating an inhospitable environment for the malaria parasites in blood cells without mitochondria but this process destroys red blood cells in affected individuals with G6PD deficiency.

Beyond these early findings, recent experimental studies have established a causal mechanism involving G6PD deficiency with alterations in vascular responses, impaired endothelium-dependent vasodilation, decreased nitric oxide bioavailability, and decreased vascular density *(15–17)*. While these findings support, in part, a molecular basis for differences in vascular and angiogenic responses between African-Americans with G6PD deficiency when compared with whites, such evidence is the most compelling to accelerate the emerging discipline of genomic medicine, which can more precisely exploit such mechanistic advances of the pathophysiology for rationale therapies in affected populations.

4.1. Health Disparities: The Role of Gender and Ethnicity

In spite of the substantial earlier literature showing gaps for heath-care access and treatment by gender or ethnicity, direct evidence that the disparities might be currently explained by biases per se is lacking and new evidence suggests evolving practices (18). In the Minnesota Heart Study, a population-based cohort of women and men admitted with acute myocardial infarction (AMI), both in-hospital diagnostic and therapeutic maneuvers were comparable between groups but women were 46% less likely than men to be referred for coronary arteriography (19). In recent studies, however, both men and women with similar severity of disease were referred for coronary revascularization procedures at equivalent rates (18,19). Prospective evaluation by angiography of patients referred with either stable angina or acute coronary syndromes (ACS) has highlighted the need to tailor clinical practice guidelines for specific subsets of at-risk population in spite of gender or ethnic differences (20).

4.2. Ethnicity-Based Therapies

As criticism has diminished for the paucity of sufficient numbers of ethnic minorities in clinical trials, the pendulum has radically shifted to the notion that treatment algorithms might be appropriate strategies for specific ethnic groups. The most widely scrutinized has been the recent African-American Heart Failure (A-HeFT), which examined a fixed dose of isosorbide dinitrate, 20 mg, plus hydralazine, 37.5 mg, added to standard therapy for heart failure in 1050 self-identified black patients with either NYHA class III or IV (21). In this placebo-controlled randomized multicenter trial, treatment with isosorbide dinitrate plus hydralazine, termed BiDil, significantly reduced mortality by 43% (95% CI, 11–63%), rate of first hospitalization and improved quality of life compared to placebo arm of the trial. Based on these provocative findings, an approval by the US Food and Drug Administration (FDA), for the fixed combination for treating heart failure in black patients, has came under considerable criticism (22). Critics argued that the data lacked reproducibility in whites, for example, the pathophysiological mechanisms remained poorly defined, and the "race-based" approach circumvented the lengthy expensive evaluation for a drug. While heralded as a novel approach, this marketing strategy with a proprietary label for race-based management has drawn considerable scrutiny ranging form the scientific community to the public at large. Among the most important lessons were that (i) BiDil's efficacy was not independently confirmed in other racial or ethnic groups, (ii) therapeutic distinctions based are fundamentally flawed constructs, and (iii) the failure to address the scientific basis such as genetic markers for predicting the response in blacks to BiDil therapy. Investigations such as A-HeFT may now serve as a powerful reminder for us to avoid similar missed opportunities to explore the emerging disciplines such as pharmacogenetics in the genomic era.

5. PHARMACOGENETICS

The emerging discipline of pharmacogenomics holds great promise for using genetic determinants to predict an individual's drug response and outcomes. Common polymorphisms account for substantial phenotypic heterogeneity and the variability of responses to pharmacologic agents among individuals. Recent lessons from studies of human heart failure illustrate handsomely both the enormous potential and the challenges for pharmacogenomics. For example, blockade of the β-adrenergic receptors (β-ARs), members of the seven membrane-spanning receptor superfamily, is now standard therapy for ischemia and heart failure, validating the hypothesis that excess catecholamines causes increased mortality.

In the β-Blocker Evaluation of Survival Trial (BEST), the DNA Study Group evaluated the β blocker bucindolol for the treatment of class III/IV hoping to uncover insights into the mechanisms for pharmacogenomic phenotypes involving the Arg/Gly polymorphism of the β_1-AR (23). Liggett and coworkers have demonstrated that stimulatory interactions between non-synonymous single-nucleotide polymorphisms of β_1-AR and heterotrimeric G proteins G_s mediate both beneficial and deleterious signal transduction pathways in heart failure. Phosphorylation of β-ARs by G protein-coupled receptor kinase (GRKs) desensitizes the receptor, leading to improve clinical outcomes. The GRK5 variant in which leucine is substituted for glutamine at position 41 is common among African-Americans and this polymorphism has been shown in human association studies to significantly decrease the morality from either cardiac ischemia or heart failure. Biochemical studies of GRK5-Leu41 revealed uncoupling to isoproterenol stimulation, both in cultured cells and in transgenic mice to catecholamine-induced cardiomyopathy (24). Further, prospective follow-up of 375 African-Americans with the GRK5-Leu41 revealed significant protection against cardiac transplantation or death, supporting the hypothesis that "genetic beta-blockade" confers a survival benefit. Therefore, the future guidelines on beta-adrenergic blockade for patients will heart failure or cardiac ischemia will inevitably be revised when the genetic information is available utilizing pharmacogenetics.

6. FUTURE DIRECTIONS

Without doubt, advances in medical genetics and genomics have the best chances to eliminate the notion to cardiovascular diseases in ethnic minorities. Knowledge of the genetic influence on disease process finds uses in predicting and understanding the manifestations of diseases, employing most appropriate diagnostic tools, and the selection of specific therapies. Specific knowledge of an individual's genetic composition will eliminate existing proxies using skin color for phenotyping disease susceptibility or resistance, while enabling adequate monitoring and surveillance measures to be instituted. The International HapMap Project is an international scientific collaboration designed to collect and report on all the common genetic variation in populations worldwide. Such efforts will inevitably lead us to understand how differences in human populations might predict susceptibility and resistance to disease and environmental exposures (e.g., drugs, toxins). The foresight of BEST investigators, for example, to recognize the power of genetic haplotyping underscores the importance for all future well-designed human trials to include contingencies for pharmacogenomics in an era of genomic medicine.

7. CONCLUSIONS AND RECOMMENDATIONS

How individuals respond to pharmacologic agents in health and disease are undoubtedly a function of their genetic make-up. Current models for individual therapies, which are based on data derived from whole population studies, are often based on marginal differences with highly variable efficacy. When would drug therapies be dictated by specific knowledge of the individual's metabolism? In the ensuing years, the convergence of pharmacology and genetics will increase efficacy, decrease the side effects, and reduce the morbidity and mortality of cardiovascular diseases in all populations.

GLOSSARY

Haploinsusufficiency Loss of function mutation often results in 50% protein product but with enough function in the heterozygote state leading to a recessive disorder. However, in the situation where 50% of the protein product is insufficient for normal function (haploinsufficiency), a dominant disorder results.

Hardy–Weinberg principle Describes the relationship between gene frequency and genotype frequency. This relationship combines both the multiplication and the addition rules of basic probability and is determined by whether a gene is dominance or recessive. The principle is used to estimate the frequencies of gene and genotype in a given population where dominant homozygote and heterozygote are indistinguishable. Knowledge of disease prevalence in the population is required; and principle or assumption of random mating (panmixia) needs to be satisfied.

Karyotypes are the ordered display of chromosomes according to length. Such visualization of chromosomes is best achieved during metaphase but is enhanced by hypotonic nuclear rupture and staining techniques. Molecular analysis of DNA polymorphisms allow for more detailed study of chromosomal abnormalities and the tracking of parental chromosomal derivation. Gene-mapping techniques have been used to pinpoint a gene to its specific location (or locus) on a chromosome and to determine the relative distances between genes on the chromosome. This can be accomplished through *chromosomal mapping* in which the frequency of meiotic crossovers between loci is used to estimate inter-locus distances. Gene mapping can also by accomplished through *physical mapping*, which uses cytogenetic and molecular techniques to determine the actual physical location of genes on chromosomes.

ACKNOWLEDGMENTS

We appreciate the helpful suggestions and comments over the many years from our many colleagues who have contributed to the much needed transition in our understanding about race and cardiovascular genomic medicine. Jennifer Schroff provided expert editorial assistance during preparation of this manuscript

REFERENCES

1. Bell J. Predicting disease using genomics. *Nature* 2004; 429(6990):453–456.
2. Liu PP, Mason JW. Advances in the understanding of myocarditis. *Circulation* 2001; 104(9):1076–1082.
3. Humphries SE, Ridker PM, Talmud PJ. Genetic testing for cardiovascular disease susceptibility: a useful clinical management tool or possible misinformation? *Arterioscler Thromb Vasc Biol* 2004; 24(4):628–636.
4. Budoff MJ, Nasir K, Mao S, Tseng PH, Chau A, Liu ST, Flores F, Blumenthal RS. Ethnic differences of the presence and severity of coronary atherosclerosis. *Atherosclerosis* 2006; 187(2):343–350.
5. Takasu J, Katz R, Nasir K, Carr JJ, Wong N, Detrano R, Budoff MJ. Relationships of thoracic aortic wall calcification to cardiovascular risk factors: the Multi-Ethnic Study of Atherosclerosis (MESA). *Am Heart J* 2008; 155(4):765–771.
6. Nasir K, Katz R, Takasu J, Shavelle DM, Detrano R, Lima JA, Blumenthal RS, O'Brien K, Budoff MJ. Ethnic differences between extra-coronary measures on cardiac computed tomography: multi-ethnic study of atherosclerosis (MESA). *Atherosclerosis* 2008; 198(1):104–114.
7. Benjamin IJ, Arnett DK, Loscalzo J. Discovering the full spectrum of cardiovascular disease: Minority Health Summit 2003: report of the Basic Science Writing Group. *Circulation* 2005; 111(10):e120–123.
8. Kahn DF, Duffy SJ, Tomasian D, Holbrook M, Rescorl L, Russell J, Gokce N, Loscalzo J, Vita JA. Effects of black race on forearm resistance vessel function. *Hypertension* 2002; 40(2):195–201.
9. Lang CC, Stein CM, Brown RM, Deegan R, Nelson R, He HB, Wood M, Wood AJ. Attenuation of isoproterenol-mediated vasodilatation in blacks. *N Engl J Med* 1995; 333(3):155–160.

10. Song J, Yoon Y, Park KU, Park J, Hong YJ, Hong SH, Kim JQ. Genotype-specific influence on nitric oxide synthase gene expression, protein concentrations, and enzyme activity in cultured human endothelial cells. *Clin Chem* 2003; 49(6 Pt 1):847–852.
11. Tanus-Santos JE, Desai M, Flockhart DA. Effects of ethnicity on the distribution of clinically relevant endothelial nitric oxide variants. *Pharmacogenetics* 2001; 11(8): 719–725.
12. Hooper WC, Lally C, Austin H, Benson J, Dilley A, Wenger NK, Whitsett C, Rawlins P, Evatt BL. The relationship between polymorphisms in the endothelial cell nitric oxide synthase gene and the platelet GPIIIa gene with myocardial infarction and venous thromboembolism in African Americans. *Chest* 1999; 116(4):880–886.
13. Marks PA, Gross RT. Erythrocyte glucose-6-phosphate dehydrogenase deficiency: evidence of differences between Negroes and Caucasians with respect to this genetically determined trait. *J Clin Invest* 1959; 38:2253–2262.
14. Butler T. G-6-PD deficiency and malaria in Black Americans in Vietnam. *Mil Med* 1973; 138(3):153–155.
15. Jain M, Brenner DA, Cui L, Lim CC, Wang B, Pimentel DR, Koh S, Sawyer DB, Leopold JA, Handy DE, Loscalzo J, Apstein CS, Liao R. Glucose-6-phosphate dehydrogenase modulates cytosolic redox status and contractile phenotype in adult cardiomyocytes. *Circ Res* 2003; 93(2):e9–e16.
16. Leopold JA, Walker J, Scribner AW, Voetsch B, Zhang YY, Loscalzo AJ, Stanton RC, Loscalzo J. Glucose-6-phosphate dehydrogenase modulates vascular endothelial growth factor-mediated angiogenesis. *J Biol Chem* 2003; 278(34):32100–32106.
17. Leopold JA, Zhang YY, Scribner AW, Stanton RC, Loscalzo J. Glucose-6-phosphate dehydrogenase overexpression decreases endothelial cell oxidant stress and increases bioavailable nitric oxide. *Arterioscler Thromb Vasc Biol* 2003; 23(3):411–417.
18. Kilaru PK, Kelly RF, Calvin JE, Parrillo JE. Utilization of coronary angiography and revascularization after acute myocardial infarction in men and women risk stratified by the American College of Cardiology/American Heart Association guidelines. *J Am Coll Cardiol* 2000; 35(4):974–979.
19. Nguyen JT, Berger AK, Duval S, Luepker RV. Gender disparity in cardiac procedures and medication use for acute myocardial infarction. *Am Heart J* 2008; 155(5):862–868.
20. Shaw LJ, Shaw RE, Merz CN, Brindis RG, Klein LW, Nallamothu B, Douglas PS, Krone RJ, McKay CR, Block PC, Hewitt K, Weintraub WS, Peterson ED. Impact of ethnicity and gender differences on angiographic coronary artery disease prevalence and in-hospital mortality in the American College of Cardiology-National Cardiovascular Data Registry. *Circulation* 2008; 117(14):1787–1801.
21. Taylor AL, Ziesche S, Yancy C, Carson P, D'Agostino R, Jr., Ferdinand K, Taylor M, Adams K, Sabolinski M, Worcel M, Cohn JN. Combination of isosorbide dinitrate and hydralazine in blacks with heart failure. *N Engl J Med* 2004; 351(20):2049–2057.
22. Temple R, Stockbridge NL. BiDil for heart failure in black patients: The U.S. Food and Drug Administration perspective. *Ann Intern Med* 2007; 146(1):57–62.
23. Liggett SB, Mialet-Perez J, Thaneemit-Chen S, Weber SA, Greene SM, Hodne D, Nelson B, Morrison J, Domanski MJ, Wagoner LE, Abraham WT, Anderson JL, Carlquist JF, Krause-Steinrauf HJ, Lazzeroni LC, Port JD, Lavori PW, Bristow MR. A polymorphism within a conserved beta(1)-adrenergic receptor motif alters cardiac function and beta-blocker response in human heart failure. *Proc Natl Acad Sci U S A* 2006; 103(30):11288–11293.
24. Liggett SB, Cresci S, Kelly RJ, Syed FM, Matkovich SJ, Hahn HS, Diwan A, Martini JS, Sparks L, Parekh RR, Spertus JA, Koch WJ, Kardia SL, Dorn GW, II. A GRK5 polymorphism that inhibits beta-adrenergic receptor signaling is protective in heart failure. *Nat Med* 2008; 14(5):510–517.

6

Hypertension and Stroke in Racial/Ethnic Groups

K.A. Jamerson, MD
and T.L. Corbin, MD

CONTENTS

Abstract

The impact of hypertension is a major contributor to the largely uncontrolled, global disease burden across all racial/ethnic groups. African-Americans have a higher incidence and prevalence of hypertension compared with Caucasians. End-organ manifestations continue to be multi-factorial and have been closely associated with salt sensitivity, obesity, and overactivity of the sympathetic nervous system as well as environmental influences. Despite the advances in the treatment of hypertension, there continues to be a disproportionate burden among racial and ethnic minorities. There is compelling evidence that African-Americans are more susceptible to increased salt load compared to Caucasians, resulting from alterations in kidney function that requires higher arterial pressure to maintain steady-state, causing a shift to the right of the pressure–natriuresis curve. In molecular genetic studies on salt sensitivity, several molecu-

From: Contemporary Cardiology: Cardiovascular Disease in Racial and Ethnic Minorities
Edited by: K.C. Ferdinand and A. Armani, DOI 10.1007/978-1-59745-410-0_6
© Humana Press, a part of Springer Science+Business Media, LLC 2009

lar variants have been identified by single strand nucleotides polymorphisms to be more exclusive in blacks than in whites. As a result of having sympathetic overactivity from obesity, there is a compensatory mechanism to burn fat and decrease weight gain, but in exchange for an increased sympathetic discharge to the peripheral vasculature which may predispose on to hypertension.

The African American Heart Failure Trial (A-HeFT) suggested that African-Americans with congestive heart failure demonstrated improvement in morbidity and mortality when added to a fixed-combination therapy of isosorbide dinitrate and hydralazine. This study also supports the implications of a nitric oxide deficiency contribution to a higher cardiovascular burden in African-Americans. The Antihypertensive and Lipid Lowering Treatment to Prevent Heart Attack Trial (ALLHAT) was also one of the first to compare the effectiveness of different classes of antihypertensive therapy; a calcium channel blocker (amlodipine), ACE inhibitor (lisinopril), or an alpha-blocker (doxazosin) were individually compared to a diuretic (chlorthalidone) to reduce fatal or non-fatal coronary heart disease on a diverse population (40,386 study participants) with sufficient power to analyze ethnic groups, especially blacks. The African-American Study of Kidney Disease (AASK) examined the effect of aggressive blood pressure control on progression of renal failure in 1094 African-Americans. One of the largest cohort studies addressing African-Americans and lifestyle modification occurred in the Dietary Approach to Stop Hypertension (DASH) designed to assess the effects of dietary pattern on blood pressure. The Heart and Stroke Statistical Update 2007 states that 70 million people experience a new or recurrent stroke each year. African-Americans may be prone to a higher risk of lacunars infarctions and large artery intracranial occlusive disease, whereas whites may be prone to cerebral embolism, and transient ischemic attack.

Key Words: Salt sensitivity; Hypertension; Sympathetic overactivity; Vascular risk factors; Endothelial dysfunction.

1. INTRODUCTION

Hypertension affects 72 million individuals in the United States. The impact of hypertension is a major contributor to the global disease burden that is largely uncontrolled across all racial/ethnic groups. In non-Hispanic whites, according to the National Health and Nutrition Examination Survey (NHANES), only 24% of treated hypertensives are uncontrolled, similar to non-Hispanic blacks. The level of uncontrolled hypertension is greatest in the Mexican American population, with only 15% of the treated hypertension controlled to a blood pressure (BP) of less than 140/90 mmHg. Furthermore, Mexican Americans have the largest percentage of patients unaware of their hypertension, 41% versus 27% of non-Hispanic blacks and 31% of non-Hispanic whites *(1)*.

Nevertheless, across all racial/ethnic groups, African-Americans have a higher incidence and prevalence of hypertension compared with Caucasians: 41.1% of blacks affected compared to 28.1% of Caucasians *(2)*. It is the single largest disease burden of cardiovascular disease in African-Americans. The morbidity attributable to hypertension – such as heart disease, stroke, peripheral vascular, and end-stage renal disease – is also highest among African-Americans. The degree of racial differences in the pathogenesis of these end-organ manifestations continues to be multi-factorial and has been closely associated with salt sensitivity, obesity, and overactivity of the sympathetic nervous system as well as environmental influences. As a result of these racial differences, the control rate of BP in the United States is equally poor for African-Americans compared with Caucasians, ultimately requiring more aggressive antihypertensive medication utilization as well as non-pharmacological management. Data presented in the Seventh Report of the Joint National Committee on Prevention, Detection, Evaluation, and Treatment of High Blood Pressure (JNC 7) showed a continued poor BP control rate <35% in US hypertension, far below the Healthy People 2010 goal of 50% *(2)*.

Stroke, the third leading cause of death in the United States, also disproportionately affects African-Americans, with excess burden of disease and mortality. The racial disparities in stroke have documented a higher prevalence of severe stroke events, hospitalization, more disability, and a lower quality of life in blacks compared with Caucasians *(3)*. Similar to hypertension, the goal to lower the incidence of stroke and to meet the Healthy People 2010 objectives to eliminate health disparities requires additional programs to address risk factors, management of acute, and treatment options *(4)*. Due to a larger database in blacks versus other racial/ethnic groups, this chapter will explore the racial/ethnic differences in hypertension and stroke in this population.

2. EPIDEMIOLOGY

Hypertension is the most striking vascular disease in the United States and continues to be a major contributor to the leading cause of premature death *(1)*. Data from the NHANES 1999–2004 overall estimated prevalence of high blood pressure (BP) was 72 million (33 million males and 39 million females), concluding that nearly one of three US adults have hypertension defined as >140/90 mmHg or are taking antihypertensive medication *(1)*. Despite the advances in the treatment of hypertension, there continues to be a disproportionate burden among racial and ethnic minorities. When compared to whites at all age ranges from 18 to greater than 60 years of age, blacks have greater hypertension prevalence versus whites, Hispanics, and others. This disparity in hypertension prevalence for African-Americans appears to be greatest in the middle age years from 40 to 59 *(1)*.

Compared to Caucasians, African-Americans have 1.3 greater rates of non-fatal stroke, 1.8 greater rate fatal strokes, 1.5 greater rate of coronary heart disease, and 4.2 greater rate of end-stage kidney disease *(5)*. In the analyses of race/gender specific trends, the prevalence of hypertension from

NHANES ascertained that although over the last three decades there has been increased patient awareness of hypertension in all racial/ethnic groups, high BP increased from 35 to 41.4% among blacks, highest among African-American women 44%, African-American males 39% versus 28.5% for non-Hispanic white males, and 28% for non-Hispanic white females. Data from the 2004 National Center for Health Statistics mortality data and National Heart, Lung, and Blood Institute survey indicate that the overall death rate of African-Americans was significantly higher than that of Caucasians (5).

3. PATHOPHYSIOLOGY

3.1. Salt Sensitivity

Changes in BP salt sensitivity occurs approximately 30% in normotensive and over 50% of hypertensive persons. Additionally, there is some compelling evidence that African-Americans are more susceptible to increased salt load compared to Caucasians. This salt sensitivity results from alterations in kidney function that requires higher arterial pressure to maintain steady-state, causing a shift to the right of the pressure–naturesis curve (6). Molecular genetics studies on salt sensitivity and increased sodium absorption studies have been aimed at African-American population involving the renal sodium transport (7). In these studies, several molecular variants have been identified by single-strand nucleotides polymorphisms to be more exclusive in blacks than in whites (T334A and C168F in β-ENaC and G442V and T5994M in β-ENaC). This establishes an increased reabsorption of sodium, leading to hypertension that is often severe, hypokalemia, and suppression of renin and aldosterone secretion (8). One γ-subunit of the epithelial sodium channel (ENaC) mutation described in black South Africans with low-renin salt sensitivity hypertension is the Liddle Syndrome, a variant to primary hypertension found more commonly in person of African Ancestry with the gene T594m (substitution of threonine to methionine). Patients with T594M have been successfully treated with amiloride, a diuretic that specifically blocks epithelial sodium channel reabsorption (9). These changes in allele frequency suggest the need for continued genome-wide studies to identify genes that influence mechanisms contributing higher BPs in blacks than in whites.

3.2. Obesity and Sympathetic Nervous System

An additional salient factor contributing to salt sensitivity hypertension in all population studies is obesity. Most recently, obesity has significantly impacted the prevalence of hypertension, notably African-Americans, but particularly African-American women compared to whites. Moreover, data from the Framingham Study showed obesity as a risk factor linked directly with several disease processes, particularly hypertension *(10)*. Other risk factors that tend to accompany hypertension include glucose intolerance, diabetes, and dyslipidemia, otherwise defined as metabolic syndrome. Of particular importance is the role of the sympathetic nervous system (SNS) association with adiposity, which increases the peripheral vascular tone leading to hypertension. Several studies have linked adiposity-related sympathetic overactivity to an increased sympathetic discharge of to skeletal muscle, a main site for energy expenditure. In one of the first studies to explore whether being overweight produces sympathetic overactivity in African-Americans, findings showed sympathetic discharge closely correlated with body mass index (BMI) after adjustments for age, arterial pressure, and family history of hypertension (Fig. 1) *(11)*. There was also significant correlation between BMI and sympathetic discharge in Caucasian men and women. Unlike in African-American women, sympathetic discharge in black men was overall higher than in white men, but there was a dissociated relationship from BMI and other indices of adiposity. In lean black men, the discharge rates are 20–40% higher than those in lean black women, lean white men and women of comparable BMI. These findings suggest that central sympathetic activity may explain why black men suffer from the highest overall cardiovascular mortality rates compared to all other ethnic/gender groups (Fig. 1). Illustrative recordings of sympathetic nerve discharge in three young black

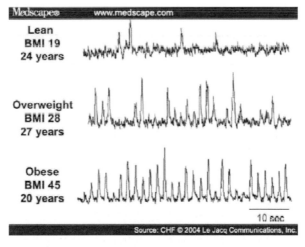

Fig. 1. Illustrative neurograms from three overtly healthy, normotensive, young adult African-American women who varied in body mass index (BMI, measured as weight in kilograms/height in m^2). On these mean voltage displays, the sympathetic nerve activity is proportional to the frequency of these spontaneous neural bursts, which is shown to increase with increasing BMI *(11)*.

women, who are lean (top), obese (middle), and very obese (bottom). The
narrow-based peaks are spontaneous bursts of post-ganglionic sympathetic
nerve discharge (SND) targeted to the skeletal muscle vasculature. The rate
of nerve firing increases progressively with increasing BMI (Fig. 1).

As result of having sympathetic overactivity from obesity, it can be the-
orized that there is a compensatory mechanism to burn fat and decrease
weight gain, but in exchange for an increased sympathetic discharge to the
peripheral vasculature which may predispose on to hypertension. Clearly,
SNS response to obesity causes a marker change in the autonomic regulation. Abate and colleagues' scatterplot showed the relationship between
individual's values of BMI and SND for four ethnic/gender groups *(11)*.

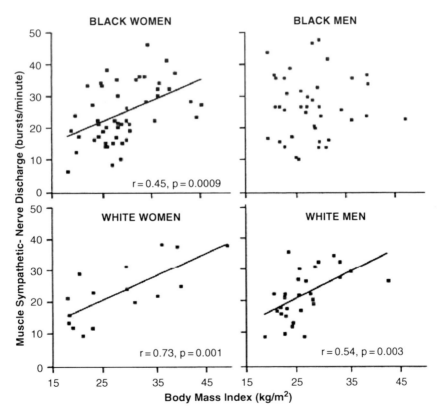

Fig. 2. Scatterplots showing the relationship between individual values of BMI and
SND for the four ethnic/gender groups. Significant correlations were evident for all
groups except black men. The average age, mean arterial pressure, heart rate, and BMI
are 30 ± 2 years, 80 ± 2 mmHg, 67 ± 3 bpm, and 28 ± 2 kg/m^2, respectively, for white
women and 28 ± 1 years, 84 ± 2 mmHg, 65 ± 2 bpm, and 26 ± 1 kg/m^2, respectively,
for white men *(11)*.

3.3. Endothelial Dysfunction

Endothelial dysfunction is an early stage in the development of coronary atherosclerosis and has been implicated in the pathogenesis of hypertension and heart failure *(12)*. The ethnic differences between African-Americans and Caucasians regarding factors regulating vascular tone control and endothelial function have been suggested to contribute to poor outcomes observed in African-Americans with congestive heart failure (CHF). Existing data suggest that a higher incidence of endothelial dysfunction in African-Americans can potentially result from abnormalities of nitric oxide (NO) synthesis, release, and/or clearance *(13)*. This damaging effect of reactive oxygen species is caused by smooth muscle cell proliferation, endothelial cell apoptosis, DNA damage, and monocyte/macrophage adhesion to endothelial cells *(13)*. A recent study by Kalinowski et al. *(12)* using nanotechnology demonstrated that African-Americans have an inherent imbalance of NO, superoxide (O_2^-), and peroxynitrite ($ONOO^-$) production in the endothelium and this overproduction triggers the release of aggressive radicals, which exerts diminished levels of nitric oxide and increased oxidative stress, precursors for cardiovascular disease. Mason et al. *(13)* suggest that nebivolol, a new generation of β-blockers, is favorable on African-Americans by its action on the level of oxidants lining the cardiovascular system and its ability to restore levels of NO and reduce oxidative stress. Regarding CHF, the African American Heart Failure Trial (A HeFT) suggested that African-Americans with CHF demonstrated improvement in morbidity and mortality when added to a fixed-combination therapy of isosorbide dinitrate and hydralazine. Results for the A-HeFT demonstrated a 39% reduction in hospitalization, improvement in quality of life, and 43% reduction in morality. This study also supports the implications of an NO deficiency contribution to a higher cardiovascular burden in African–Americans *(14)*. Additionally, a study done by Suthanthiran and colleagues demonstrated that transforming growth factor $β_1$ (TGF-$β_1$), a mediator of hypertension, is hyperexpressed in hypertensives compared with normotensives and that TGF-$β_1$ overexpression is more frequent in blacks compared to whites (Fig. 3) *(15)*. Figure 3 compared TGF-$β_1$ protein levels across diagnosis (hypertensive or normotensive) and race (black and white). TGF-$β_1$ levels were the highest in black's hypertensives. These findings support the ideal that TGF-$β_1$ overexpression is a risk factor for hypertension and hypertensive complications such as cardiovascular and renal disease as well as providing a mechanism for the excess burden of hypertension in blacks.

Heart disease from left ventricular hypertrophy, renal disease, and stroke are manifestations of target organ damage from hypertension that predicts more adverse cardiovascular events in African-Americans compared to Caucasians. The prevalence of hypertension in African-Americans is at least 3–7 times higher than in Caucasians *(16)*. The rate of end-stage renal disease

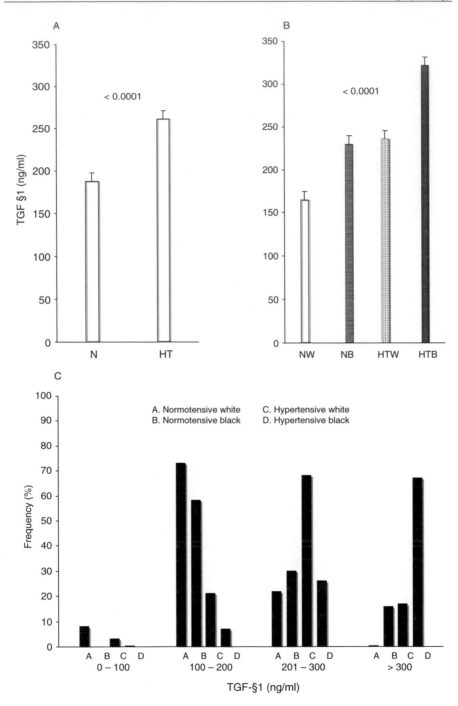

Fig. 3. (Continued)

resulting from hypertension is 2000% higher, and the rate of stroke and associated fatality is even higher. In the review of many clinical trials focused on target organ damage, the representation of African-Americans has been inconsistent *(17)*. Previously, many studies addressing target organ damage in African-Americans have been mainly retrospective, resulting in inaccuracies associated in the data analyses. Although, most recently, a few landmarks trials have been designed specifically for African-Americans and have shown to be of clear benefit for therapy in African-Americans: the A-HeFT *(14)* and the African American Study of Kidney Disease (AASK) *(18)*. The need for these studies stems from the reality of African-Americans at higher risk for more malignant hypertension and a continuum of disease burden associated with numerous cardiovascular complications. The A-HeFT was able to demonstrate that African-Americans who frequently present with different etiology and drug response compared to Caucasians by a higher prevalence, earlier onset, increased risk for hospitalization and mortality demonstrate improvement when the combination of hydralazine and isosorbide dinitrate is added to standard therapy, with a 39% reduction in hospitalization, improvement in quality of life or functional status, and a 43% reduction in mortality *(14)*. The Antihypertensive and Lipid Lowering Treatment to Prevent Heart Attack Trial (ALLHAT) was also one of the first to compare the effectiveness of different classes of antihypertensive therapy; a calcium channel blocker (amlodipine), ACE inhibitor (lisinopril), or an alpha-blocker (doxazosin) were individually compared to a diuretic (chlorthalidone) to reduce fatal or non-fatal coronary heart disease on a diverse population (40,386 study participants). After a 4.9 year study, the results of the ALLHAT indicated that thiazide diuretics (chlorthalidone) are reasonable first-line pharmacologic therapy option for patients with hypertension. They are superior in lowering BP, reducing clinical events and tolerability, and are less costly. Finally, the results inferred that diuretics were reasonable to include in all regimens when more than one drug therapy is required *(19)*. The AASK trial examined the effect of aggressive BP control on progression of renal failure in 1094 African-Americans. The results

---

Fig. 3. Serum TGF-$_1$ protein levels. Circulating levels of TGF-$_1$ protein were quantified by using a TGF-$_1$-specific sandwich ELISA. TGF-$_1$ protein levels distinguished by diagnosis (hypertensive versus normotensive) are shown in **A**. The mean $\pm$ SEM TGF-$_1$ level was 188 ± 7 ng/ml in normotensives (N) and was 261 ± 9 ng/ml in hypertensives (HT). TGF-$_1$ protein levels, distinguished by diagnosis as well as by race, are illustrated in **B**. The mean $\pm$ SEM TGF-$_1$ concentrations were 165 ± 6, 221 ± 12, 235, and 322 ng/ml in normotensive whites (NW), normotensive blacks (NB), hypertensive whites (HTW), and hypertensive blacks (HTB), respectively ($P < 0.0001$, ANOVA). The frequency distribution of TGF-$_1$ levels, distinguished by race and diagnosis is shown in **C** *(15)*.

showed evidence that antihypertensive treatment plays a critical role in reducing the rate of deteriorating renal function and AASK was one of the first trials to demonstrate 80% of the study patients were able to lower their BP to <140/90 mmHg. Moreover, an ace inhibitor (ramipril) reduced the decline in kidney function to a significantly greater effect than did therapies based on amlopidine or metoprolol in patients with proteinuria *(18)*.

4. MANAGEMENT OF HYPERTENSION

4.1. Non-drug Therapy

Hypertension in African-American adults appears to be more then 50% higher than for white Americans and the rate of morbidity and morality from hypertension and its associated diseases are also substantially higher *(20)*. Disparities in hypertension partly due to a higher prevalence and severity of several risk factors impacting African-Americans have been focused on psychological stress, obesity, alcohol consumption, physical inactivity, and dietary sodium–potassium ratio. One of the largest cohort studies addressing African-Americans and lifestyle modification occurred in the Dietary Approach to Stop Hypertension (DASH). The DASH diet was designed to assess the effects of dietary pattern on BP. The results provided evidence that a diet rich in fruits, vegetables, and low-fat diary foods and with reduced saturated fats, lowered BP in blacks *(21)*. This study definitely showed a positive association between sodium restriction, weight maintenance, and BP reduction in African-Americans. Clearly, the cornerstone to treating hypertension is addressing lifestyle modifications attributable to changes in behavior, participation in educational programs, and compliance with pharmacological therapy, as well as better excess to primary-care providers.

5. NEW TREATMENT FOR HYPERTENSION

As a result of blacks being at a higher risk for hypertension and its associated complications, they require more aggressive treatment strategies to optimally reduce cardiovascular and renal morbidity and mortality. Recently, clinical trials have focused on racial differences in response to various classes of antihypertensive medications, as well the use of combination therapy as an initial therapeutic regimen. The JNC 7 issued recommendations on the prevention and management of hypertension beginning with lifestyle modification and thiazide-type diuretics either alone or in combination with other classes of drugs, including β-blockers, angiotensin-converting enzyme inhibitors (ACEI), angiotensin receptor blockers (ARB), all instrumental in a reduction of cardiovascular and renal complications in randomized controlled outcome trials *(2)*.

5.1. Hypertension in Hispanics

"Hispanic" is a demographic term denoting a Spanish or Latin family ancestry. Mexican Americans are the largest single Hispanic group, followed by Central and South Americans, Puerto Ricans, and Cuban Americans. Hispanic Americans are a heterogeneous group, composed of various races, including black, white, and Native American populations and hypertension in Hispanics specifically varies by gender and country of origin. Despite an apparent great prevalence of obesity and diabetes, the prevalence of hypertension in Hispanic Americans appears to be somewhat similar or lower than that seen in the general population. According to the National Health Interview Survey of 2000–2002, there is a health disparity between blacks and white adults of Hispanic descent. Black Hispanics are at slightly greater risk that white Hispanics, although non-Hispanic black adults have by far the highest rate of high BP. Additionally, in the analysis of self-identified Hispanic subgroups, there appears to be an increase in the risk for stroke in certain populations. For instance, versus the overall Hispanic population, the risk for stroke is somewhat increased in Puerto Rican and Mexican American males. The cause of these differences based on geographic origin remains unclear (1).

5.2. Hypertension in Asians

Cardiovascular disease is the leading cause of death in Asian-Americans. However, hypertension in Asian patients does not appear to be significantly increased compared to the general population. It should be recognized that similarly to Hispanics, Asian are extremely heterogeneous. Nevertheless, those identified as South Asians appear to have an increased number of coronary heart disease events, potentially related to the metabolic syndrome, i.e., insulin resistance, truncal obesity, and dyslipidemia. An increased prevalence of high BP with excessive abdominal obesity may potentially increase cardiovascular mortality rate seen in Asian-Americans. Prevalence of hypertension in Asia itself is low in rural compared to urban population. However, in the Indian subcontinent itself, hypertension looms as the major public health consideration, and among South Asians living in Western societies including the United States, it is suggested that the prevalence of hypertension, along with CHD, will increase. Another Asian population demonstrating high rates of hypertension prevalence is the Native Hawaiians.

Much of the variations across the population defined as "Asian" may be related to sodium intake and decreased physical activity, instead of clearly identified genetic patterns. Overall, although data are limited in regards to pharmacologic therapy, antihypertensive agents appear to be as effective in Asians as whites. Interesting drug side effects with ACEI, including cough and flushing, may be greater among certain Asian subgroups. American

Indians as a group are also heterogeneous. Although inactivity and obesity are seen in higher frequency in many American Indians communities, the prevalence rates of hypertension are similar or perhaps lower than seen in the general population (1).

6. EPIDEMIOLOGY OF STROKE

Stroke is the third leading cause of death in the United States for African-Americans and one of the leading causes of adult disabilities (22). The Heart and Stroke Statistical Update 2007 states that 70 million people experience a new or recurrent stroke each year (3). Recently, epidemiological studies are focusing on the difference in stroke incidence between racial/ethnic groups. Data from the Northern Manhattan Study (NOMAS) indicate that age-adjusted incidence of first stroke in African-Americans is twice that of whites. The incidence rates (per 100,000) for first ever stroke are 323 for black males and 260 for black females compared to 167 for white males and 138 for white females. Across various geographic regions of the United States, the excess burden of stroke continues to have a relatively higher prevalence in the southeastern regions (23). African-Americans have the highest age-adjusted prevalence of stroke in both southeastern and non-southeastern regions compared with whites from either regions. Additionally, stroke mortality is also disproportionately higher among African-Americans; in 2003, the death rates of black males and females were 78.8 and 69.1%, respectively, versus 51.9% and 50.5%, respectively, in white males and females. Two possible explanations for excess mortality of stroke in African-Americans can be attributed to strokes occurring at a younger age and the likelihood of having a higher case fatality following a stroke.

7. PATHOPHYSIOLOGY OF STROKE

7.1. Traditional Risk Factors

The development of stroke is known to be related to vascular risk factors such as hypertension, smoking, diabetes mellitus, and high cholesterol. Besides these conventional risk factors, genetic predispositions and environmental lifestyle may enhance the risk of developing cerebrovascular thrombotic events. Studies have documented racial differences in stroke subtypes. There are disproportions in the incidence of more severe hemorrhagic stroke, with blacks having twice the rate of subarachnoid hemorrhages as whites and a 2.3 higher incidence of intracerebral hemorrhage (20). A number of studies have attempted to demonstrate gene association as strong predictors of the type of stroke most prevalent among African-Americans.

7.2. Novel Risk Factors

Although it has been established that hypertension is the most common risk factor for intracerebral hemorrhage (ICH), one study focused on a single specific gene, e4 allele. Researchers found blacks with a single e4 allele inherited from one parent were twice as likely to have ICH when compared to whites and were eight times more likely to have an ICH if they inherited two alleles *(24)*. Currently, research is directed at genetic vulnerability in explaining the excess burden of stroke in African-Americans. A group of investigators studied 48 African-American women and 48 Caucasian women between the ages of 15 and 49 to identify a novel single-nucleotide polymorphism (SNP) on the PDE4D human gene locus on stroke risk among young adults. Results demonstrated SNP rs918592 to be highly associated with all stroke subtypes particularly among smokers: (OR = 3.22, $P = 0.75$) smokers, (OR = 1.16, $P = 0.66$) former smokers, and (OR = 0.93, $P = 0.75$) never smoked. Of particular interest from this group, the high risk for SNP rs918592 was present in about 18% of Caucasians and 55% of African-Americans *(25)*. Additionally, another gene investigated, GNβ3, has shown significant association with higher incidence of ischemic strokes subtypes and race. African-Americans may be prone to a higher risk of lacunars infarctions and large artery intracranial occlusive disease, whereas whites may be prone to cerebral embolism and transient ischemic attack *(25)*. These studies underscore the need for further genomic studies to address the early need to identify individuals at increased risk for stroke.

7.3. Risk of Stroke

The most confounding risk factors for stroke are hypertension, heart disease, diabetes, and cigarette smoking *(26)*. For most patients, these factors are especially important because lifestyle modification can result in significant reduction in a recurrent stroke. Strategies to motivate behavioral modification to address include improving quality of health care, insurance coverage for post-stroke care, access to rehabilitation, transport to local health-care providers, as well as access to current medication regimens *(26)*. Evidence has shown minorities who are less educated and older are significantly less likely to use physical therapy or occupational therapy, resulting in a greater residual disability.

7.4. Treatment of Stroke

Considering that African-Americans are at higher risk for stroke treatment, further recommendations and drug strategies must address patients' awareness of early signs and symptoms and timely access to emergency stroke care to minimize the effects.

Table 1
Stroke Deaths in Non-Hispanic Blacks and Non-Hispanic
Whites, 1999–2000

Population	Overall death rate (%)
African-American males	49.9
African-American females	40.6
Caucasian males	15.6
Caucasian females	14.3

Adapted from (5).

Table 2
Landmark Clinical Trials and Classes/Agents Comparisons

Study	Drug Class	Population	Benefits
AASK	ARB	African-Americans with nephrosclerosis	Ramipril provided best renal protection
IDNT	ARB	Type 2 DM and nephropathy	Irbesartan delays the progression of nephropathy due to diabetes
IRMA-2	ARB	BP, type 2 DM, normal GFR, microalbuminuria	Irbesartan-delayed progression of nephropathy due to type 2 DM
LIFE	ARB	BP > 174/98 LVH (diabetes 13%, blacks 5.8%)	Losartan more effective that atenolol in prevent stroke in hypertensive with LVH
Val-HeFT	ARB	Heart failure classes II–IV	Valsartan benefit ACE-inhibitor-intolerant HF patients
ALLHAT	ACEI	High BP and one other risk factor	Chlorthalidone (diuretic) tolerated, cost effective

For acute care, one thrombolytic agent tissue plaminogen activator (tPA) is used to treat ongoing strokes within 3 hours of presentation *(27)*. Other drug therapies most commonly used to prevent or treat stroke are antithrombotics (antiplatelet agents and anticoagulants). Anticoagulants (heparin and coumadin) prevent the risk of strokes by reducing the clotting properties; and antiplatelet drugs (ASA) prevent clotting by decreasing the activity of clotting properties. The most widely use ASA are aspirin and ticlopidine. The African-American Antiplatelet Stroke Prevention Study (AAASPS) is the first clinical trial to address the disproportionate stroke burden among non-whites. In a subset analysis of 603 non-white participants, results showed a 24.1% risk reduction for stroke and death at 2 years with ticlopidine relative to aspirin, but no statistical differences in the prevention of recurrent strokes *(28)*.

8. CONCLUSIONS

There yet remains some well-described ethnic variations in the prevalence, pathophysiology, and management of hypertensive disease, particularly pertaining to African-Americans and Caucasians. Although our understanding of hypertension continues to evolve, especially with the introduction of clinical trials designed for specific ethnic groups, early detection for diagnosis, new antihypertensive agents, and lipid lowering agents and antithrombolytic, there is continued need to explore additional strategies to meet the goal for Healthy People 2010.

REFERENCES

1. Burt VL, Cutler JA, Higgins M, et al. Trends in the prevalence, awareness, treatment, and control of hypertension in the adult US population. ata from the Health Examination Surveys, 1960 to 1991. *Hypertension* 1995; 26:60–69.
2. Joint National Committee on Prevention, Disease, Detection, Evaluation and Treatment of High Blood Pressure. The sixth report of the Joint National Committee on Prevention, Detection, Evaluation, and Treatment of High Blood Pressure. *Arch Intern Med* 1997; 157:2413–2446.
3. The AHA Statistic Update Writing Group. Heart Disease and Stroke Statistics 2007 Update. A Report from the American Heart Association Committee and Stroke Statistics Subcommitte. *Circulation* 2007; 115:e69–171.
4. Gu Q, Paulose-Ram R, Dillion C, et al. Antihypertensive medication use among U.S. adults with hypertension. *Circulation* 2006; 113:213–221.
5. Centers for Disease Control. Health Disparities experienced by Blacks or African Americans – United States. *MMWR* 2005; 54(1):1–3.
6. Peters RM, Flack JM. Salt sensitivity and hypertension in African Americans: implications for cardiovascular nurses. *Prog Cardiovasc Nurs* 2000; 15 (4):138–144.
7. Ambrosius WT, Bloem LJ, Zhou L, et al. Genetic variants in the epithelial sodium channel in relation to aldosterone and potassium excretion and risk for hypertension. *Hypertension* 1999; 34:631–637.
8. Pratt HJ. Central role for ENaC in development of hypertension. *J Am Soc Nephrol* 2005; 16:3154–3159.

9. Pratt HJ, Ambrosius WT, Agarwal R, et al. Racial difference in the activity of the amiloride-sensitive epithelial sodium channel. *Hypertension* 2002; 40:903–908.
10. Eslami P, Tuck M. The role of sympathetic nervous system in linking obesity with hypertension in whites versus black Americans. *Curr Hypertens Rep* 2003; 5:269–272.
11. Abate NI, Mansour YH, Meryem T, et al. Overweight and sympathetic overactivity in Black Americans. *Hypertension* 2001; 38:379–383.
12. Kalinowski L, Dobrucki IT, Malinski T. Race-specific differences in endothelial function: predisposition of African American to vascular diseases. *Circulation* 2004; 109:2511–2517.
13. Mason, PR, Kalinowski L, Jacob RF, et al. Nebivolol reduces nitric stress and restores nitric oxide bioavailability in endothelium of Black Americans. *Circulation* 2005; 112:3795–3801.
14. Taylor AL, Zieche S, Yancy C, et al., for the African American Heart Failure Trial Investigators. Combination of isosorbide dinitrate and hydralizine in blacks with heart failure. *N Engl J Med* 2004; 351:2049–2057.
15. Suthanthriran M, Li B, Song JO, et al. Transforming growth factor-β_1 hyperexpression in African American hypertensives: a novel mediator of hypertension and/or target organ damage. *Proc Natl Acad Sci USA* 2000; 97:3479–3448.
16. Douglas J, Bakis G, Epstein M, et al., the Hypertension in African Americans Working Group. Management of high blood pressure in African Americans. *Arch Intern Med* 2003; 163:525–540.
17. Ferdinand KC. African American heart failure trial: role of endothelial dysfunction and heart failure in African *Americans. Am J Card* 2007; 99:3d–6d.
18. Agodoa LY, Appel L, Bakris GL, et al., African American Study of Kidney Disease and Hypertension (AASK) Study Group. Effect of ramipril vs. amlodipine on renal outcomes in hypertensive nephroscelorsis: a randomized controlled trial. *JAMA* 2001; 285(21): 2719–2728.
19. Davis BR, Culter JA, Gordon DJ, et al., for the ALLHAT Research Group. Rationale and design for the Antihypertensive and Lipid Lowering Treatment to Prevent Heart Attack Trial (ALLHAT). *Am J Hypertens* 1999; 9:342–362.
20. Gillum RF. Stroke mortality in blacks. *Stroke* 1999; 30:1711–1715.
21. Appel LJ, Moore TJ, Obarzanek E, et al., for the DASH Collaborative Group. A clinical trial of the effects of dietary patterns on blood pressure. *N Engl J Med* 1997; 336: 1117–1124.
22. Stansbury JP, Jia H, Williams LS, et al. Ethnic disparities in stroke epidemiology, acute care, and postacute outcomes. *Stroke* 2005; 36:374–387.
23. Hauser WA, Paik MC, Shea S. Race-ethnic disparities in the impact of stroke risk factors: the Northern Manhattan Stroke Study. *Stroke* 2001; 32:1725–1731.
24. Duke Med News. Study finds gene is associated with higher risk of one kind of stroke among African Americans; 1998, Feb 6 (http://www.dukemednews.org/news/article. php?id=623).
25. Song Q, Cole JW, O'Connel JR, et al. Phosphodiesterase 4D polymorphisms and the risk of cerebral infarction in a biracial population: the Stroke Prevention in Young Women Study. *Hum Mol Gene* 2006; 15:2468–2478.
26. Kissela B, Schneider A, Kleindorfer D, et al. Stroke in a biracial population. The excess burden of stroke among blacks. *Stroke* 2004; 35:426–431.
27. Katzan IL, Hammer MD, Furlan AJ, et al., on behalf of the Cleveland Clinic Health System Stroke Quality Improvement Team. Quality improvement and tissue-type plasminogen activator for acute ischemic stroke. A Cleveland update. *Stroke* 2003; 34:799–800.
28. Gorelick PB, Richardson D, Kelly M, et al. on behalf of the African American Antiplatelet Stroke Prevention Study Investigators. Aspirin and ticlopidine for prevention of recurrent stroke in black patients: a randomized trial. *JAMA* 2003; 289 M(22):2947–2957.

7

Dyslipidemia in Racial/Ethnic Groups

L. T. Clark, MD
and S. Shaheen, MD

CONTENTS

Abstract

Some population groups in the United States have excess burdens of major risk factors for cardiovascular disease (CVD) and are more likely to have more risk factors than their white counterparts. Although the reasons for the excess CVD mortality among African-Americans remain controversial, it is evident that the high prevalence and suboptimal control of coronary risk factors and a greater degree of clustering of certain coronary risk factors contribute importantly. The predictive value of most conventional CVD risk factors appears to be similar for African-Americans and whites. Most population-based

From: *Contemporary Cardiology: Cardiovascular Disease in Racial and Ethnic Minorities*
Edited by: K.C. Ferdinand and A. Armani, DOI 10.1007/978-1-59745-410-0_7
© Humana Press, a part of Springer Science+Business Media, LLC 2009

studies report that African-Americans have lower total serum cholesterol levels and a lower prevalence of hypercholesterolemia, but low-density lipoprotein cholesterol (LDL-C) levels were similar. Although African-Americans achieve a similar lowering of LDL-C with statin therapy, they are less likely to have increased cholesterol treated. Although low HDL as a CHD risk factor has been known for decades, only recently has clinical trial evidence addressed the benefits of raising high-density lipoprotein (HDL)-C.

On an average, higher levels of HDL-C are observed in African-American adults compared to white adults. Low hepatic lipase activity leads to increased plasma HDL-C concentrations in African-American men. Triglyceride levels in African-American men and women are generally lower than in white men and women, either with or without CHD. When African-Americans have elevated lipoprotein(a) levels in conjunction with small apolipoprotein(a) isoforms, a significant association with CHD has been found. Hispanics have lower mortality rates than non-Hispanic whites and blacks, referred to as the "Hispanic Paradox," although a recent study provided evidence against the Hispanic Paradox in a population of diabetic individuals. Like African-Americans and other ethnic minorities, Hispanics have been under-represented in lipid clinical trials. South Asian Indians have a two- to three-fold higher prevalence of diabetes and a higher prevalence of metabolic syndrome than in whites. Premature atherosclerosis in young Asian Indians also appears to be related in part to the commonly observed dyslipidemia tetrad of elevated triglycerides, low HDL, small dense LDL-C, and elevated lipoprotein(a). High prevalence of modifiable risk factors provides great opportunity for prevention, risk reduction, reducing and ultimately eliminating disparities in cardiovascular care and outcomes.

Key Words: Dyslipidemia; Coronary risk factors; LDL-cholesterol; HDL-cholesterol; Triglycerides; Metabolic syndrome; Undertreatment.

1. INTRODUCTION

Cardiovascular disease (CVD), and in particular, ischemic heart disease, is the leading cause of death in the United States for both males and females and for Americans of all racial and ethnic backgrounds. Some population groups in the United States – African-Americans, Hispanics, South Asian Indians – have excess burdens of major risk factors for CVD and are more likely to have risk multiple risk factors than their white counterparts. The increased risk factor burden plus the combination of lower screening and less effective treatment of risk factors, all contribute to worse outcomes and health disparities. Although the reasons for the disparities in CVD outcomes in US ethnic minorities – compared to Caucasians – have not been fully elucidated, this can be accounted for, at least in part, by high rates of dyslipidemia and other coronary risk factors. The high prevalences of dyslipidemia and other modifiable risk factors provide great opportunities for the prevention of CVD and patients at high risk should be targeted for intensive risk reduction measures.

2. DYSLIPIDEMIA AND CVD IN AFRICAN-AMERICANS

African-Americans have the highest CVD mortality rate of any racial/ethnic group, particularly out-of-hospital deaths, and especially at younger ages *(1–3)*. In addition, compared with whites, African-Americans have a higher annual rate of first myocardial infarction at all ages (Fig. 1). The earlier age of onset of CHD in African-Americans creates striking African-American/white differences in years of potential life lost for both total and ischemic heart disease *(2)*. Although the reasons for the excess CVD mortality among African-Americans remain controversial, it is evident that the high prevalence and suboptimal control of coronary risk factors – and a greater degree of clustering of certain coronary risk factors in blacks than in whites (Table 1) *(3–5)* contribute importantly. The predictive value of most conventional risk factors for CVD appears to be similar for African-Americans and whites. However, the risk of death and other seque lae attributable to some risk factors (i.e., hypertension, diabetes) is disproportionately greater for African-Americans *(3,6–8)*.

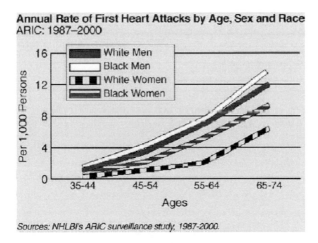

Fig. 1. Annual rate of first heart attacks by age, sex, and race. (From Annual rate of first heart attacks by age, sex, and race, ARIC: 1987–2000. American Heart Association. Heart disease and stroke statistics 2005 update. Available at: http://www.american-heart.org.

Table 1
Cardiovascular risk factors more prevalent in
African Americans than in whites

Associated with increased risk
  Hypertension
  Type 2 diabetes mellitus
  Obesity
  Cigarette smoking
  Physical inactivity
  Left ventricular hypertrophy
Associated with decreased risk
  Higher leves of high-density lipoprotein
    cholesterol
Association with coronary heart disease risk
  unclear
  Higher lipoprotein(a)

2.1. Dyslipidemia

Dyslipidemia is one of the most common contributors to increased risk
for the development of CHD. Increased levels of total cholesterol (TC),
low-density lipoprotein cholesterol (LDL-C), and triglycerides (TG) are
associated with increased risk as are low levels of high-density lipoprotein
(HDL-C). Approximately 25% of adult African-Americans in the general
population have high-risk lipid profiles. Differences in the burdens of dyslipidemia between blacks and whites may explain some of the observed differences in CVD risk burden.

2.2. Total and Low-Density Lipoprotein (LDL) Cholesterol

In population studies, elevated total or LDL cholesterol levels are established independent risk factors for CHD, and reductions in LDL cholesterol
have been demonstrated to decrease the risk for CHD events in several large
clinical outcome trials (9–15). Most population-based studies report that
African-Americans have lower total serum cholesterol levels than whites
and a lower prevalence of hypercholesterolemia (2). However, in young
to middle-aged adults in the Coronary Artery Risk Development in Young
Adults (CARDIA) study, the prevalence of LDL cholesterol levels was similar in African-American and white women and in African-American and
white men (16). The relationship between total cholesterol levels and CHD
mortality was the same among the 23,490 black and 325,384 white men

followed for an average of 12 years in the Multiple Risk Factor Intervention Trial (MRFIT) *(17)*. In the Atherosclerosis Risk in Communities (ARIC) study, LDL cholesterol was similarly predictive of CHD events in all races and in both sexes *(18)*. In some other studies, the relationship between total or LDL cholesterol, atherosclerotic plaque formation, and CHD events appears to be somewhat weaker in African-Americans *(2,19)*. For example, total cholesterol was not predictive of CHD incidence and mortality in analyses of the combined Charleston and Evans County cohorts *(19)*.

In the ongoing Dallas Heart Study *(20)*, a greater proportion of black men had elevated total cholesterol when compared to their white counterparts, but fewer black men had low HDL levels, no ethnic differences were observed in the frequency of elevated LDL-C levels, and for both genders, high plasma levels of triglycerides were less common in blacks.

2.3. Undertreatment of Dyslipidemia in African-Americans

Although African-Americans achieve a similar lowering of LDL cholesterol when compared with whites following statin therapy in clinical trials, African-American adults are less likely than whites to have increased cholesterol treated *(2, 3, 21–26)*. Furthermore, among patients treated for dyslipidemia, African-American patients are less likely to achieve treatment goals, are more likely to be in the highest risk category, and less likely to be using lipid drug therapy, taking high-efficacy statins and receiving care from a subspecialist *(22,27,28)*. In the Antihypertection in CHD event rates was obsnsive and Lipid Lowering Treatment to Prevent Heart Attack Trial (ALLHAT), a statistically significant 27% reduction in CHD event rates was observed only in African-American study participants (treated with pravastatin sodium) compared to those subjected to usual care in the community *(29)* The major contributor to this isolated positive outcome was that African-American hypertensive patients with concomitant hypercholesterolemia were less likely to be treated with lipid-lowering drugs than were white patients. Suboptimal control of dyslipidemia may therefore contribute to the overall higher rates of cardiovascular death and morbidity in African-American patients.

2.4. High-Density Lipoprotein Cholesterol (HDL-C)

Low HDL cholesterol levels increase the risk for development of CHD independent of LDL levels and other risk factors, whereas elevated HDL cholesterol levels appear to be protective. The NCEP ATP III guidelines define low HDL-C as <40 mg/dL in men and women *(3)*. However, for a diagnosis of the metabolic syndrome, HDL-C <40 mg/dL in men or

<50 mg/dL in women is considered abnormal and one of the diagnostic criteria.

Low HDL-C may be caused by factors associated with insulin resistance, such as elevated triglycerides (TG), type 2 diabetes, excess weight, physical inactivity, a high level of carbohydrate consumption, cigarette smoking, and certain drugs (β-blockers, anabolic steroids, and progesterone).

The precise mechanism of HDL's protective action is not completely understood, but is thought to be multifactorial and likely includes promotion of reverse cholesterol transport from macrophages to the liver, as well as an anti-inflammatory and antioxidant activity, induction of NO synthesis, and possibly an effect on platelet aggregation.

2.4.1. HDL-Raising as a Therapeutic Target

Although low HDL as a CHD risk factor has been known for decades, only recently has clinical trial evidence emerged which address the benefits of raising HDL-C. *Statins* are used primarily to lower LDL-C. However, they also increase HDL levels by 5–10%. *Fibrates* another group of lipid-modifying therapies, raise HDL-C by 5–20% while also decreasing the levels of triglycerides. In the Veteran Affairs High Density Lipoprotein Intervention Trial (VA-HIT) study, HDL-C levels increased on an average about 6% and were associated with a reduction in cardiovascular events *(30)*. *Niacin* increases HDL-C by 15–30% in some studies, making it the most potent HDL-C-raising therapy currently available. Data from Coronary Drug Project demonstrated that niacin reduced the incidence of cardiovascular events *(31,32)*. Its mechanism of action is probably multifactorial and includes slowing of HDL metabolism by the liver cells, reduction in hepatic LDL and very low-density lipoprotein (VLDL) production, inhibition of adipose tissue lipolysis, stimulation of lipoprotein lipase activity, and possibly a direct effect on the macrophages. Unfortunately, many patients have difficulties related to the drugs side effects of flushing and pruritus, which precludes its more widespread use. *ApoA-1 Milano* is a mutated variant of ApoA-1 lipoprotein that was identified in a small population in the Northern Italy. This variant differs from the wild type protein by arginine for cysteine substitution at position 173, allowing for dimer formation. Patients with this mutation characteristically have very low levels of HDL-C, longevity, and low incidence of atherosclerotic heart disease. A randomized, multicenter study comparing the effects of intravenous recombinant ApoA-1 Milano phospholipid complex on coronary atheroma volume in patients with known coronary disease and acute coronary syndromes demonstrated a statistically significant reduction in the volume of coronary atheromas as measured by coronary intravascular ultrasound following a 5-week course of ApoA-1 Milano infusion *(33)*.

2.4.2. TORCETRAPIB

The cholesterol ester transfer protein (CETP) is a plasma glycoprotein that facilitates the exchange of cholesterol esters for triglycerides from HDL to ApoB-containing lipoproteins. Physiologically, inhibition of CETP results in an increase of HDL-C. Despite considerable evidence suggesting that HDL-C should be a therapeutic target for treatment and prevention of atherosclerosis, the hypothesis that raising levels of HDL cholesterol by the inhibition of CETP was dealt a considerable blow by the Investigation of Lipid Level Management to Understand its Impact in Atherosclerotic Events (ILLUMINative AmericanTE) trial in which torcetrapib therapy resulted in an increased risk of cardiovascular mortality and morbidity despite a mean increase in HDL-C of 72% and a decrease in LDL-C of 25% *(34)*. The investigators presented evidence that the adverse effect on CVD outcomes in this study was due to an off-target effect of torcetrapib, although adverse effects related to CETP inhibition cannot be ruled out *(34)*.

2.4.3. NCEP RECOMMENDATIONS FOR LOW HDL-C

According to the NHLBI National Cholesterol Education Program (NCEP), in individuals with low HDL-C levels, the primary therapeutic objective is to achieve the recommended LDL-C goal *(3)*. After this has been achieved, emphasis shifts to weight reduction and increased physical activity. If the TG level is elevated, reduction of non-HDL-C is the secondary target. If the TG level is not elevated (<200 mg/dL), specific therapies to increase HDL-C may be considered (fibrates and nicotinic acid). Drug therapy solely for raising the HDL-C level when the TG level is <200 mg/dL is generally reserved for very high-risk patients, such as those with CHD or CHD equivalents. In some high-risk patients with the metabolic syndrome, combination therapy with statins and fibrates, or statins and niacin, can be considered, although the risk for the development of myositis with some of the combinations may be increased. Additional therapeutic options are currently being investigated and may be available in the near future.

2.4.4. MECHANISM OF HIGHER HDL LEVELS IN AA

On an average, higher levels of HDL cholesterol are observed in African-American adults compared to white adults. National data and data from the Multiple Risk Factor Intervention Trial (MRFIT) participants demonstrate an inverse relationship between HDL levels and education, income, and measures of socioeconomic status that is common to both African-Americans and whites *(17)*. In ARIC, there is a similar, though slightly less protective, effect of HDL in African-American than in white persons *(4)*.

The mechanism of higher HDL levels in African-American men was recently studied by Vega et al., who found that the difference in plasma

HDL-C concentrations between African-American and white men reflects racial/ethnic differences in hepatic lipase activity *(29)*. Low hepatic lipase activity leads to increased plasma HDL-C concentrations in African-American men. The low hepatic lipase activities in African-American men are likely to be genetically determined and are due in part to polymorphism in the hepatic lipase gene – higher frequency of the -514T allele in African-American men *(35)*.

3. ELEVATED TRIGLYCERIDES

Elevated serum triglyceride (TG) levels (>150 mg/dL) are an independent risk factor for CHD *(36)*. Although a number of older studies demonstrated a univariate association between serum triglyceride levels and CHD risk in men and women, multivariate analyses did not document elevated triglyceride levels as an independent risk factor for CHD. However, recent studies, including a meta-analysis *(36)*, have demonstrated an independent correlation of elevated triglyceride levels with CHD, suggesting that triglyceride-rich lipoproteins, such as very low–density lipoprotein (VLDL) remnants, are independently atherogenic. In addition, elevated triglyceride levels are associated with low HDL cholesterol levels, small LDL particles, procoagulant effects, hypertension, and insulin resistance – factors known to increase the risk of developing atherosclerosis.

Hypertriglyceridemia can be caused by obesity and overweight status, physical inactivity, a high-carbohydrate diet (>60% of calories), diabetes mellitus, certain drugs (estrogens and corticosteroids), excessive alcohol intake, and genetic disorders.

3.1. Management of Hypertriglyceridemia

The goal of therapy in patients with elevated TGs is a level of <150 mg/dL *(3)*. The treatment strategy for reducing TGs should take into consideration the severity and the cause of TG elevation. In patients with borderline high TG levels (150–199 mg/dL), dietary modification, weight reduction, and increased physical activity are the first-line therapies. Drug therapy, in addition to lifestyle changes, is often necessary in individuals with TG levels of >200 mg/dL. It is recommended that very low-density lipoprotein cholesterol (VLDL-C) be targeted by setting non-HDL-C goals 30 mg/dL higher than the LDL-C goal *(3)*. The non-HDL-C level refers to the concentration of LDL-C plus VLDL-C and can be determined by subtracting the HDL-C level from the total cholesterol level – measurements that can be obtained with the patient in a fasting or a non-fasting state. The non-HDL-C goal can be achieved by intensifying the therapy to reduce the LDL-C or VLDL-C level. For patients requiring drug therapy, the cautious addition of fibrate or

nicotinic acid to a low-fat diet (<15% of daily calories) is usually beneficial. Patients with very high TG levels (>500 mg/dL) are at risk for acute
pancreatitis and lowering the TG level should be the primary objective.

Triglyceride levels in African-American men and women are generally lower than in white men and women, either with or without CHD
(20,37–39). The metabolic syndrome (characterized by hypertension; obesity; diabetes mellitus; hyperinsulinemia; elevated triglycerides; small,
dense LDL; and low HDL), however, is relatively common in both African-
Americans and whites *(40)*.

4. LIPOPROTEIN(a)

Lipoprotein(a) or Lp(a) s structurally similar to LDL, with an additional
disulfide-linked glycoprotein termed apolipoprotein(a). Apolipoprotein(a)
has extensive structural homology with plasminogen but varies in size due to
variations in the number of plasminogen kringle-IV repeats. Lipoprotein(a)
levels are two to three times higher in African-Americans than in whites
(41–48). Prospective studies evaluating the role of Lp(a) levels as a predictor of cardiovascular events demonstrate conflicting results. Some studies have reported that Lp(a) levels are an independent risk factor for CHD,
whereas others have demonstrated no significant association. In whites, ele
vated Lp(a) levels have been shown to be an independent risk factor for CHD
while several recent trials in African-Americans, evaluating the relationship
of Lp(a) levels and atherosclerosis, failed to detect an association *(41–48)*.
The explanation for this apparent paradox appears to be in the size distribution of Lp(a). The size of an individual Lp(a) particle can vary substantially
due to the genetic size polymorphisms of apo(a). The small apo(a) isoforms
(with fewer kringle-IV repeats) have been associated with CHD, regardless
of total Lp(a) level. The majority of whites with elevated Lp(a) possess at
least one small apo(a) isoform, whereas the majority of African-Americans
with elevated Lp(a) do not. However, when African-Americans have elevated Lp(a) levels in conjunction with small apo(a) isoforms, a significant
association with CHD has been found *(49)*.

5. RISK FACTOR CLUSTERING

African-Americans are 1.5 times more likely to have multiple risk factors
than whites *(39,40,50–52)*. The presence of multiple risk factors increases
CHD risk synergistically. Although the etiology of risk factor clustering is unknown, both genetic and environmental factors have been implicated. Insulin resistance and hyperinsulinemia appear pivotal to risk factor
clustering and contribute to the pathogenesis of coexistent hypertension, diabetes, dyslipidemia, and atherosclerosis.

6. METABOLIC SYNDROME

The metabolic syndrome – also known as insulin resistance syndrome, metabolic syndrome X, and dysmetabolic syndrome – is a specific clustering of cardiovascular risk factors in the same person (abdominal obesity, atherogenic dyslipidemia, elevated blood pressure, insulin resistance, a prothrombotic state, and a proinflammatory state) *(39,40,53)*. Patients with the metabolic syndrome are at increased risk for the development of diabetes and cardiovascular disease.

According to a recent analysis of data from the Third National Health and Nutrition Examination Survey (NHANES III), approximately 47 million Americans (23.7% of the population) have the metabolic syndrome *(40)*. The highest rates were observed in Mexican American women and men. The prevalence of the metabolic syndrome was approximately 57% higher in African-American women than in African-American men, and it was approximately 26% higher in Hispanic women than in Hispanic men (Fig. 2). In older persons, the prevalence of the metabolic syndrome is currently approximately 44%, and as the population of the United States continues to age, the prevalence rate of the metabolic syndrome will continue to increase among men and women.

Although a high degree of association between individual components of the metabolic syndrome and CVD risk exists, several recent analyses have confirmed that the cluster of risk factors in the metabolic syndrome is associated with an increased risk of cardiovascular morbidity and mortality. Because of the strong relationship of obesity to the metabolic syndrome, the rising prevalence of obesity in the United States is cause for particular concern. The metabolic syndrome is closely associated with insulin resistance, although the mechanisms of the association between insulin resistance and metabolic risk factors have not been fully elucidated.

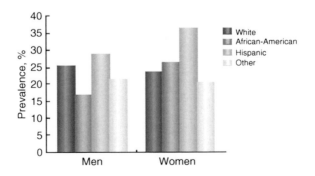

Fig. 2. Age-adjusted prevalence of the metabolic syndrome in US adults by gender and race or ethnicity (modified from *(40)*).

Susceptibility to the specific risk factors for the metabolic syndrome varies among racial/ethnic groups *(3,39,53)*. Whites of European ancestry are more predisposed to atherogenic dyslipidemia, whereas blacks of African descent are more prone to hypertension, type 2 diabetes, and obesity. Hypertension is less likely to develop in Hispanics and Native Americans than in blacks, but Hispanics and Native Americans appear to be particularly susceptible to type 2 diabetes. In the Jackson Heart Study *(54)*, more than a third (37.2%) of the 5302 men and women in the population-based study of African-Americans met the criteria for metabolic syndrome. Of the five components comprising the syndrome, increased WC and high BP were most prevalent (65.3 and 63.7%, respectively).

6.1. Management of the Metabolic Syndrome

Because the root causes of the metabolic syndrome (overweight/obesity and physical inactivity) are reversible and the individual components of the metabolic syndrome are modifiable, recognition of the metabolic syndrome provides a great opportunity for risk reduction. Management of the metabolic syndrome consists primarily of two strategies: modification or reversal of the root causes, including weight reduction and increased physical activity, and direct treatment of the metabolic risk factors, including atherogenic dyslipidemia, elevated blood pressure, the prothrombotic state, and underlying insulin resistance. All of the components of the metabolic syndrome may be improved with weight reduction and increased physical activity. Treatment of several of the individual risk factors associated with the metabolic syndrome has been shown to decrease CVD risk, although no randomized clinical trials are yet available to show a decrease in clinical events or increased survival following treatment of the metabolic syndrome per se. In an analysis of the benefits of treating elevated blood pressure and dyslipidemia in individuals with the metabolic syndrome, Wong et al. *(55)* found that aggressive treatment of risk factors and control to optimal levels could, at least theoretically, result in the prevention of ≥80% of cardiovascular events. Recognition, diagnosis, and treatment of the metabolic syndrome in African-Americans have the potential for reducing cardiovascular morbidity and mortality.

7. CLINICAL TRIALS

A number of clinical trials have demonstrated that lipid-lowering therapy with the statins reduces CHD risk in patients with and without established CHD *(3)*. African-Americans are absent or under-represented in most of these clinical trials. However, several studies did include sufficient AA to allow meaningful analysis. Several older studies demonstrated that the magnitude of LDL cholesterol reduction with the statins is similar in African-Americans and whites treated with lovastatin *(24)* or pravastatin *(23,25)*. More recent studies include ALLHAT, ARIES, and NEPTUNE II.

7.1. ALLHAT

The Antihypertensive and Lipid-Lowering Treatment to Prevent Heart Attack Trial (ALLHAT) was a study designed to *(1)* assess the relative benefits of newer antihypertensive agents compared to diuretics in high-risk hypertensive subgroups, such as the elderly, black patients, and diabetic patients; and *(2)* evaluate the impact of large, sustained cholesterol reduction on all-cause mortality, CHD event rates, and other CVD outcomes in a hypertensive cohort with at least one other CHD risk factor *(29)*. The study population comprised 42,418 hypertensive patients, 55 years of age or older, with at least one additional CHD risk factor. The study population was diverse, consisting of 36% black patients, 47% women, 36% patients with diabetes, 22% smokers, 19% Hispanic patients, and 47% patients with existing cardiovascular diseases.

The ALLHAT-LLT included 10,355 treated hypertensives who had moderate hypercholesterolemia and who were randomized to receive open-label pravastatin 40 mg daily, or usual care provided by their primary-care physician *(29)*. The ALLHAT-LLT is the largest trial of lipid-lowering therapy in blacks and the still the only clinical trial of lipid lowering therapy sufficiently powered to address cardiovascular outcomes in a black cohort.

After a mean follow-up of 4.8 years, total cholesterol levels were reduced to 17% in the pravastatin group and 8% in the usual care group. Among the random sample that had LDL-cholesterol levels measured, levels were reduced by 28% in the pravastatin group compared to 11% in the usual care group. All-cause mortality was similar in the two groups (14.9% in the pravastatin group versus 15.3% with usual care), and there was no significant difference in CHD event rates between the groups (9.3% for pravastatin and 10.4% for usual care). However, blacks in the pravastatin-treated group had a 27% reduction in CHD events compared to the usual care group ($p = .03$). Because there was no difference for combined cardiovascular events overall, the ALLHAT investigators concluded that the "biological significance of the racial differences for CHD and stroke is unclear." The observed differences in the treated and usual care cohorts of blacks appear to have resulted from the undertreatment of blacks in the usual care group compared to non-blacks.

7.2. ARIES

The African American Rosuvastatin Investigation of Efficacy and Safety (ARIES) trial *(26)* compared the efficacy and safety of rosuvastatin and atorvastatin treatment for 6 weeks in 774 hypercholesterolemic African-American adults. After 6 weeks of therapy, significantly greater reductions in low-density lipoprotein cholesterol, total cholesterol, non-high-density lipoprotein cholesterol, and apolipoprotein B concentrations, as well as lipoprotein and apolipoprotein ratios, were seen with rosuvastatin versus milligram-equivalent atorvastatin doses.

Although the ARIES trial was conducted exclusively in African-Americans and comparisons with other similarly designed trials in other patient populations should be done with great caution, it is noteworthy that the mean LDL cholesterol reductions seen with both rosuvastatin and atorvastatin were smaller than those observed previously in the US-based, 6-week trials comparing these two therapies across their dose ranges in largely white hypercholesterolemic populations (56,57). The reasons for this finding are unclear and may reflect differences in patient compliance with therapy or perhaps the dampening effect of a higher dietary fat consumption in this population. Furthermore, this observation suggests the need for more aggressive therapy and particularly diligent monitoring to insure achieving of the desired therapeutic effect.

7.3. NEPTUNE II

The National Cholesterol Education Program Evaluation Project Utilizing Novel E-Technology (NEPTUNE) II surveyed patients with treated dyslipidemia to assess achievement of treatment goals established by the Adult Treatment Panel III of the National Cholesterol Education Program (22), US physicians working in primary care or relevant subspecialties. Patient data were recorded in Personal Digital Assistants and uploaded to a central database via the Internet. Among 4,885 patients receiving treatment for dyslipidemia, 79.7% were non-Hispanic white (NHW) and 8.4% were AA. Non-Hispanic white and AA patients had significantly different frequencies of treatment success, with 69.0 and 53.7%, respectively, having achieved their LDL-C goal (p <0.001). African-American patients were more likely to be in the highest risk category and less likely to be using lipid drug therapy, taking high-efficacy statins, and receiving care from a subspecialist, but the difference in goal achievement remained significant (p <0.001) after adjustment for these and other predictors of treatment success. Thus, the frequency of treatment success in dyslipidemia management was significantly lower in AA than non-Hispanic white patients. This study did not elucidate the reasons for this disparity but did highlight the need for better strategies for improving treatment efficacy and goal achievement among African-American patients receiving therapy for dyslipidemia.

8. HISPANIC AMERICANS

Hispanics are the largest and fastest growing minority group in the United States. Hispanics are a heterogeneous population with national origins or ancestry that may include Puerto Ricans, Cubans, Mexicans, Spaniards, and other Latinos. Approximately 66% of the US Hispanics are of Mexican origin, 15% South and Central American, 9% Puerto Rican, and 4% Cuban *(58)*. In the NHANES III analysis, Mexican American males (28.3%) and females (35.6%) had the highest prevalence of metabolic syndrome *(40)*. However, despite their higher rates of metabolic syndrome, diabetes, obesity, lower HDL-C and higher TG levels, lower socioeconomic status (SES), and barriers to health care, several studies have suggested that Hispanics have lower all-cause and cardiovascular mortality rates than non-Hispanic whites and non-Hispanic blacks *(40,59–61)*. This observation has been referred to by some as the "Hispanic Paradox" *(60)*, although a recent study provided evidence against the Hispanic Paradox in a population of diabetic individuals.

Hispanic patients like African-Americans and other racial/ethnic minorities have been under-represented in clinical trials of lipid-lowering therapies. The limited available data on achievement of lipid-lowering goals in Hispanic patients have indicated that goal achievement is suboptimal *(27)*. The Study Assessing Rosuvastatin in Hispanic Population (STARSHIP) demonstrated that statin therapy produces LDL cholesterol lowering in Hispanics similar to those in largely non-Hispanic white populations with hypercholesterolemia *(62)*.

Even though Hispanics may have lower than expected mortality rates than non-Hispanic blacks and non-Hispanic whites, heart disease and stroke still remain the leading cause of death, both in Hispanic males and in Hispanic females. Thus, one should not conclude that Hispanics are protected from CHD or that they should be treated less aggressively than other groups.

9. SOUTH ASIANS

According to the 2000 Census, there are approximately 2 million people in the United States who identify themselves as Asian-Indians or Indian-Americans – first- and second-generation immigrants or those whose ancestors migrated to the United States from India *(63–65)*. South Asians appear to be at heightened risk of CHD both in Asia – especially urban settings – and in North America *(59–63)*. South Asian Indians have a 50–100% higher risk of dying from CHD compared with Caucasians, especially at younger ages, and often in the absence of traditional risk factors *(65–69)*. Although the prevalence of obesity is not high in Asian Indians, the higher CHD risk appears to be related largely to a higher prevalence of insulin resistance, the metabolic syndrome, and diabetes *(65,66)*.

The Coronary Artery Disease in Asian Indians (CADI) Study *(69)* was the first major study of Asian Indians in the United States. This study showed that approximately one-third of the excess CVD in South Asian Indians can be accounted for by their two- to three-fold higher prevalence of diabetes and a higher prevalence of metabolic syndrome than in whites.

Premature atherosclerosis in young Asian Indians also appears to be related in part to the commonly observed dyslipidemia tetrad of elevated triglycerides, low HDL, small dense LDL-C, and elevated lipoprotein(a) *(70)*. South Asians, like other racial/ethnic minorities in the United States, have been historically under-represented in clinical trials. The Investigation of Rosuvastatin in South Asians (IRIS) Study evaluated the lipid-modifying effects of rosuvastatin and atorvastatin in South Asians with hypercholes-terolemia residing in the United States and Canada *(71)*. IRIS was the first large-scale randomized lipid-lowering trial in an exclusively South-Asian population in North America. The trial showed that statins (rosuvastatin and atorvastatin) are effective in decreasing LDL cholesterol, non-HDL, and total cholesterol in South-Asian patients with similar efficacy to that seen in other population groups.

Efforts to reduce cholesterol and other CHD risk factors in individuals with South Asian Indian ancestry appear to be especially important and these individuals should be targeted for aggressive therapeutic lifestyle change and CVD risk reduction.

10. NATIVE AMERICANS (AMERICAN INDIANS)

There is limited information on the risks of dyslipidemia and the benefits of lipid management for reduction of CHD and CVD in this population. Cardiovascular disease mortality rates vary among the Native American communities in the United States. However, Native Americans have the highest prevalence of diabetes in the United States and CVD in Native American communities – unlike for other US racial/ethnic groups – is increasing *(72–74)*.

The Honolulu Heart Program is an ongoing prospective study of CHD and stroke in a cohort of Japanese American men living in Hawaii *(75,76)*. In this study, CHD and CVD mortality rates are lower than in the general US population, and the Framingham risk scoring system appears to overestimate actual risk.

11. SUMMARY AND CONCLUSIONS

Cardiovascular disease (in particular, CHD) is the leading cause of death in the United States for Americans of both sexes and of all racial and racial/ethnic backgrounds. Some groups, in particular African-Americans and South Asian Indians, are disproportionately impacted. The greater CVD burden in these populations can be accounted for in part by a high prevalence of dyslipidemia and other coronary risk factors – and their frequent occur-rence in clusters. The high prevalence of modifiable risk factors provides great opportunity for prevention, risk reduction, reducing and ultimately eliminating disparities in cardiovascular care and outcomes

One of the major barriers to CVD prevention, especially in racial/ethnic minorities, is lack of patient compliance with therapy. Important contributors to lack of compliance include problems with doctor–patient communications, cost, and medication side effects *(3,21)*. Poor communication between physicians and patients may be the most important impediment to effective adherence to treatment. Improvement in physician–patient interaction requires mutual participation and commitment. Physicians must convey interest in controlling the patient's risk factors and a commitment to overcoming obstacles. Physicians must spend time educating patients about the importance of risk factor control, taking their medications, and the goals of therapy. Patient responsibilities include keeping follow-up appointments, following non-pharmacologic recommendations, and alerting the physician to other prescribed medications or problems with medicines.

Furthermore, CVD prevention should begin in childhood. The epidemic of obesity in adults in the United States has been accompanied by an increase in the proportion of children who are overweight *(5)* due to an increase in caloric intake and a decrease in physical activity. Thus, it is important that preventive measures focus on adults and children. Individual measures to decrease sedentary lifestyles (e.g., less television hours, and so forth) are extremely important, as are community and public health measures (e.g., increasing the number and safety of walking areas, eliminating high-calorie fast-food specials, providing simple nutrition information on food labels, increasing school-based physical activity programs, and other measures).

Disparities in cardiovascular health and outcomes continue to exist in the United States. Excessive risk factor burdens and undertreatment of high-risk individuals are important contributors. Reduction and ultimate elimination of disparities requires dedicated commitment and better strategies to minimize racial/ethnic differences in prevention and effective treatment of high risk individuals.

REFERENCES

1. American Heart Association. Heart Disease and Stroke Statistics—2005 Update. Dallas, TX: American Heart Association; 2005.
2. Clark LT, Ferdinand KC, Flack JM, et al. Coronary heart disease in African Americans. *Heart Dis* 2001; 3:97–108.
3. The Expert Panel. Third Report of the National Cholesterol Education Program (NCEP) Expert Panel on Detection, Evaluation, and Treatment of High Blood Cholesterol in Adults (Adult Treatment Panel III): final report. *Circulation* 2002; 106:3146–3421.
4. Hutchinson RG, Watson RL, Davis CE, et al. Racial differences in risk factors for atherosclerosis: The ARIC Study. *Angiology* 1997; 48:279–290.
5. Hall WD, Clark LT, Wenger NK, et al. The metabolic syndrome in African Americans: a review. *Ethn Dis* 2003; 13:414–428.
6. Cooper RS, Liao Y, Rotimi C. Is hypertension more severe among U.S. blacks, or is severe hypertension more common? *Ann Epidemiol* 1996; 6:173–180.

7. Liao Y, Cooper RS, McGee DL, Mensah GA, Ghali JK. The relative effects of left ventricular hypertrophy, coronary artery disease, and ventricular dysfunction on survival among black adults. *JAMA* 1995; 273:1592–1597.
8. Gavin JR III. Diabetes in minorities: reflections on the medical dilemma and the health-care crisis. *Trans Am Clin Climatol Assoc* 1995; 107:213–223.
9. Scandinavian Simvastatin Survival Study Group. Randomized trial of cholesterol lowering in 4444 patients with coronary heart disease: the Scandinavian Simvastatin Survival Study (4S). *Lancet* 1994; 334:1383–1389.
10. Sacks FM, Pfeffer MA, Moye LA, et al. The effect of pravastatin on coronary events after myocardial infarction in patients with average cholesterol levels. *N Engl J Med* 1996; 335:1001–1009.
11. Long-term Intervention with Pravastatin in Ischaemic Disease (LIPID) Study Group. Prevention of cardiovascular events and death with pravastatin in patients with coronary heart disease and a broad range of initial cholesterol levels. *N Engl J Med* 1998; 339:1349–1357.
12. Shepherd J, Cobbe SM, Ford I, et al., for the West of Scotland Coronary Prevention Study Group. Prevention of coronary heart disease with pravastatin in men with hypercholesterolemia. *N Engl J Med* 1995; 333:1301–1307.
13. Downs JR, Clearfield M, Weis S, et al. Primary prevention of acute coronary events with lovastatin in men and women with average cholesterol levels: results of AFCAPS/TexCAPS. Air Force/Texas Coronary Atherosclerosis Prevention Study. *JAMA* 1998; 279:1615–1622.
14. Heart Protection Study Collaborative Group. MRC/BHF Heart Protection Study of cholesterol lowering with simvastatin in 20,536 high-risk individuals: a randomised placebo controlled trial. *Lancet* 2002; 360:7–22.
15. Cannon CP, Steinberg BA, Murphy SA, Mega JL, Braunwald E. Meta-analysis of cardiovascular outcomes trials comparing intensive versus moderate statin therapy. *J Am Coll Cardiol* 2006; 48(3):438–445.
16. Gidding SS, Liu K, Bild DE, et al. Prevalence and identification of abnormal lipoprotein levels in a biracial population aged 23 to 35 years (the CARDIA study). The Coronary Risk Development in Young Adults study. *Am J Cardiol* 1996; 78: 304–308.
17. Watkins LO, Neaton JD, Kuller LH. Racial differences in high-density lipoprotein cholesterol and coronary heart disease incidence in the usual care group of the Multiple Risk Factor Intervention Trial. *Am J Cardiol* 1986; 57:538–545.
18. Hutchinson RG, Watson RL, Davis CE, et al. Racial differences in risk factors for atherosclerosis. The ARIC study. *Angiology* 1997; 48:279–290.
19. Keil JE, Sutherland SE, Haines CG, et al. Coronary disease mortality and risk factors in black and white men. Results from the combined Charleston, SC, and Evans County, Georgia, heart studies. *Arch Intern Med* 1995; 155:1521–1527.
20. Jain T, Peshock R, McGuire DK, et al.; the Dallas Heart Study Investigators. African Americans and Caucasians have a similar prevalence of coronary calcium in the Dallas Heart Study. *J Am Coll Cardiol* 2004; 44:1011–1017
21. Clark LT. Issues in minority health: atherosclerosis and coronary heart disease in African Americans. *Med Clin N Am* 2005; 89(5):977–1001.
22. Clark LT, Maki KC, Galant R, Maron DJ, Pearson TA, Davidson MH. Racial/ethnic differences in achievement of cholesterol treatment goals: results from the National Cholesterol Education Program Evaluation Project Utilizing Novel E-Technology (NEPTUNE) II. *J Gen Intern Med* 2006; 21(4):320–326.
23. LaRosa JC, Applegate W, Crouse JR III, et al. Cholesterol lowering in the elderly. Results of the Cholesterol Reduction in Seniors Program (CRISP) pilot study. *Arch Intern Med* 1994; 154:529–539.

24. Prisant LM, Downton M, Watkins LO, et al. Efficacy and tolerability of lovastatin in 459 African-Americans with hypercholesterolemia. *Am J Cardiol* 1996; 78:420–424.
25. Jacobson TA, Chin MM, Curry CL, et al. Efficacy and safety of pravastatin in African Americans with primary hypercholesterolemia. *Arch Intern Med* 1995; 155:1900–1906.
26. Ferdinand KC, Clark LT, Watson KE, et al.; the ARIES Study Group. Comparison of efficacy and safety of rosuvastatin versus atorvastatin in African-American patients in a six-week trial. *Am J Cardiol* 2006; 97:229–235.
27. Pearson TA, Laurora I, Chu H, Kafonek S. The lipid treatment assessment project (L-TAP): a multicenter survey to evaluate the percentages of dyslipidemic patients receiving lipid-lowering therapy and achieving low density lipoprotein cholesterol goals. *Arch Intern Med* 2000; 28:459–467.
28. Williams ML, Morris MT, Ahmad U, Yousseff M, Li W, Ertel N. Racial differences in compliance with NCEP II recommendations for secondary prevention at a veterans affairs medical center. *Racial/Ethn Dis* 2002;12: S1-58–62.
29. ALLHAT Officers and Coordinators of the ALLHAT Collaborative Research Group. Major outcomes in moderately hypercholesterolemic, hypertensive patients randomized to Pravastatin versus usual care. The Antihypertensive and Lipid-Lowering Treatment to Prevent Heart Attack Trial (ALLHAT-LLT). *JAMA* 2002; 288:2988–3007.
30. Robins SJ, Collins D, Wittes JT, et al.; VA-HIT Study Group. Veterans Affairs High-Density Lipoprotein Intervention Trial. Relation of gemfibrozil treatment and lipid levels with major coronary events: VA-HIT: a randomized controlled trial. *JAMA* 2001; 285:1585–1591.
31. Coronary Drug Project Research Group. Clofibrate and niacin in coronary heart disease. *JAMA* 1975; 231:360–381.
32. Canner PL, Berge KG, Wenger NK, Stamler J, Friedman L, Prineas RJ, Friedewald W. Fifteen year mortality in Coronary Drug Project patients: long-term benefit with niacin. *J Am Coll Cardiol* 1986; 8:1245–1255.
33. Nissen SE, Tsunoda T, Tuzcu EM, et al. Effect of recombinant ApoA-I Milano on coronary atherosclerosis in patients with acute coronary syndromes: a randomized controlled trial. *JAMA* 2003; 290:2292–2300.
34. Barter PJ, Caulfield M, Eriksson M, et al. Effects of torcetrapib in patients at high risk for coronary events. *N Engl J Med* 2007; 357:2109–2122.
35. Vega GL, Clark LT, Tang A, Marcovina S, Grundy SM, Cohen JC. Hepatic lipase activity is lower in African American men than in white American men: effects of 5′ flanking polymorphism in the hepatic lipase gene (LIPC). *J Lipid Res* 1998; 39:228–232.
36 ustin MA, Hokanson JE, Edwards KL. Hypertriglyceridemia as a cardiovascular risk factor. *Am J Cardiol* 1998; 81(4A):7B–12B.
37. Rowland ML, Fulwood R. Coronary heart disease risk factor trends in blacks between the First and Second National Health and Nutrition Examination Surveys, United States, 1971–1980. *Am Heart J* 1984; 108:771–779.
38. Hutchinson RG, Watson RL, Davis CE, et al. Racial differences in risk factors for atherosclerosis. The ARIC study. *Angiology* 1997; 48:279–290.
39. Hall WD, Clark LT, Wenger NK, et al. The metabolic syndrome in African Americans: a review. *Ethn Dis* 2003; 13:414–428.
40. Ford ES, Giles WH, Dietz WH: Prevalence of the metabolic syndrome among US adults: findings from the Third National Health and Nutritional Examination Survey. *J Am Med Assoc* 2002; 287:356–359.
41. Watson KE, Topol EJ. Pathobiology of atherosclerosis: are there racial and racial/ethnic differences? *Rev Cardiovasc Med* 2004; 5(Suppl 3):S14–S21.
42. Moliterno DJ, Jokinen EV, Miserez AR, et al. No association between plasma lipoprotein(a) concentrations and the presence or absence of coronary atherosclerosis in African-Americans. *Arterioscler Thromb Vasc Biol* 1995; 15:850–855.

43. Guyton JR, Dahlen GH, Patsch W, et al. Relationship of plasma lipoprotein Lp(a) levels to race and to apolipoprotein B. *Arteriosclerosis* 1985; 5:265–272.
44. Sorrentino MJ, Vielhauer C, Eisenbart JD, et al. Plasma lipoprotein(a) protein concentration and coronary artery disease in black patients compared with white patients. *Am J Med* 1992; 93:658–662.
45. Schreiner PJ, Heiss G, Tyroler HA, et al. Race and gender differences in the association of Lp(a) with carotid artery wall thickness. The Atherosclerosis Risk in Communities (ARIC) study. *Arterioscler Thromb Vasc Biol* 1996; 16:471–478.
46. Stein JH, Rosenson RS. Lipoprotein Lp(a) excess and coronary heart disease. *Arch Intern Med* 1997; 157:1170–1176.
47. Kostner GM, Avogaro P, Cazzolato G, et al. Lipoprotein Lp(a) and the risk for myocardial infarction. *Atherosclerosis* 1981; 38:51–61.
48. Moliterno DJ, Lange RA, Meidell RS, et al. Relation of plasma lipoprotein(a) to infarct artery patency in survivors of myocardial infarction. *Circulation* 1993; 88:935–940.
49. Paultre F, Pearson TA, Weil HF, et al. High levels of Lp(a) with a small apo(a) isoform are associated with coronary artery disease in African American and white men. *Arterioscler Thromb Vasc Biol* 2000; 20:2619–2624.
50. Rowland ML, Fulwood R. Coronary heart disease risk factor trends in blacks between the First and Second National Health and Nutrition Examination Surveys, United States, 1971–1980. *Am Heart J* 1984; 108:771–779.
51. Cutter GR, Burke GL, Dyer AR, et al. Cardiovascular risk factors in young adults. The CARDIA baseline monograph. *Control Clin Trials* 1991;12: 1S–25S, 51S–77S.
52. Hutchinson RG, Watson RL, Davis CE, et al. Racial differences in risk factors for atherosclerosis. The ARIC study. *Angiology* 1997; 48:279–290.
53. Grundy SM. Obesity, metabolic syndrome, and coronary atherosclerosis. *Circulation* 2002; 105:2696–2698.
54. Taylor H. Metabolic syndrome in African Americans, elderly. Jackson Heart Study and Metabolic Syndrome. AHA Scientific Sessions; 2005.
55. Wong ND, Pio JR, Franklin SS, L'Italien GJ, Kamath TV, Williams GR. Preventing coronary events by optimal control of blood pressure and lipids in patients with the metabolic syndrome. *Am J Cardiol* 2003; 91:1421–1426.
56. Schneck DW, Knopp RH, Ballantyne CM, McPherson R, Chitra RR, Simonson SG. Comparative effects of rosuvastatin and atorvastatin across their dose ranges in patients with hypercholesterolemia and without active arterial disease. *Am J Cardiol* 2003; 91:33–41.
57. Jones PH, Davidson MH, Stein EA, et al; the STELLAR Study Group. Comparison of the efficacy and safety of rosuvastatin versus atorvastatin, simvastatin, and pravastatin across doses (STELLAR trial). *Am J Cardiol* 2003; 92.152–160.
58. The Hispanic Population in the United States: March 2000. U.S. Census Bureau, Population Division, Racial/ethnic & Hispanic Statistics Branch. Available at: http://www.census.gov/population/www/socdemo/hispanic/ho00.html
59. Hunt KJ, Williams K, Resendez RG, et al. All-cause and cardiovascular mortality among diabetic participants in the San Antonio Heart Study: evidence against the Hispanic Paradox. *Diabet Care* 2002; 25(9):1557–1563.
60. Markides KS, Coreil J. The health of Hispanics in the southwestern United States: an epidemiologic paradox. *Public Health Rep* 1986; 101:253–265.
61. Liao Y, Cooper RS, Cao G, et al. Mortality from coronary heart disease and cardiovascular disease among adult U.S. Hispanics: findings from the National Health Interview Survey (1986 to 1994). *J Am Coll Cardiol* 1997; 30:1200–1205.
62. Lloret R, Ycas J, Stein M, Haffner S for the STARSHIP Study Group. Comparison of rosuvastatin versus atorvastatin in Hispanic-Americans with hypercholesterolemia (from the STARSHIP Trial). *Am J Cardiol* 2006; 98:768–773.

63. The Asian Population: 2000 (Census 2000 Brief). Issued February 2002. Available at: http://www.census.gov/prod/2002pubs/c2kbr01-16.pdf.
64. Enas EA. Clinical implications: dyslipidemia in the Asian Indian population. Monograph was adapted from material presented at the 20th Annual Convention of the American Association of Physicians of Indian Origin, Chicago, IL, 2002. Available at: http://www.cadiresearch.com/downloads/AAPImonograph.pdf
65. Singh V, Prakash D. Dyslipidemia in special populations: Asian Indians, African Americans, and Hispanics. *Curr Atheroscler Rep* 2006; 8:32–40.
66. Vikram NK, Pandey RM, Misra A, et al. Non-obese (body mass index $<25 \text{ kg/m}^2$) Asian Indians with normal waist circumference have high cardiovascular risk. *Nutrition* 2003; 19(6):503–509.
67. Deedwania PC, Gupta R. Prevention of coronary heart disease in Asian populations. In: Wong ND, ed. Preventive cardiology. New York, New York: McGraw-Hill, 2000: 503–516.
68. Gupta M, Singh N, Verma S. South Asians and cardiovascular risk: what clinicians should know. *Circulation* 2006; 113:e924–e929.
69. Enas EA, Garg A, Davidson MA, et al. Coronary heart disease and its risk factors in first-generation immigrant Asian Indians to the United States of America (CADI Study). *Indian Heart J* 1996; 48:343–353.
70. Kulkarni KR, Markovitz JH, Nanda NC, Segrest JP. Increased prevalence of smaller and denser LDL particles in Asian Indians. *Arterioscler Thromb Vasc Biol* 1999; 19: 2749–2755.
71. Deedwania CP, Gupta M, Stein M, Joseph Y, Gold A; IRIS Study Group. Comparison of rosuvastatin versus atorvastatin in South-Asian patients at risk of coronary heart disease (from the IRIS Trial). *Am J Cardiol* 2007; 99:1538–1543.
72. Resnick HE, Jones K, Ruotolo G, et al., for the Strong Heart Study. Insulin resistance, the metabolic syndrome, and risk of incident cardiovascular disease in non-diabetic American Indians: the Strong Heart Study. *Diabet Care* 2003; 26:861–867.
73. Lee ET, Howard BV, Savage PJ, et al. Diabetes and impaired glucose tolerance in three American Indian populations aged 45–74 years: the Strong Heart Study. *Diabet Care* 1995; 18:599–610.
74. Howard BV, Lee ET, Cowan LD, et al. Rising tide of cardiovascular disease in American Indians: the Strong Heart Study. *Circulation* 1999; 99:2389–2395.
75. Goldberg RJ, Burchfiel CM, Benfante R, Chiu D, Reed DM, Yano K. Lifestyle and biologic factors associated with atherosclerotic disease in middle-aged men: 20-year findings from the Honolulu Heart Program. *Arch Intern Med* 1995; 155:686–694.
76. Abbott RD, Sharp DS, Burchfiel CM, et al. Cross-sectional and longitudinal changes in total and high-density-lipoprotein cholesterol levels over a 20-year period in elderly men: the Honolulu Heart Program. *Ann Epidemiol* 1997;7:417–424.

8

Novel & Emerging Risk Factors in Racial/Ethnic Groups

K.E. Watson, MD

CONTENTS

INTRODUCTION
HOMOCYSTEINE
LIPOPROTEIN(A)
INFLAMMATORY MARKERS
CONCLUSIONS
REFERENCES

Abstract

Over the last decade, the increased research focus on cardiovascular imaging for the identification of patients at risk for and with significant coronary artery disease (CAD) has augmented clinician awareness and ability to properly risk stratify and categorize patients. Cardiac imaging has now become a technique not only for assessing patients with established CAD but also for the identification of patients with subclinical CAD who are at risk for ischemic heart disease and cardiac events of death and myocardial infarction. The Multi-Ethnic Study of Atherosclerosis (MESA) is a 10-year longitudinal study supported by the National Heart, Lung, and Blood Institute with the goals of identifying and quantifying risk factors for subclinical atherosclerosis and for transition in patients from subclinical disease to clinically apparent events. Cardiac imaging findings from MESA with respect to racial/ethnic differences reveal that the incidence and prevalence of CAD differ among some racial and ethnic groups in the United States. The large number of patients affected by CAD has driven the development of effective, non-invasive methods to identify and

From: *Contemporary Cardiology: Cardiovascular Disease in Racial and Ethnic Minorities*
Edited by: K.C. Ferdinand and A. Armani, DOI 10.1007/978-1-59745-410-0_8
© Humana Press, a part of Springer Science+Business Media, LLC 2009

risk-stratify patients with and at risk for CAD. When patients are properly identified, the appropriate treatment strategies can be applied to individual patients
to prevent future events, such as death or myocardial infarction. Historically,
exercise treadmill testing (ETT) with electrocardiogram (ECG) monitoring was
the initial test applied to patients suspected of having CAD. Today, non-invasive
cardiovascular testing with imaging has become the gold standard for the diagnostic and prognostic assessment of patients with suspected or known cardiovascular disease.

Most of the diagnostic non-invasive imaging tests currently available are
based on assessment of regional and global function (echocardiography,
radionuclide angiography, magnetic resonance imaging [MRI]), myocardial perfusion (single-photon emission computed tomography [CT], contrast-enhanced
MRI), or coronary anatomy (CT angiography, magnetic resonance angiography) under resting conditions, stress conditions, or both. Diagnostic techniques
such as electron beam CT, multi-slice cardiac CT scanning, and measurement
of carotid intimal–medial thickness have emerged in recent years for detecting
asymptomatic coronary or carotid atherosclerosis. Recent data on the assessment of long-term prognosis based upon the results of imaging tests to define
false results have been shown to be reliable and helpful in risk prediction of
cardiac events. In daily clinical practice, the assessment of risk allows for the
identification of subsets of patients.

Key Words: Homocysteine; B vitamin; Lipoprotein(a); Inflammatory
markers; C-reactive protein; Interleukin-6.

1. INTRODUCTION

The relationship between ethnicity and cardiovascular diseases is highly
complex and is additionally complicated by a number of other variables,
such as the effects of migration, generation gaps, and socioeconomic status. While classic cardiovascular risk factors undoubtedly explain much
of the excess risk faced by certain ethnic minorities, other ethnic groups
have apparently decreased cardiovascular risk for a given risk factor burden.
There is increasing interest in a number of newer or "emerging" cardiovascular risk markers as possibly explaining some of the cardiovascular risk
faced by all patients including ethnic minorities and this remains an active
area of research. In the current chapter, three "emerging" cardiovascular risk
markers will be discussed: homocysteine, Lp(a), and inflammatory markers.

2. HOMOCYSTEINE

Elevated plasma homocysteine levels are associated with an increased risk
of atherothrombotic vascular disease and increased mortality in individuals
with previously diagnosed vascular disease *(1–8)*. Impaired enzyme function as a result of genetic mutation or deficiency of the essential B vitamins

folic acid, B_{12}, and B_6 can lead to hyperhomocysteinemia. Although there is uncertainty as to whether increased homocysteine is causal or merely a marker for cardiovascular disease risk, several lines of evidence suggest that it may play a role in the pathophysiology of atherothrombotic disease. Homocysteine appears to alter the anticoagulant properties of endothelial cells to a procoagulant phenotype. Furthermore, elevated homocysteine levels causes dysfunction of the vascular endothelium. Plasma homocysteine concentrations differ among ethnic groups *(9,10)* but the actual effect of these differences on cardiovascular morbidity and mortality is not known. Furthermore, the contribution of diet (rather than race/ethnicity) to these differences makes defining the role of ethnicity difficult *(11)*. In certain ethnic groups, for instance, homocysteine concentrations may be very high and this may partly be explained by dietary intakes. Refsum and colleagues found that in a group of presumed healthy Asian Indians, homocysteine levels were markedly elevated in 77% of the total population, with a median of nearly 20 µmol/L, a finding that was at least partly explained by their low cobalamin status *(11)*. These investigators also noted that a substantial proportion of the population of India adheres to a vegetarian diet for cultural and religious reasons and a strict vegetarian diet has been associated with an increased risk of cobalamin deficiency which can lead to elevated homocysteine concentrations *(12,13)*. Plasma homocysteine levels can be lowered with the B complex vitamins. However, until recently intervention trials had not been undertaken to define whether or not homocysteine lowering would decrease morbidity and mortality from cardiovascular disease; thus The Heart Outcomes Prevention Evaluation (HOPE) 2, the Norwegian Vitamin trial, and the Western Norway B-Vitamin Intervention Trial were undertaken.

In the HOPE 2 trial *(14)*, 5522 patients 55 years of age or older who had vascular disease or diabetes were randomized to receive daily treatment with the combination of 2.5 mg of folic acid, 50 mg of vitamin B_6, and 1 mg of vitamin B_{12}, or with placebo for an average of 5 years. The primary outcome was a composite of death from cardiovascular causes, myocardial infarction, and stroke.

The investigators found that mean plasma homocysteine levels decreased by 0.3 mg/L in the active-treatment group and *increased* by 0.1 mg/L in the placebo group. As compared with placebo, active treatment did not significantly decrease the risk of death from cardiovascular causes (relative risk, 0.96; 95% confidence interval, 0.81–1.13), myocardial infarction (relative risk, 0.98; 95% confidence interval, 0.85–1.14), or any of the secondary outcomes. Fewer patients assigned to active treatment than to placebo had a stroke (relative risk, 0.75; 95% confidence interval, 0.59–0.97), however, more patients in the active-treatment group were hospitalized for unstable angina (relative risk, 1.24; 95% confidence interval, 1.04–1.49). From these results, the authors concluded that supplements combining folic acid and vitamins B_6 and B_{12} did not reduce the risk of major cardiovascular events in patients with vascular disease.

In the Norwegian Vitamin trial (15), the investigators randomized 3749 men and women who had had an acute myocardial infarction within the prior 7 days to receive therapy. Participants were randomly assigned, in a two-by-two factorial design, to receive one of the following four treatments:

– 0.8 mg of folic acid, 0.4 mg of vitamin B_{12}, and 40 mg of vitamin B_6
– 0.8 mg of folic acid and 0.4 mg of vitamin B_{12}
– 40 mg of vitamin B_6
– or placebo

Study medication was given in a single capsule, taken once per day. For the first 2 weeks after enrollment, the combination-therapy groups received a loading dose of 5 mg of folic acid per day, whereas the other two groups received placebo for the first 2 weeks. The primary end point was a composite of new nonfatal and fatal myocardial infarction, nonfatal and fatal stroke, and sudden death attributed to CHD. In this trial, the investigators found that the mean total homocysteine level was lowered by 27% among patients randomized to receive folic acid plus vitamin B_{12}. Despite this effective reduction in homocysteine levels, however, such treatment had no significant effect on the primary end point (risk ratio, 1.08; 95% confidence interval, 0.93–1.25; $P = 0.31$). Also, treatment with vitamin B_6 alone did not show significant benefit with regard to the primary end point (relative risk of the primary end point, 1.14; 95% confidence interval, 0.98–1.32; $P = 0.09$). Also, of concern, in the group randomized to receive combined therapy with folic acid, vitamin B_{12}, and vitamin B_6, there was a statistically significant increase in risk. From these results, the authors concluded that treatment with B vitamins did not lower the risk of recurrent cardiovascular disease after acute myocardial infarction, and in fact, they noted a harmful effect from combined B vitamin treatment in these post-myocardial infarction patients. They further concluded that such treatment should not be recommended.

The most recent large-scale clinical trial of homocysteine lowering, the Western Norway B-Vitamin Intervention Trial (WENBIT), was recently presented and details of the trial design have been previously published (16). In this trial, 3090 CHD patients were randomized (in a 2×2 factorial design) to four groups to receive a daily oral dose of folic acid 0.8 mg (with vitamin B_{12} 0.4 mg) and vitamin B_6 40 mg, folic acid (with vitamin B_{12}) alone, vitamin B_6 alone, or placebo. After a median follow-up of 38 months, there was no significant difference in the risk of death or major cardiovascular events among the four groups.

These three strikingly similar clinical trials lead to the conclusion that there is no clinical benefit in reduction of coronary heart disease to the use of folic acid and vitamin B_{12} (with or without the addition of vitamin B_6) in patients with established vascular disease and that in some cases there may be harm. It is not clear why homocysteine lowering with B complex vitamins does not reduce the risk of coronary heart disease (CHD), given the epidemiologic evidence associating elevated serum homocysteine levels with adverse cardiovascular outcomes. Possibilities include the higher risk nature of these patients, already having vascular disease; the possibility that combination therapy with B vitamins is not the optimal way to reduce homocysteine, or perhaps that other complicated metabolic consequences of lowering homocysteine levels in this way ensued, or a complicated interaction with other cardiovascular risk factors – like smoking – may have ensued. Several studies have reported that smokers have higher plasma homocysteine concentrations compared to non-smokers *(17–20)*. One study has also shown that in smokers, the risk of a cardiovascular event is greatly increased if there is also concomitant hyperhomocysteinemia *(21)*. O'Callaghan and colleagues used data from the European Concerted Action Project case–control study of 750 cases and 800 age- and sex-matched controls aged less than 60 years from 19 centers in 10 European countries. The investigators found that smokers were at increased risk of vascular disease and that this risk was greatly increased in the presence of a raised plasma homocysteine. Cigarette smokers with a plasma homocysteine above 12 µmol/L had a 12-fold increased risk of cardiovascular disease (OR 12.4 95% confidence interval 7.3–21.2) compared with non-smokers with a normal plasma homocysteine. In both cases and controls, the current smokers had a higher plasma homocysteine level than the never smokers. Current smokers also tended to have lower levels of folate, and vitamin B6 and vitamin B12 than never smokers, possibly explaining the elevated homocysteine levels. For the time being, however, the use of combination B vitamin therapy to homocysteine, and thereby, lower coronary heart disease risk, remains unproven.

3. LIPOPROTEIN(A)

Lipoprotein(a) is structurally similar to LDL, with an additional disulfied linked glycoprotein termed apolipoprotein(a) [apo(a)] *(22)*. Apo(a) shares extensive structural homology with plasminogen but varies in size, which is due to the variation in the number of Kringle 4-like domains (Type 2 repeats) of plasminogen. Due to the size heterogeneity, apo(a) exhibits a genetic size polymorphism with apparent molecular weights of isoforms ranging from 300 to 800 kDa *(22,23)*. There are considerable differences in the mean of plasma Lp(a) concentrations between different populations and ethnic groups *(24)*. Many, though not all, epidemiologic and case–control studies have shown that when Lp(a) is present in high level in the plasma, it is an independent risk factor for CHD *(25–28)*. In addition to high Lp(a) levels, the presence of small apo(a) isoforms (with fewer kringle

IV Type 2 repeats) has been associated with CHD in Caucasians *(29,30)*. Interestingly, although mean Lp(a) levels are more than twice as high in African-Americans compared with Caucasians, some studies have failed to establish a significant association between elevated Lp(a) levels and CHD among African-Americans *(31,32)*. The majority of Caucasians with high Lp(a) levels possesses at least 1 small apo(a) isoform; however, the majority of African-Americans with high Lp(a) levels have no small apo(a) isoforms *(33)*. To try to understand why studies had failed to establish a significant association between elevated Lp(a) levels and CHD in African-Americans, Paultre and colleagues hypothesized that CHD was associated specifically with the presence of an elevated level of Lp(a) in concert with a small apo(a) isoform *(34)*. They, therefore, compared Lp(a) levels, apo(a) sizes, and the level of Lp(a) particles carrying small apo(a) sizes in African-American and Caucasian patients undergoing coronary angiography. Elevated Lp(a) levels with small apo(a) isoforms were significantly associated with CAD ($P<0.01$) in African-American and Caucasian men but not in women. This association remained significant after adjusting for multiple variables. The authors concluded that elevated levels of Lp(a) with small apo(a) isoforms independently predict risk for CAD in African-American and Caucasian men. This study, by determining the predictive power of Lp(a) levels combined with apo(a) isoform size, may provide an explanation for the apparent lack of association of Lp(a) levels alone with CHD in African-Americans.

In regards to Lp(a) levels in Hispanics, available data suggest somewhat higher values in Hispanics as compared to non-Hispanic Caucasians. In a study by Chiu et al., 390 non-Hispanic Caucasians and 214 Hispanics from San Luis Valley, Colorado, were studied *(35)*. Mean ($\pm$SD) and median Lp(a) levels were 9.6 $\pm$ 12.5 and 3.8 mg/dl, respectively, in non-Hispanic Caucasians and 12.1 $\pm$ 15.6 and 4.9 mg/dl, respectively, in Hispanics.

Lp(a) levels in American Indians were measured in participants in the Strong Heart Study *(36)*. Median Lp(a) concentration in American Indians was 3.0 mg/dl. This was almost half of that in Caucasians and one-sixth the level found in African-Americans. Correlation analysis showed lower Lp(a) levels were significantly correlated with the degree of Indian heritage.

Higher serum lipoprotein(a) concentrations have also been reported in Asian Indians. In a study, of young Asian Indian patients (age less than 45 years) who had suffered a myocardial infarction, the mean lipoprotein (a) level was 22.28 $\pm$ 5.4 mg/dl in patients and 9.28 $\pm$ 22.59 mg/dl in controls *(37)*. Also, a study by Velmurugan and colleagues evaluated carotid intimal–medial thickness (IMT) in Type 2 diabetic Asian Indian subjects *(38)*. They found that the prevalence of carotid atherosclerosis (as detected by IMT) among subjects with elevated Lp(a) levels >20 mg/dl was significantly higher compared with those with Lp(a) levels = 20 mg/dl (26.9% vs. 16.3%, $P=0.003$). Furthermore, multiple logistic regression analysis of carotid IMT with other cardiovascular risk factors showed that only age

(P=0.010), LDL-cholesterol (P=0.032), and Lp(a) (P=0.021) were significantly associated with carotid atherosclerosis.

4. INFLAMMATORY MARKERS

It is now recognized that atherosclerosis is an inflammatory disease *(39)*. Chronic, subclinical inflammation appears to be one pathophysiologic mechanism explaining the increased risk of atherosclerotic disease regardless of the amount of obstruction produced by that coronary disease. In the inflammatory model of atherosclerosis, it is the degree of inflammation not the degree of obstruction that causes acute coronary syndromes and increased CHD mortality. Cytokines are key mediators of the inflammatory response and have been implicated in the development of atherosclerosis. There are significant ethnic differences in cytokine levels. Studies have shown, for instance, that African-Americans are more likely than White Americans to carry allelic variants demonstrated to increase production of inflammatory cytokines *(40)*. Two of the most studied inflammatory cytokines are C-reactive protein and interleukin-6.

4.1. C-Reactive Protein (CRP)

There is now accumulating evidence that markers of subclinical inflammation may indeed predict future CHD events. One of the most studied markers is C-reactive protein (CRP) *(41)*. Elevation of CRP is associated with several major coronary heart disease risk factors and increased projected 10-year coronary heart disease risk in both men and women *(41,42)*, and CRP levels have been shown to vary by race–ethnicity *(43)*. In one study, utilizing the National Health and Nutrition Examination Survey (NHANES) database, highly sensitive CRP levels (hs-CRP) were found to be highest among non-Hispanic black men and Mexican American women. According to multiple logistic regression analysis, cigarette smoking, increased age, body mass index, and systolic blood pressure in men, and body mass index and diabetes in women, were strongly associated with a greater likelihood of CRP levels of greater than or-equal to 1.0 mg/dl (p<0.001). While hs-CRP levels have been shown to be related to cardiovascular risk factors, public health approaches to modifying hs-CRP levels have been less well studied. One recent study *(44)*, however, addresses physical fitness and its relation to hs-CRP by ethnicity. LaMonte and colleagues hypothesized that physical fitness might protect against high levels of hs-CRP. They analyzed data from a subset of 44 African-American, 45 Native-American, and 46 Caucasian women who were part of the Cross-Cultural Activity Participation Study (CAPS) in the mid-1990s.

In CAPS, physical fitness was determined by exercise on a treadmill while both speed and incline were increased, and the women continued on the treadmill until they reached their point of exhaustion. Each woman's tread-mill time was adjusted for her age and women in each of the three ethnic groups were divided into three levels of fitness – low, moderate, and high – on the basis of their treadmill tests, and the researchers assessed CRP levels by race, fitness, obesity, and waist size. They found that

- CRP levels were 4.3 mg/L in African-American women, 2.5 mg/L in Native American, and 2.3 mg/L in Caucasian women.
- Women with low fitness had significantly higher CRP levels (4.3 mg/L) than those in the moderate (2.6 mg/L) and high (2.3 mg/L) fitness categories.
- CRP was also significantly elevated in women with the highest body mass index (BMI). Women with BMI values from 18.5 to 24.9 had hs-CRP levels of 1.9 mg/L, in overweight women (BMI 25–29.9) 3.4 mg/L and in obese women (BMI = 30) 4.2 mg/L.
- Women whose waists measured more than 35 in. had CRP concentrations of 4.2 mg/L, while those with waist circumference of less than 35 in. had CRP levels of 2.5 mg/L.

4.2. Interleukin-6 (IL-6)

Overproduction of IL-6, a proinflammatory cytokine, is associated with a wide variety of diseases including cardiovascular disease. Researchers have found evidence of ethnic differences in IL-6, with African-Americans having higher IL-6 levels than non-African-Americans (45).

The reasons for these differences are not known but may be related to lifestyle factors, genetics, or other variables. Researchers have demonstrated that higher plasma IL-6 levels are associated with adverse health habits: values are higher in smokers than non-smokers, in individuals who report less physical activity, in those whose sleep is impaired, and in those with a higher BMI (46–49).

A growing body of evidence suggests that inflammatory markers like IL-6 may be modulated by stress. IL-6 levels are normally very low and increase during infection, trauma, or stress, and increased IL-6 is associated with increased mortality (50). Elevated levels of IL-6 are associated with an increased risk of death from cardiovascular A recent longitudinal community study was performed to describe the pattern of change in IL-6 over 6 years among older adults undergoing a chronic stressor (51). In this study, the chronic stressor they studied was caregiving for a spouse with dementia, and the investigators assessed the relationship between this chronic stressor and IL-6 production. There were 119 men and women who were caregivers and 106 participants who were non-caregivers, with a mean age at study entry of 71 years. Levels of IL-6 and health behaviors associated with IL-6 were measured across 6 years. Caregivers' average rate of increase in IL-6 was about four times as large as that of non-caregivers. Moreover, the mean annual changes in IL-6 among former caregivers did not differ from that of current caregivers even several years after the death of the impaired spouse. These data provide evidence of a key mechanism through which chronic stressors may accelerate atherosclerosis which may have important implications for certain race–ethnic populations.

5. CONCLUSIONS

The increased focus on risk factors for the prevention and treatment of cardiovascular disease has greatly improved outcomes. Public health campaigns to decrease cigarette smoking, elevated serum cholesterol, and high blood pressure have resulted in steady declines in atherosclerotic diseases in all populations, including ethnic minorities. Despite these initiatives, however, cardiovascular diseases remain the leading causes of death in the developed world and are rapidly becoming the leading causes of death worldwide. In an effort to continue to combat cardiovascular diseases, researchers have focused on identifying additional "emerging" risk factors for cardiovascular disease. While these factors have promise in terms of helping us understand atherosclerosis, the focal point of future research must be on clarifying the role of these factors in atherosclerotic disease, including the role they play in ethnic minorities.

REFERENCES

1. Ueland PM, Refsum H, Brattström L. Plasma homocysteine and cardiovascular disease. In: Francis RBJ, ed. Atherosclerotic cardiovascular disease, hemostasis, and endothelial function. New York: Marcel Dekker, Inc; 1992:183–236.
2. Stampfer MJ, Malinow MR, Willett WC, et al. A prospective study of plasma homocyst(e)ine and risk of myocardial infarction in US physicians. *JAMA* 1992; 268: 877 881.
3. Arnesen E, Refsum H, Bonna KH, Ueland PM, Forde OH, Nordrehaug JE. Serum total homocysteine and coronary heart disease. *Int J Epidemiol* 1995; 24:704–109.
4. Perry IJ, Refsum H, Morris RW, Ebrahim SB, Ueland PM, Shaper AG. Prospective study of serum total homocysteine concentration and risk of stroke in middle-aged British men. *Lancet* 1995; 346:1395–1398.
5. Perry IJ, Refsum H, Morris RW, Ebrahim SB, Ueland PM, Shaper AG. Serum total homocysteine and coronary heart disease in middle-aged British men. *Heart* 1996; 75(Suppl 1):P53 (abstr).
6. Malinow MR, Nieto FJ, Szklo M, Chambless LE, Bond G. Carotid artery intimal-medial wall thickening and plasma homocyst(e)ine in asymptomatic adults: the Atherosclerosis Risk in Communities Study. *Circulation* 1993; 87:1107–1113.
7. Selhub J, Jacques PF, Bostom AG, et al. Association between plasma homocysteine concentrations and extracranial carotid-artery stenosis. *N Engl J Med* 1995; 332: 286–291.
8. Nygard O, Nordrehaug JE, Refsum H, Ueland PM, Farstad M, Vollset SE. Plasma homocysteine levels and mortality in patients with coronary artery disease. *N Engl J Med* 1997; 337:230–236.

9. Jacques PF, Rosenberg IH, Rogers G, et al. Serum total homocysteine concentrations in adolescent and adult Americans: results from the Third National Health and Nutrition Examination Survey. *Am J Clin Nutr* 1999; 69:482–489.

10. Ubbink JB, Vermaak WJ, Delport R, van der Merwe A, Becker PJ, Potgieter H. Effective homocysteine metabolism may protect South African blacks against coronary heart disease. *Am J Clin Nutr* 1995; 62:802–808.

11. Refsum H, Yajnik CS, Gadkari M, et al. Hyperhomocysteinemia and elevated methylmalonic acid indicate a high prevalence of cobalamin deficiency in Asian Indians. *Am J Clin Nutr* 2001; 74:233–241.

12. Sanders TA. The nutritional adequacy of plant-based diets. *Proc Nutr Soc* 1999; 58: 265–269.

13. Herbert V. Staging vitamin B-12 (cobalamin) status in vegetarians. *Am J Clin Nutr* 1994; 59(Suppl):1213S–1222S.

14. The Heart Outcomes Prevention Evaluation (HOPE) 2 Investigators. Homocysteine lowering with folic acid and B vitamins in vascular disease. *N Engl J Med* 2006; 354: 1567–1577.

15. Bønaa KH, Njølstad I, Ueland PM, et al. Homocysteine lowering and cardiovascular events after acute myocardial infarction. *N Engl J Med* 2006; 354:1578–1588.

16. B-Vitamin Treatment Trialists' Collaboration. Homocysteine-lowering trials for prevention of cardiovascular events: a review of the design and power of the large randomized trials. *Am Heart J* 2006; 151(2):282–287.

17. Reis RP, Azinheira J, Reis HP, Pina JE, Correia JM, Luis AS. Influence of smoking on homocysteinemia at baseline and after methionine load. *Rev Port Cardiol* 2000; 19: 471–474.

18. Pagan K, Hou J, Goldenberg RL, Cliver SP, Tamura T. Effect of smoking on serum concentrations of total homocysteine and B vitamins in mid-pregnancy. *Clin Chim Acta* 2001; 306:103–109.

19. McCarty MF. Increased homocysteine associated with smoking, chronic inflammation and aging may reflect acute-phase induction of pyridoxal phosphatase activity. *Med Hypotheses* 2000; 55:289–293.

20. Nygard O, Refsum H, Ueland PM, Vollset SE. Major lifestyle determinants of plasma total homocysteine distribution: the Hordaland Homocysteine Study. *Am J Clin Nutr* 1998; 67:263–270.

21. O'Callaghan P, Meleady R, Fitzgerald T, Graham I; European COMAC Group. Smoking and plasma homocysteine. *Eur Heart J* 2002; 23(20):1580–1586.

22. Uterman G. The mysteries of lipoprotein(a). *Science* 1989; 246:904–910.

23. Gunther MF, Catherin AR, Angelo MS. Heterogeneity of human lipoprotein(a). *J Biol Chem* 1984; 259:11470–11478.

24. Para HG, Luyey I, Buramoue C, et al. Black-white differences in serum lipoprotein(a) levels. *Clin Chim Acta* 1987; 167:27–31.

25. Scanu AM. Lipoprotein(a): a genetic risk factor for premature coronary heart disease. *JAMA* 1992; 267:3326–3329.

26. Macovina SM, Koshchinsky ML. Lipoprotein(a) as a risk factor for coronary artery disease. *Am J Cardiol* 1998; 82(12A):57U–66U.

27. Rim L, Ali B, Slim BA, Bechir Z. Lipoprotein(a): a new risk factor for coronary artery disease. *Tunis Med* 2000; 78(11):648–652.

28. Ridker PM. An epidemiologic reassessment of lipoprotein(a) and atherothrombotic risk. *Trends Cardiovasc Med* 1995; 5:225–229.

29. Wild SH, Fortmann SP, Marcovina SM. A prospective case-control study of lipoprotein(a) levels and apo(a) size and risk of coronary heart disease in Stanford Five-City Project participants. *Arterioscler Thromb Vasc Biol* 1997; 17:239–245

30. Sandholzer C, Saha N, Kark JD, Rees A, Jaross W, Dieplinger H, Hoppichler F, Boerwinkle E, Utermann G. Apo(a) isoforms predict risk for coronary heart disease: a study in six populations. *Arterioscler Thromb* 1992; 12:1214–1226.

31. Moliterno DJ, Jokinen EV, Miserez AR, Lange RA, Willard JE, Boerwinkle E, Hillis LD, Hobbs HH. No association between plasma lipoprotein(a) concentrations and the presence or absence of coronary atherosclerosis in African-Americans. *Arterioscler Thromb Vasc Biol* 1995; 15:850–855.

32. Sorrentino MJ, Vielhauer C, Eisenbart JD, Fless GM, Scanu AM, Feldman T. Plasma lipoprotein(a) protein concentration and coronary artery disease in black patients compared with white patients. *Am J Med* 1992; 93:658–662.

33. Marcovina SM, Albers JJ, Wijsman E, Zhang ZH, Chapman NH, Kennedy H. Differences in Lp(a) concentrations and apo(a) polymorphs between black and white Americans. *J Lipid Res* 1996; 37:2569–2585.

34. Paultre F, Pearson TA, Weil HF, et al. High levels of Lp(a) with a small apo(a) isoform are associated with coronary artery disease in African American and white men. *Arterioscler Thromb Vasc Biol* 2000; 20(12):2619–2624.

35. Chiu L, Hamman RF, Kamboh MI. Apolipoprotein A polymorphisms and plasma lipoprotein(a) concentrations in non-Hispanic Whites and Hispanics. *Hum Biol* 2000; 72(5):821–835.

36. Wang W, Hu D, Lee ET, Fabsitz RR, Welty TK, Robbins DC, J L Yeh, Howard BV. Lipoprotein(a) in American Indians is low and not independently associated with cardiovascular disease. The Strong Heart Study. *Ann Epidemiol* 2002; 12(2): 107–114.

37. Isser HS, Puri VK, Narain VS, Saran RK, Dwivedi SK, Singh S. Lipoprotein (a) and lipid levels in young patients with myocardial infarction and their first-degree relatives. *Indian Heart J* 2001; 53:463–466.

38. Velmurugan K, Deepa R, Ravikumar R, Lawrence JB, Anshoo H, Senthilvelmurugan M, Enas EA, V. Mohan. Relationship of lipoprotein(a) with intimal medial thickness of the carotid artery in Type 2 diabetic patients in south India. *Diabet Med* 2003; 20(6): 455–461.

39. Ross R. Atherosclerosis: an inflammatory disease. *N Engl J Med* 1999; 340:115–126.

40. Ness RB, Haggerty CL, Harger G, Ferrell R. Differential distribution of allelic variants in cytokine genes among African Americans and White Americans. *Am J Epidemiol* 2004; 160(11):1033–1038.

41. Ridker PM. High-sensitivity C-reactive protein: potential adjunct for global risk assessment in the primary prevention of cardiovascular disease. *Circulation* 2001; 103: 1813–1818.

42. Ridker PM, Glynn RJ, Hennekens CH. C-reactive protein adds to the predictive value of total and HDL cholesterol in determining risk of first myocardial infarction. *Circulation* 1998; 97: 2007–2011.

43. Wong, ND, Pio J. Valencia R, Thakal G. Distribution of C-reactive protein and its relation to risk factors and coronary heart disease risk estimation in the National Health and Nutrition Examination Survey (NHANES) III. *Prev Cardiol* 2001; 4(3):109–114.

44. LaMonte MJ, Durstine JL, Yanowitz FG, Lim T, DuBose KD, Davis P, Ainsworth BE. Cardiorespiratory fitness and C-reactive protein among a tri-ethnic sample of women. *Circulation* 2002; 106(4): 403–406.

45. Hassan MI, Aschner Y, Manning CH, et al. Racial differences in selected cytokine allelic and genotypic frequencies among healthy, pregnant women in North Carolina. *Cytokine* 2003; 21:10–16.

46. Reuben DB, Judd-Hamilton L, Harris TB, Seeman TE. MacArthur Studies of Successful Aging. The associations between physical activity and inflammatory markers in

high-functioning older persons: MacArthur Studies of Successful Aging. *J Am Geriatr Soc* 2003; 51(8):1125–1130.

47. Roytblat L, Rachinsky M, Fisher A, et al. Raised interleukin-6 levels in obese patients. *Obes Res* 2000; 8(9):673–675.

48. Tappia PS, Troughton KL, Langley-Evans SC, Grimble RF. Cigarette smoking influences cytokine production and antioxidant defences. *Clin Sci (Lond)* 1995; 88(4): 485–459.

49. Okun ML, Hall M, Coussons-Read ME. Sleep disturbances increase interleukin-6 production during pregnancy: implications for pregnancy complications. *Reprod Sci* 2007; 14(6):560–567.

50. Harris TB, Ferrucci L, Tracy RP, et al. Associations of elevated interleukin-6 and C-reactive protein levels with mortality in the elderly. *Am J Med* 1999; 106:506–512.

51. Kiecolt-Glaser JK, Preache KJ, MacCallum RC, Atkinson C, Malarkey WB, Glaser R. Chronic stress and age-related increases in the proinflammatory cytokine IL-6. *Proc Natl Acad Sci U S A* 2003; 100(15):9090–9095.

9

Weight Loss Interventions to Control Blood Pressure in an Increasingly Overweight, Multi-ethnic Society

L.J. Appel, MD, MPH,
M.E. Gauvey-Kern, BA, and
C.A.M. Anderson, PhD

CONTENTS

From: *Contemporary Cardiology: Cardiovascular Disease in Racial and Ethnic Minorities*
Edited by: K.C. Ferdinand and A. Armani, DOI 10.1007/978-1-59745-410-0_9
© Humana Press, a part of Springer Science+Business Media, LLC 2009

Abstract

This chapter will review the epidemiology of overweight and obesity, summarize the relationship of weight with blood pressure (BP), examine the effectiveness of lifestyle intervention trials in achieving weight loss, review differences in weight loss success by racial/ethnic groups, and explore factors that might explain observed differences in racial/ethnic responses to lifestyle interventions. Worldwide, obesity is one of the most common and important public health problems. In the U.S., approximately one third of adults are obese and another third are overweight. In men, the prevalence of obesity in Whites, African-Americans, and Hispanic Americans is similar. In women, however, African-Americans are more likely to be obese compared to Whites and Hispanic Americans. Asian-Americans represent the one racial/ethnic minority group for which the prevalence of overweight and obesity does not exceed that of their white counterparts.

Clinical trials have documented that lifestyle interventions can achieve weight loss and that weight loss reduces BP. However, recidivism is commonplace, and there is substantial variability across and within trials. On average, African-Americans, particularly women, achieve less weight loss than Caucasians. Culturally adapted interventions, including church-based programs that target African Americans, have likewise had mixed results. Explanations for the limited success of weight loss programs in African-Americans include social-cultural-environmental factors as well as physiologic factors. The paucity of weight loss studies in Hispanic Americans, Native Americans, and Native Hawaiian/Pacific Islander populations is striking. The magnitude of the obesity epidemic in combination with the lack of effective interventions in minority populations argues strongly for additional research.

Key Words: Lifestyle interventions; Obesity; Blood pressure; Weight loss interventions; Church and faith-based interventions; Black women.

1. INTRODUCTION

Lifestyle modification is an essential component of population-based strategies to prevent blood pressure (BP)-related cardiovascular diseases. The high prevalence of hypertension (27% of the US adult population) *(1)*, the relentless rise in systolic BP with age (beginning in childhood) *(2)*, and the high (90%) lifetime risk of developing hypertension *(3)* provide a compelling rationale for population-based lifestyle modifications that lower BP. In addition to excess weight, other dietary factors (high sodium intake, insufficient potassium intake, a poor quality diet, and high alcohol intake) adversely affect BP *(4)*. However, given the dramatic increase in obesity over the past few decades, the problem of excess weight is now a foremost concern *(5)*.

Obesity has emerged as one of the most important public health problems in the United States and throughout most of the world. In the United States, approximately two-thirds of the adult population are overweight or obese, and one-third of all children and adolescents are overweight or at risk for overweight *(6)*. In certain racial and ethnic minority populations[1], the problem is even more pronounced.

The health and financial costs attributable to obesity are enormous. Excess weight strongly and adversely affects several risk factors for cardiovascular disease and increases the risk of several non-cardiovascular diseases, including breast cancer and osteoarthritis. It has been estimated that each year, obesity contributes to 300,000 US deaths and leads to approximately $100 billion in direct medical costs and indirect costs *(7)*.

This chapter will *(1)* review the epidemiology of overweight and obesity, *(2)* summarize the relationship of weight (and weight change) with BP, *(3)* examine the effectiveness of lifestyle intervention trials in achieving weight loss, *(4)* review differences in weight loss success by racial/ethnic groups, and *(5)* explore factors that might explain observed differences in racial/ethnic responses to lifestyle interventions.

2. EPIDEMIOLOGY OF OBESITY

Several metrics have been used to classify individuals based on excess weight, including percent body fat, waist circumference, and body mass index (BMI). This chapter will use the contemporary classification scheme, based on BMI, which is calculated as weight in kilograms divided by height in meters squared (see Table 1).

3. PREVALENCE OF OVERWEIGHT AND OBESITY

Data from the Third National Health and Nutrition Examination Survey (NHANES) highlight the extent to which unhealthy body weight is pervasive in US society *(6)*. As of 2004, two-thirds (66.3%) of US adults were overweight or obese and 32.2% were obese. Data for children and young adults from the same 2004 survey document that one-third (33.6%) of US children were overweight or at risk for overweight and that over half (17.1%) were already overweight. The following sections provide an overview of the prevalence of overweight and obesity by demographic characteristics (age, sex, and race–ethnicity).

---

[1] In the medical literature, the nosology and terminology that are used to describe race–ethnicity populations is inconsistent. In particular, there are multiple terms for the same race–ethnic group (e.g., African-American, Blacks, persons of color). Whenever possible, we use the terminology as presented in cited publications.

Table 1
Classification of Weight Status Based on Body Mass Index (BMI)

	Category	BMI (kg/m^2)
Adults (20+)	Underweight	<18.5
	Normal/healthy body weight	$18.5 \leq BMI \leq 24.9$
	Overweight	$25.0 \leq BMI \leq 29.9$
	Obesity	$BMI \geq 30$
	Extreme obesity	$BMI \geq 40$
Children and Adolescents	At risk for overweight	$BMI \geq$ 85th percentile
	Overweight	$BMI \geq$ 95th percentile

3.1. Age

Over the lifespan, from birth through adult's ages, individuals steadily gain weight, except at advanced ages. Hence, the prevalence of overweight and obesity increases with age. Elderly adults are an exception – the prevalence of obesity among those over 80 does not differ significantly from those of 20- to 39-year olds *(6)*.

3.2. Sex

The prevalence of overweight and obesity also varies by sex, but the pattern is complex, in part because the associations vary by race–ethnicity. Sex differences are particularly apparent for extreme obesity – the most recent NHANES data showed that 6.9% of females compared to only 2.8% of males can be categorized as extremely obese (Fig. 1) *(6)*. Sex differences in overall obesity prevalence are less clear. Analysis of 1999–2002 NHANES data showed that obesity prevalence was significantly higher for women than men *(8)*. However, analysis of the 2003–2004 NHANES data found no significant sex difference *(6)*.

Although data on sex and obesity risk in the general population are equivocal, significant sex–race interactions are consistently observed. Among whites, obesity rates are similar in men and women; however, in minority groups, the prevalence of obesity is much higher in women than men.

3.3. Race/Ethnicity

The prevalence of overweight and obesity varies considerably by race/ethnicity. It is well documented that the prevalence of overweight or obesity is higher in several minority populations (Hispanics and African-Americans) in comparison to whites. In the United States, national surveys

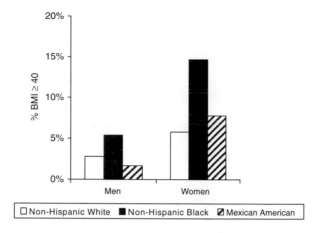

Fig. 1. Prevalence of extreme obesity (BMI > 40 kg/m^2) in adults by race–sex group. Source: NHANES 2003–2004. Adapted from *(6)*.

focus on three race–ethnic groups: non-Hispanic whites/Caucasians, non-Hispanic blacks/African-Americans, and Hispanics/Mexican Americans. With a prevalence of 30%, whites are least likely to be obese, while blacks are most likely to be obese (prevalence of 45%). The prevalence of obesity in Mexican Americans is intermediate at 36%.

Asian Americans represent the one racial/ethnic minority group for which the prevalence of overweight and obesity does not exceed that of their white counterparts. However, the standard BMI weight class definitions may be inappropriate for the average Asian body type. Since Asians have smaller frames, they have a higher percent body fat for a given BMI relative to other racial/ethnic groups. In light of these findings, the World Health Organization's International Obesity Task Force recently recommended that overweight status for Asian adults should be defined as a BMI of 23.0–24.9 and obesity defined by a BMI of ≥ 25. Because few surveys have reported prevalence data using these cutpoints, the existing literature most likely underestimates obesity and overweight prevalence in Asian Americans *(6)*.

Data on the prevalence of obesity in Native Americans (American Indians), Native Alaskans, and Native Hawaiians are limited. According to a review by Broussard *(9)*, overweight and obesity have emerged as a substantial public health problem among Native Americans (Fig. 2). However, there is substantial variation by tribal affiliation and region. For example, while the prevalence of overweight and obesity in the Navajo tribe only slightly exceeded that of whites, members of the Zuni, Pueblo, and Pima tribes were roughly one and a half times as likely to be overweight.

Importantly, the relationship between racial/ethnic group and weight varies substantially by age and sex (Fig. 3). In adult men, the prevalence of obesity in whites, blacks, and Hispanic Americans is similar *(10)*. However,

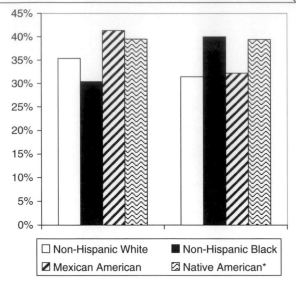

Fig. 2. Prevalence of overweight or at risk for overweight in children by race–sex group (*data for Native Americans lags that of other races by 10+ years).
Source: Adapted from *(6,9)*.

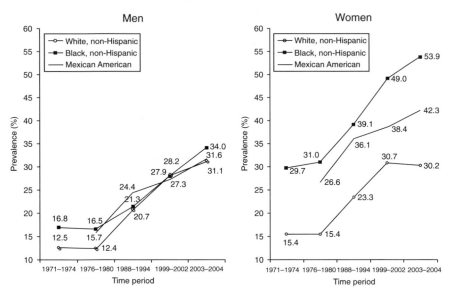

Fig. 3. Trends in the prevalence of obesity by race–ethnicity in men (left panel) and women (right panel).
Source: Reprinted with permission from *(10)*.

significant racial/ethnic differences in overweight prevalence are evident for male children and adolescents. Mexican American boys have significantly higher incidence of overweight than their black and white counterparts *(6,8)*.

The most consistent racial/ethnic disparities in overweight and obesity prevalence are evident in women. White women and girls are more likely to have a normal weight than Mexican American and black women. With a prevalence rate of 14.7%, black women are two to three times more likely to be extremely obese when compared to their white (5.8%) and Hispanic (7.8%) counterparts *(8)*.

3.4. Trends in Obesity Prevalence

While the high prevalence of overweight and obesity is certainly disturbing, trend data are of even greater concern. Between 1980 and 2002, the proportion of US adults classified as obese doubled, and the prevalence of overweight among children and adolescents (age 6–19 years) tripled. In recent years, substantial increases in the prevalence of overweight for children and adolescents continued – between 1999 and 2004, the percentage of overweight boys increased from 14.0 to 18.2% and that of girls from 13.8 to 16.0% *(6)* (Fig. 4). In the same time period, the prevalence of obesity among adult males also increased significantly from 27.5 to 31.1%. As displayed in Fig. 3, the prevalence of obesity increased in a similar fashion in men, irrespective of race–ethnicity. Among women, the prevalence of obesity increased in blacks and Mexican Americans. For white women, prevalence appeared to level off between the 1999–2002 and the 2003–2004 survey periods *(10)*.

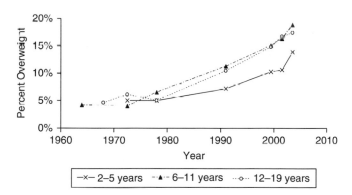

Fig. 4. Trends in child and adolescent overweight by age group, 1963–2004.
Source: http://www.cdc.gov/nchs/products/pubs/pubd/hestats/overweight/overwght_child_03.htm.

4. WEIGHT AND BLOOD PRESSURE

4.1. Observational Epidemiology

Observational studies have repeatedly documented a direct relationship of weight, and other measures of body fat, with BP. Over 40 years ago, the Framingham Heart Study reported that both the average BP and the prevalence of hypertension increase with weight *(11)*. In both men and women, there is a direct progressive relationship between BMI and incident hypertension *(12)* (Fig. 5). More recently, the Atherosclerosis Risk in Communities Study (ARIC) documented that weight loss is associated with reduced systolic and diastolic BP levels as well as remission of hypertension *(13)*. Persuasive evidence on the relationship between weight and BP comes from randomized clinical trials which have consistently documented that weight reduction lowers BP, improves hypertension control, and can prevent hypertension.

4.2. Behavioral Interventions to Accomplish Weight Loss

A large number of clinical trials have tested the effects of behavioral, weight loss interventions on BP, or a related outcome. These trials typically focus on achieving a net calorie deficit through reduced calorie intake and/or increased physical activity. It has been estimated that in order to achieve weight loss of 1 pound per week, a daily calorie deficit of 500 kcal is required. Such a calorie deficit is difficult to achieve through increased physical activity alone. Hence, contemporary weight programs emphasize calorie restriction as a means to lower weight.

Typical weight loss interventions emphasize behavioral counseling rather than provision of information. Counseling is done in group settings with

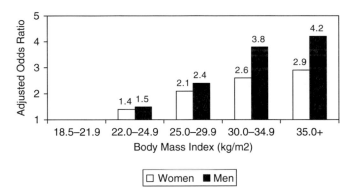

Fig. 5. Risk of developing hypertension over 10 years of follow-up according to initial BMI level for female and male health professionals, adjusted for age, smoking status, and race.
Source: Adapted from *(12)*.

periodic one-on-one counseling sessions. Group sessions foster accountability, provide social support, and are less costly than individual counseling *(14)*. Counselors include a wide spectrum of allied health professionals,
including registered dietitians, health educators, and clinical psychologists.
Ideally, counselors are trained in behavioral techniques that motivate individuals to make and sustain lifestyle changes.

Most weight loss programs consist of two phases – an initial, intensive
phase in which interventionist–participant contact occurs roughly weekly
for up to 6 months. During this period, individuals attempt to lose approximately 5–10 kg (or approximately 7–10%) of body weight. A second or
weight maintenance phase then occurs in which individuals attempt to sustain weight loss. The weight maintenance phase is typically less intensive
than the initial weight loss phase. Intervention features that are associated
with weight loss include increased duration of intervention, self-monitoring
of calories and weight, use of group sessions, and promotion of diets with
reduced portion size, reduced caloric density, and high intake of fiber and
whole grains *(14,15)*. Based on data from the Weight Loss Registry, factors associated with sustained weight loss include ongoing self-monitoring,
restrained eating and caloric reduction, high levels of physical activity, and
comparatively small amounts of television time *(16,17)*.

4.3. Effects of Behavioral Interventions on Weight Loss

Randomized controlled trials have documented that lifestyle interventions
can achieve weight loss. However, recidivism is commonplace, and there is
substantial variability across and within trials. During the initial weight loss
period, average weight loss in trials was typically 4–6 kg *(18)*, but the range
was wide (0.6–11.9 kg).

The extent of weight loss varies by demographic factors. Women generally lose less total weight than men, though the difference may be explained
by differences in baseline bodyweight *(19)*. Age also appears to impact
weight loss. Individuals over age 60 generally lose more weight initially
and more effectively maintain weight reductions than their younger counterparts *(20)*. Race/ethnicity is a predictor of weight loss outcomes; specifically,
members of minority populations generally lose less weight than their white
counterparts. As discussed subsequently, the discrepancy is greatest for non-
Hispanic black women who tend to lose less weight than members of other
race/ethnic groups *(21)*.

4.4. Effects of Behavioral Weight Loss Interventions
on Blood Pressure

The modest weight loss that is achieved through lifestyle interventions
is nonetheless sufficient to improve health outcomes. Such levels of weight

loss reduces the risk of diabetes *(22)*, lowers BP *(18)*, and can prevent hypertension *(23)*. In the Framingham Heart Study, weight loss of only 5 pounds (2.3 kg) reduced cardiovascular risk by 40% *(24)*.

In a meta-analysis by Neter, the average net reduction in weight of 5.1 kg lowered mean systolic and diastolic BP by 4.4 and 3.6 mmHg, respectively. On an average, systolic and diastolic BP decreased by roughly 1 mmHg/kg of weight reduction. In dose–response analyses, persons who lost more weight had greater reduction in BP. Specifically, populations with an average weight loss greater than 5 kg achieved reductions in systolic/diastolic BP of 6.2/5.0 mmHg compared with average reductions of only 2.4/2.0 mmHg for those who lost less weight. Those taking antihypertensive medication experienced 7.0/5.5 mmHg average reductions in systolic/diastolic BP compared to 3.8/3.0 mmHg achieved by non-medicated counterparts with similar weight loss. No differences in BP response to weight loss were evident in subgroups defined by initial BMI, sex, age, intervention component, or initial BP. There was a non-significant trend such that Asians had greater reductions in both systolic and diastolic BP for a given weight loss than did their black and white counterparts.

Whether weight loss retards the age-related rise in systolic BP is uncertain. Data from Phase 2 of the Trials of Hypertension Prevention (TOHP-Phase 2) (Fig. 6) suggest that BP continues to rise over time even in persons who maintained long-term weight loss *(25)*. In this trial, those individuals who sustained a >10 pound weight loss achieved a lower BP that nonetheless rose over time

BP reduction of the magnitude observed in weight loss trials should have substantial public health benefits. It has been estimated that a

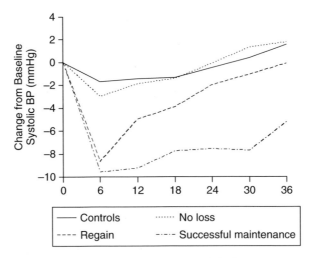

Fig. 6. Mean change in systolic blood pressure by weight loss status. Source: Adapted from *(25)*.

population-wide 3 mmHg reduction in the systolic BP should lead to 5 and 8% decreases in annual coronary and stroke deaths respectively *(26)*. A 2 mmHg average decrease in diastolic levels among white 35- to 64-year olds alone would result in a 17% reduction of US hypertension prevalence, a 5.6% drop in coronary artery disease, and a 13.8% decrease in stroke events *(27)*.

4.5. Weight Loss as a Means to Prevent Hypertension

Clinical trials also document that weight loss can prevent hypertension among individuals with pre-hypertension. Of the seven non-pharmacologic interventions tested in Phase 1 of the Trials of Hypertension Prevention (Phase 1-TOHP) *(28)*, only weight loss and sodium reduction significantly reduced BP. Compared to controls, the weight loss intervention group experienced an average weight loss of 3.9 kg, resulting in net systolic and diastolic BP reductions of 2.9 and 2.4 mmHg, respectively. The relative risk of incident hypertension was 0.49.

TOHP-Phase 2 investigated the long-term effects of weight loss and sodium reduction, alone and combined, on BP and hypertension over a 3-year study period *(23)*. In the weight loss intervention group, average weight loss was 4.4, 2.0, and 0.2 kg at 6, 18, and 36 months, respectively. The control group on average gained 1.8 kg of weight over the 3-year period, leading to a net difference in weight of approximately 2.0 kg at the end of the trial. Race/ethnicity substantially and significantly impacted weight loss in the first half of the study – blacks lost 1.8 kg less than whites at both the 6- and the 18-month assessments, but no significant racial/ethnic differences in weight loss were observed at 36 months *(25)* (Fig. 7). Women achieved significantly less weight loss than men throughout the study. Differences in baseline weight explained the sex disparity in weight change at 6 months but did not explain disparity at 18 months.

Blood pressure and hypertension findings were similar in Phases 1 and 2 of TOHP. A linear dose–response relationship was again observed with weight loss, as systolic and diastolic BP levels decreased 0.45 and 0.35 mmHg, respectively, per kilogram reduction in weight. Race/ethnicity had no effect on the extent of reduction per unit change in weight. However, sex apparently exerted a significant influence on diastolic response to weight loss; specifically, women experienced a 0.15 mmHg/kg smaller reduction than their male counterparts.

Observed risk ratios for the onset of hypertension again support findings for the protective effect of weight loss. Relative to the control, the relative risk of incident hypertension among those in the weight loss intervention was 0.58 at 6 months and roughly 0.8 from 18 months through the end of the study. Stratified analysis showed that reduction in risk for hypertension was proportional to the amount of weight loss achieved and maintained.

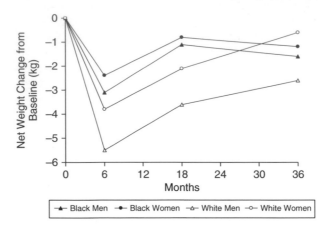

Fig. 7. Net weight change in TOHP-2 by race–sex group.
Source: Adapted from *(25)*.

4.6. Maintenance of Weight Loss

Weight loss interventions have improved considerably over the past 30 years. Indeed, well-designed intervention programs typically result in clinically significant weight loss for one-half to two-thirds of the participants over the initial 6 months. Despite short-term success, weight regain is commonplace. Generally, attendance at interventions and adherence with behavioral recommendations diminish over time. Observational studies suggest that continued intervention contacts; self-monitoring of dietary intake, physical activity and weight; accountability; and regular physical activity lead to sustained weight loss *(16,29)*.

This tendency toward weight regain has raised concern regarding the potential for adverse effects from weight cycling. Some observational studies suggest that weight variation is associated with increased rates of morbidity and mortality *(30,31)*. However, these studies often fail to differentiate between intentional and unintentional weight loss, as well as between overweight or obese and normal-weight individuals. Studies which do take these factors into account find no significant association between cycling due to intentional weight loss and mortality or morbidity. Field's 1999 analysis of the Nurses Health Study II showed that BMI and weight gain were independently associated with hypertension, but such an association was not evident for either mild or severe weight cycling *(32)*. Wing et al. similarly found no negative effects of weight cycling on cardiovascular risk factors; those who intentionally lost weight and then regained it appear no worse off than counterparts who never lost weight *(33)*.

4.7. Strategies to Reduce BP in the Absence of Weight Loss

In view of the well-recognized challenges of sustaining weight loss, it is appropriate to highlight the effects of other lifestyle interventions that reduce BP. Indeed, multiple dietary factors affect BP *(4)*. In addition to weight loss, other dietary modifications that lower BP are reduced salt intake, increased potassium intake, moderation of alcohol consumption (among those who drink), and consumption of dietary patterns similar to the DASH diet. The DASH diet emphases fruits, vegetables, and low-fat dairy products and is reduced in saturated fat and cholesterol. Results from the DASH–Sodium trial, a feeding study in which weight was held constant, document that obese individuals, on average, achieve similar BP reductions as non-obese individuals from sodium reduction and the DASH diet (see Fig. 8) *(34)*. In contrast, African-Americans are especially sensitive to the BP lowering effects of a reduced salt intake, increased potassium intake, and the DASH diet *(4)*.

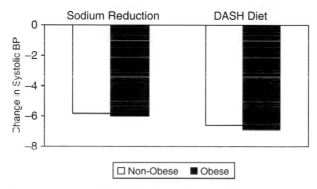

Fig. 8. BP effects of sodium reduction and the DASH diet in non-obese and obese individuals with pre-hypertension or stage 1 hypertension: Subgroup results from the DASH–Sodium Trial.
Source: Adapted from *(34)*.

5. EFFECTS OF BEHAVIORAL WEIGHT LOSS INTERVENTIONS IN AFRICAN-AMERICANS

The following section describes the weight loss experience of African-Americans in trials of behavioral interventions. Initially, we discuss their experience in large trials that enrolled multi-ethnic populations. Such trials provide an opportunity to compare the weight loss experiences of different race–ethnic groups that received comparable interventions. Subsequently, we discuss the effects of interventions that were culturally adapted for African-Americans.

5.1. Multi-ethnic Randomized Controlled Trials
of Weight Loss Interventions

Several large randomized controlled trials have examined the effects of lifestyle interventions on weight loss in multi-ethnic populations (Table 2). In these trials, African-Americans tend to lose less weight than Caucasians *(21)*. Among men, racial/ethnic differences attenuate and lose statistical significance after the first 12–18 months. In contrast, differentials in weight loss are more pronounced among women. A partial explanation appears to be the weight trajectory of control groups in these studies; African-American control participants tend to gain more weight than Caucasians *(35)*. Thus, examination of weight change, net of control, somewhat attenuates observed racial/ethnic differences in intervention effects that appear more pronounced when examining just the active-intervention group.

Two trials documenting differential weight loss in whites and African-Americans, as well as weight gain in African-Americans under control conditions, are the Hypertension Prevention Trial (HPT) *(35)* and TOHP-Phase 1 *(35)*. HPT was a 3-year trial that enrolled 236 participants (aged 25–49 years, 22% African-American) with pre-hypertension or hypertension. In the short-term, there was a significant difference in weight loss by race; African-Americans lost 1.4 and 2.7 kg less than their white counterparts. For male participants, racial differences decreased after the first year with no significant difference at 36 months. For black women weight regain occurred. All initial weight was regained by 18 months; by 36 months, there was a net gain of 2.3 kg from baseline.

Other major trials have noted a similar pattern *(25,36)*. In TOHP-Phase 2, whites lost 1.8 kg more than blacks at both 6 and 18 months, however, weight loss did not vary significantly by race/ethnicity at 36 months *(25)*. In a review of HPT and TOHP- Phase 1, Kumanyika notes that greater weight gain for black control subjects compared to whites somewhat attenuates the racial/ethnic differences observed in intervention effect *(35)*. However, significant racial/ethnic discrepancy in net weight loss remains, particularly among female participants.

Differences in weight loss among African-Americans and non-African-Americans are also evident in older Americans. The Trial of Nonpharmacologic Interventions in the Elderly (TONE) *(37)* enrolled 585 overweight medication-controlled hypertensives, 28% black, aged 60–79 years. Blacks lost roughly 3 kg less than whites both at 6 months (-2.7 versus -5.9 kg, $p = 0.0002$) and the end of follow-up to 3 years later (-2.0 versus -4.9 kg, $p = 0.007$) *(38)*. Only 41% of blacks compared to 66% of white participants achieved the weight loss goals of either -4.5 kg by intervention end or at least -3.6 kg by 6 months.

The Diabetes Prevention Project (DPP), a more recent study of overweight adults at risk for diabetes, enrolled 1079 participants, 19%

Table 2

Weight Loss in Behavioral Intervention Trials that Enrolled Diverse Populations*

Trial (year**, duration)	Findings
PREMIER (2000, 18 months) $N = 810$ Pre-HTN; HTN 34% AA; 62% female **Age (y):** 50 ± 9 **Weight (kg):** 96.9 Source: Svetkey et al. (2005)	Net weight loss (established Plus DASH group – control group): **Short-term (6 months)** **End of study (18 months)** AA(f): −2.4 kg [not reported by race] AA(m): −1.6 kg Non-AA(f): −4.8 kg Non-AA(m): −6.1 kg **Attendance:** similar across subgroups. **Comment:** weight loss occurred in the control arm of all subgroups and was largest for AA(m) and non-AA(f). Because of weight loss in the control arm, weight loss in the 0.5–1.9 kg in the active intervention was greater than net weight loss.
DPP†† (1996, 3.25 year average) $\bar{N} = 1079$ high risk for diabetes 19% AA; 17% Hisp; 6% Nat. Am.; 5% Asian/Pac. Isl.; 68% female **Age (y):** 51 ± 11 **Weight (kg):** 94.1 ± 20.8 Source: Wing et al. (2004)	% achieving weight loss goal (7% of baseline weight) in **Intensive Lifestyle Intervention** **Short-term (24 weeks)** **End of study (3.25 year average)** White: 57% White: 39% AA: 34% AA: 28% Hisp: 48% Hisp: 39% Nat. Am.: 36% Nat. Am.: 30% Asian/Pac. Isl.: 44% Asian/Pac. Isl.: 38% **Attendance:** not reported by subgroup. **Comment:** ethnicity was a significant factor in weight loss success with Caucasians more successful than other groups in short-term, despite Hisp, Asian/Pac. Isl., and Nat. Am. being more likely to meet exercise goal.

Table 2
(Continued)

Trial (year**, duration)	Findings
TONE[†] (1992, 15–36 months) N = 294 HTN controlled on 1 med. 29% black; 57% female **Age (y):** 65 (60–79) **Weight (kg):** 87.3 Source: Kumanyika et al. (2002)	**Net weight loss** **Short-term (6 months)** Black (f): −3.3 kg Black (m): −4.9 kg White (f): −4.1 kg White (m): −6.1 kg **End of study (average 30 months)** Black (f): −1.9 kg Black (m): insufficient data White (f): −3.8 kg White (m): −5.7 kg **% achieving weight loss goal (3.6 kg at 6 months or 4.5 kg overall):** 41% black; 66% white. **Attendance:** somewhat lower for blacks in first 4 months ($p = 0.02$) but similar when averaged over entire follow-up. Attendance did not explain ethnic differences in weight loss. **Comment:** whites lost ~ 3 kg more than blacks. Weight regain was somewhat greater in whites than in blacks after 6 months, but differences were not statistically significant.
TOHP-II[†] (1990, 36 months) N = 1191 Pre-HTN 18% black; 34% female **Age (y):** 43 ± 6 **Weight (kg):** 93.5 Source: Stevens et al. (2001)	**Net weight loss** **Short-term (6 months)** Black (f): −2.4 kg Black (m): −3.1 kg White (f): −3.8 kg White (m): −5.5 kg **End of study (36 months)** Black (f): −1.2 kg Black (m): −1.6 kg White (f): −0.6 kg White (m): −2.6 kg **Attendance:** no racial/ethnic differences reported. **Comment:** blacks experienced net weight loss of 1.8 kg less than whites at 6 and 18 months ($p = 0.01$, $p = 0.03$) but weight loss did not vary significantly ($p>0.2$) by race at 36 months. Control group participants (especially blacks) experienced weight gain, causing net weight loss to appear substantially larger than the weight loss achieved in active intervention group.

Table 2
(Continued)

Trial (year**, duration)	Findings	
TOHP-I† (1987, 18 months) $N = 564$ Pre-HTN no meds. 21% black; 32% female **Age (y):** 43 (30–54) **Weight (kg):** 89.8 Source: Kumanyika et al. (1991)	**Net weight loss** **Short-term (6 months)** Black (f): −2.1 kg Black (m): −5.4 kg White (f): −4.6 kg White (m): −6.5 kg **Attendance:** similar across subgroups. **Comment:** in terms of actual weight loss achieved, black women lost 2.2 kg less than their white counterparts (black men lost 2.0 kg less). Black women also regained the weight loss initially achieved by 18 months. While whites in the control group experienced slight weight loss (up to -0.5 kg), blacks in the control gained about 1 kg.	**End of study (18 months)** Black (f): −1.0 kg Black (m): −4.5 kg White (f): −2.0 kg White (m): −4.8 kg
HPT† (1983, 36 months) $N = 380$ Pre-HTN 20% black; 33% female **Age (y):** 39 (25–49) **Weight (kg):** 85.0 Source: Kumanyika et al. (1991)	**Net weight loss** **Short-term (6 months)** Black (f): −4.8 kg Black (m): −3.1 kg White (f): −4.7 kg White (m): −5.7 kg	**End of study (36 months)** Black (f): − 1.5 kg Black (m): − 1.5 kg White (f): −2.6 kg White (m): −3.4 kg

Table 2
(Continued)

Trial (year**, duration)	Findings
	Attendance: not reported by subgroup. **Comment:** weight gain occurred in control groups and was especially large for black females. Black females and males lost 2.7 and 1.4 kg less respectively compared to whites. Black females regained all weight loss by 18 months and were up 2.3 kg from baseline by 36 months. Race effects were clearly significant for both sexes in the short term but only remained so for females after the first year.

* Information presented is estimated from available data.

** First year of participant enrollment

† Data presented for control and weight loss participants only.

†† Data for DPP is for Intensive Lifestyle Intervention participants only.

African-American. Despite a substantially and significantly greater tendency to meet physical activity goals, blacks remained less successful in achieving weight loss compared to their white counterparts *(39)*. As displayed in Fig. 9, blacks were roughly 65% less likely than whites to achieve the 7% weight loss goal at the end of the 24 week core and 40% less likely to be successful by the end of the 3-year study.

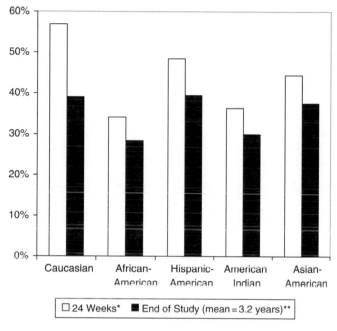

* p ≤ 0.0001 for difference in percent achieving weight-loss goal by race/ethnicity at 24 weeks.

** p = 0.11 for difference in percent achieving weight-loss goal by race/ethnicity at end of study.

Fig. 9. Percent of Diabetes Prevention Program intervention participants achieving 7% weight loss goal by race/ethnicity.
Source: Adapted from *(39)*.

The public health significance of racial disparities in weight loss as well as the potential for improved weight loss from culturally tailored interventions prompted researchers to develop and test such interventions in African-Americans.

5.2. Targeted, Culturally Adapted Weight Loss Interventions in African-Americans

Targeted interventions are generally developed based on information from all-black or racially mixed focus groups. Common adaptations include increased African-American representation among intervention staff, training local community members as interventionists, use of materials from print and broadcast media designed by and for African-Americans, cookbooks and diet plans that focus on healthier adaptations of ethnic foods, as well as efforts to integrate various aspects of the intervention into the individuals' daily life. Unfortunately, most trials that tested such interventions have been small in size; many were uncontrolled pilot studies (Table 3).

One of the largest and most rigorously conducted trials of a culturally adapted intervention was the Healthy Eating and Lifestyle Program (HELP) study. HELP tested a community-based, weight loss intervention that was specifically adapted for African-Americans. The weight loss achieved by the largely female African-American participants, though well maintained, was low. The average 1.5 kg weight loss was well below the 3–5 kg losses expected based on findings from similar programs in non-African-American population *(40)*.

Two additional studies have been conducted with notable success. The first is the Steps Study (Table 3) which had similar cultural adaptations, but had more social and interactive interventions. Women participating in this trial lost an average of 3.7 kg by the end of the 6-month study *(41)*. These results are comparable to those obtained in studies of non-African-Americans. BALI was another relatively successful targeted trial in which African-American women lost roughly 3 kg by the end of the 10-week intervention *(42)*. Both the BALI and the Steps studies achieved low program drop-out rates of only 10 and 5%, respectively.

5.3. Church and Faith-Based Targeted, Culturally Adapted Interventions

Church plays a particularly large role in African-American communities. Accordingly, several researchers have developed and tested church or faith-based lifestyle interventions *(43–45)*. These weight loss programs generally recruit through churches with predominantly black memberships, occur on church property, and are lead, at least in part, by trained church members.

The Baltimore Church High Blood Pressure Program (CHBPP), one of the earliest and largest faith-based interventions, enrolled 187 moderately overweight women (98% black) *(43)*. The study had an 8-week core and a 6-month follow-up after the intervention but no control group. Average weight loss achieved at the end of the core was 2–3% baseline weight (2.7 kg) with nearly 90% of participants losing weight. The attendance rate was 63%. Of the 41% of participants that provided 6-month data, 65% maintained or exceeded their initial weight loss. At 8 months, 95% of women with

Table 3
Weight Loss in Behavioral Intervention Studies that Focused on African-Americans (AA)*

Study (duration)	Cultural adaptations	Findings
HELP (21 month maximum)	• AA interventionists (4/9 staff members and PI)	**Weight loss**
Participants	• Logo-featured AA	**Short-term (4–5 months):**
Age (year): 25–70	• "Soul Food Pyramid" and other information on ethnic food choices and cooking styles	AA: −1.5 kg
Weight: 30 ≤ BMI ≤ 50		
Sex: Both (91% female)		**End of study (8–20 months):**
Other:	• Sister Talk, an AA-targeted cable weight loss program	AA: −1.2 kg
N = 237 (phase 1), 128 (phase 2)	• Interactive (partner/team focus)	**Other:** attendance was roughly 50% during Phase-1 and generally worse for Phase-2. No differences were observed by Phase-2 treatment group.
% Minorities: 100% AA		**Retention:** Phase-1, 57–80%; Phase-2, 68%.
Controlled: Phase-2 only		**Comment:** extent of weight loss was moderate but was well maintained throughout the study. This minimal regain was similar to that observed in TONE (the trial upon which HELP was based).
Source: Kumanyika et al. (2005)		

Table 3
(Continued)

Study (duration)	Cultural adaptations	Findings
Steps (6 months) **Participants** **Age (year):** 18+ (mean = 44) **Weight:** overweight (mean BMI =39) **Sex:** female $N = 66$ **% Minorities:** 100% AA **Controlled:** no Source: Karanja et al. (2002)	• All AA intervention team • Social support via 30–45 min socialization at start of session, group meals, and family involvement • Healthy adaptations of ethnic foods • Demonstration format • Increased program ownership • Interactive	**Weight loss** **Short-term (8 weeks):** **End of study (26 weeks):** AA(f): −1.5 kg (−1.3%) AA(f): −3.7 kg (−3.3%) **Other:** at roughly 60%, attendance was comparable to that seen in similar trials. Attendance was strongly related to weight loss: those who had attendance rates of at least 75% achieved an average −6.2 kg weight loss while those attending fewer than 75% of sessions lost only −0.9 kg. **Retention:** 95%. **Comment:** steps participants appeared to have lost more weight than AA women in other trials. Study authors attribute Steps' success to cultural adaptation in program.

Table 3
(Continued)

Study (duration)	Cultural adaptations	Findings
BALI – pilot (10 weeks) **Participants** **Age (year):** 40–64 **Weight:** $30 \leq BMI \leq 40$ **Sex:** female **Other:** earned \$1000–\$5000 per month $N = 67$ **% Minorities:** 100% AA **Controlled:** no	• Led by AA(f) nutritionist • All educational materials, recipes, and menu plans reviewed by minority advisors to ensure cultural appropriateness • Based on 1991 interview of 195 obese AA women	**Weight loss:** **Short-term/End of study (10 weeks):** AA(f): -2.95 kg (-3.5% baseline weight) **Other:** Attendance high at over 80%. **Retention:** 90%. **Comment:** weight loss achieved is better than that generally seen for minorities in similar programs. Attendance was high. The drop-out rate (attended 6 of 10 sessions) of only 10% was lower than in other minority intervention programs which had reported drop-out rates of 23–80%.

Source: Knaders et al. (1994)

Table 3
(Continued)

Study (duration)	Cultural adaptations	Findings
PATHWAYS (14 weeks) **Participants** **Age (year):** mean = 57 **Weight:** $30 \leq BMI \leq 45$ **Sex:** female **Other:** members of urban AA churches $N = 39$ **% Minorities:** 100% AA **Controlled:** yes Source: McNabb et al. (1997)	• AA Church-based • Emphasizes ethnic foods • Encourages weight loss, not "slenderness" • Lay facilitators – trained church member volunteers • Interactive • Discovery learning	**Net weight loss:** **Short-term/End of study (14 weeks):** AA(f): $-5.4\,kg$ **Other:** average weight loss among intervention participants was $-4.5\,kg$ (5% baseline weight) while members of the control gained 0.9 kg. Attendance was 71%. **Retention:** 85%. **Comment:** this intervention was particularly successful as AA women achieved higher than usual weight loss (on par with Caucasians in similar studies). The $-5.4\,kg$ average net weight loss represents a conservative estimate as control drop-outs were assigned no weight change and intervention drop-outs were attributed a 0.9 kg gain. The PATHWAYS program proved similarly successful in a previous church pilot as well as in the clinical setting where it was originally implemented.

Table 3
(Continued)

Study (duration)	Cultural adaptations	Findings
Lose Weight and Win (8 months) **Participants** **Age (year):** 18–81 **Weight:** moderate-severe overweight (at least 10–100% above ideal weight) **Sex:** female (men chose not to join) **Other:** HTN or at risk for HTN $N = 187$ **% Minorities:** 98% AA **Controlled:** no Source: Kumanyika and Charleston (1992)	• Church based • Social support	**Weight loss:** **Short-term (8 weeks):** AA(f): −2.7 kg (2–3%) **End of study (8 months):** AA(f): 65% maintained or exceeded 8-week weight loss **Other:** 53% completed the 8-week weight loss program. Almost 90% of the women lost weight at the end of the 8 week weight loss intervention. However, 95% of women in the 8 month follow-up sample lost 1 kg or less from baseline **Retention:** 41%. **Comment:** the intervention successfully induced modest weight loss in most participants.

Table 3
(Continued)

Study (duration)	Cultural adaptations	Findings
Faith on the Move (12 weeks) **Participants** **Age (year):** 21+ **Weight:** BMI $\geq$ 25 **Sex:** female **Other:** $N = 52$ **% Minorities:** 100% AA **Controlled:** no Source: Fitzgibbon et al. (2005)	• "Culturally appropriate" materials • Emphasis on family and social support • Faith-based intervention arm which included weekly scripture readings and "addressed faith/spirituality issues in a structured and systematic manner"	**Weight loss** **Short-term (12 weeks):** AA(f): • faith-based: $-2.6\,\mathrm{kg}$ (2.4%) with 78% of participants losing weight • comparison: $-1.6\,\mathrm{kg}$ (1.7%) with 61% of participants losing weight **Other:** **Retention:** uncertain **Comment:** though study findings suggest inclusion of a faith-based component positively impacts weight loss success, differences between the two intervention arms were not statistically significant

*Information presented is estimated from available data.

the follow-up data achieved only 0.9 kg weight loss or less. Another small, uncontrolled pilot study of 40 black overweight adult church members in Baton Rouge, LA, had a substantially better retention rate –95% of those starting the program provided follow-up data *(46)*. Results were somewhat more promising than those seen in CHBPP, as participants lost and maintained an average of 3.3 kg over the 6-month study period.

In PATHWAYS, a 14-week church-based trial of 39 obese African-American women, data are especially promising *(44)*. The PATHWAYS program focused on gradual calorie reduction, incorporation of less fat and more fiber, moderate exercise, and behavioral modification in weekly meetings. Cultural adaptations included encouraging weight loss but not "slenderness" while emphasizing ethnic foods. Attendance rates were roughly 70% and retention was 85%. At 14 weeks, program participants lost an average of 4.5 kg (5% baseline weight), while those in the control group gained 1.9 kg during the same period.

In aggregate, faith- and church-based weight loss programs provide some evidence that targeted, culturally adapted interventions can be successful. However, design limitations including small sample size, incomplete outcome ascertainment, short intervention duration, and lack of control groups hinder the interpretation and generalizable study findings.

5.4. Possible Reasons for Differences in Weight Loss Among Black and White Women

This section highlights potential reasons for the high prevalence of excess in weight in African-Americans and for the differential weight loss experience of African-Americans in weight loss programs (see Table 4).

Table 4
Possible Reasons for Weight Differences between Black and White Women

Environmental/Behavioral/Psychosocial Differences
Increased caloric intake
Suboptimal diet (low fiber, high fat, and high fast food)
Reduced physical activity
Body image perception and satisfaction
Socioeconomic factors
Genetic/Physiological Differences
Lower resting metabolic rate

5.4.1. MODIFIABLE BEHAVIORAL DIFFERENCES

In general, diet and exercise patterns are less favorable among African-American women compared to their Caucasian counterparts. Black females consume more calories, fat, and fast food *(47)*, as well as less fiber *(48)* than do whites. Additionally, leisure-time inactivity is twice as prevalent among blacks versus whites *(49,50)*.

Some of the differences in diet and exercise patterns and thus weight loss success may be attributable to differences in socioeconomic status (SES) and cultural norms *(51)*. The most commonly examined indicators of SES are education, income, occupation, and neighborhood. Though education is inversely related to BMI in white women, education and BMI appear unrelated among blacks *(52)*. Education moderates but does not eliminate racial/ethnic differences in leisure-time physical activity *(50)*. Education generally fails to account for the racial/ethnic discrepancy in weight loss success *(53)*. Income is inversely related to leisure-time inactivity for both black and white women *(50)*. Those who earn less are more likely to live in less safe neighborhoods which effectively discourage walking. Furthermore, low-income individuals have less money to spend on gym memberships, transportation, and childcare *(54)*. Still, accounting for income moderates but does not eliminate racial/ethnic differences in physical activity *(49,50)*. Income also likely influences dietary choices as healthier food, particularly pre-prepared, often costs more than less healthy fast-food options.

Several studies suggest cultural differences in body image and ideals may account for some racial/ethnic discrepancy in weight and weight loss success *(55)*. Such studies ask individuals to comment on silhouettes of body images. Though black and white perceptions of weight and body width appear equally accurate, the labels blacks used to describe silhouettes were "thinner" than those used by whites for the same images. Black girls and women were more likely to describe themselves as thin or normal weight than white females of similar body sizes. However, while the black female ideal weight is greater than that of white women, it still falls within the normal weight category. Overweight black girls were also more likely to consider themselves attractive and socially accepted than whites *(55)*. Open-ended in-depth interviews with 24 rural African-American women performed by Baturka et al. *(54)* indicated a strong cultural pressure toward self-acceptance of physical shape: the women emphasized a need to be "happy with what God gave you" and to make the most of one's appearance, particularly with clothes.

The extent to which differences in body image perception and satisfaction are due to differences in SES is unclear. Caldwell's 1997 study *(56)* of middle to upper class women found no significant differences in body image ideals and satisfaction by race. However, other studies report that accounting for SES only partially attenuates this racial discrepancy. Overall, studies suggest weight loss interventions with African-American women need to focus on health benefits rather than body image. For example, Annesi's *(57)* 20-week diet and exercise weight loss intervention found that while Body Area Satisfaction scores contributed significantly to and were the primary predictor of weight loss among white women, they played no such role among African-American women. Rather, only Exercise Self-Efficacy Scale scores appeared to make a significant contribution to and serve as a primary predictor for weight loss.

5.4.2. PHYSIOLOGICAL DIFFERENCES

A growing body of research cites physical differences in energy expenditure as a cause of racial/ethnic differences. While the existence of racial/ethnic differences in energy expenditure during exercise remains controversial, the literature strongly suggests that differences in resting metabolic rate (RMR) may help explain racial disparities in weight loss trials *(58–61)*. In a review by Gannon (2000), 10 of 15 studies documented that African-Americans have a RMR of 81–274 kcal/day less than their Caucasian counterparts *(61)*. A significant race–sex interaction suggests this lower RMR is particularly problematic for black women. This racial discrepancy in RMR was not explained by age, body composition, or methodological concerns *(61)*. This differential in RMR, if true, implies that black women must, on average, achieve a greater calorie deficit and hence must receive a more intense intervention in order to achieve weight loss similar to their white counterparts.

Some evidence refuting the idea of an inherent racial difference in ability to achieve weight loss comes from a study by Hong et al. *(62)*. The study examines 304 overweight women aged 18–65, matching black and white participants for age, BMI, and metabolic syndrome status. The 12-week highly structured program includes a very low calorie diet (VLCD) of 500–800 kcal/day utilizing liquid meal replacement. The total weight loss achieved by week 12 was similar in blacks (20.9 kg) and whites (23.0 kg) – see Fig. 10. Importantly, the study did not report average daily calorie levels by race. Thus, it is possible that black women had to restrict their diets more than whites to attain the same results.

6. EFFECTS OF BEHAVIORAL WEIGHT LOSS INTERVENTIONS IN OTHER RACIAL/ETHNIC MINORITY POPULATIONS

Despite the high prevalence of overweight and obesity among all racial/ethnic minorities, there is a paucity of research on weight loss interventions in racial/ethnic groups in the United States other than blacks/African-Americans.

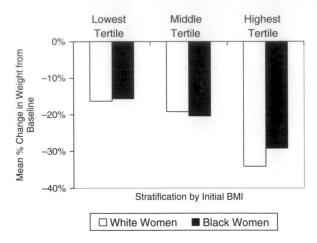

Fig. 10. Weight loss at 12 weeks in white and black women participants in a Structured Weight Loss Program at UCLA Obesity Center.
Source: Adapted from *(62)*.

6.1. Hispanic Americans

To date, the only multi-ethnic trial that reported racial/ethnic group-specific findings was the Diabetes Prevention Project *(63)*. Findings from this trial (displayed in Fig. 9) suggest that Hispanics were somewhat less likely to meet weight loss goals than whites but more likely than African-Americans. However, the difference attenuated over time.

The medical literature reports few trials that tested targeted, culturally adapted interventions in Hispanics. Our sense, based on conversations with researchers, is that the dearth of published studies reflects publication bias. Specifically, completed but unpublished studies were likely to have disappointing results. One published trial tested the effects of including a family component in a weight loss intervention that targeted Mexican American mothers *(64)*. Mexican American culture emphasizes the importance of family unity. However, while the family-oriented intervention arm achieved somewhat greater weight loss than the individual-oriented intervention, the difference was not significant. Retention was low, and only 51% of participants provided follow-up data at each of the four measurement points *(64)*.

Another culturally adapted weight loss intervention for Latinas (Table 5) focused on physical activity. By the end of the 3-month study, net weight loss was nearly 6 kg. However, this study also had problems with retention; only 45% of participants provided follow-up data *(65)*.

6.2. Asian Pacific Islanders/Native Hawaiians

Published data on weight and weight loss interventions in Asian/Pacific Islanders and Native Hawaiians are likewise sparse (Table 5). Survey data,

Table 5

Weight Loss in Behavioral Intervention Studies that Focused on Minority Populations Other than African-Americans

Study (duration)	Cultural adaptations	Findings
		Hispanic
Cousins, 1992 (12 months)	• Bilingual	**Net weight loss**
Participants	• Cookbook with low-fat	**Short-term (3 months):** **End of study (12 months):**
Age (year): 18–45	modifications of traditional	MA(f): MA(f):
Weight: 20–100% above ideal	Mexican foods	• individual: −1.5 kg • individual: −1.4 kg
weight	• One family-oriented	• family oriented: −2.1 kg • family oriented: −2.1 kg
Sex: female	intervention arm	**Other:** an average weight loss of −0.9 and −0.7 kg was seen in
Other: healthy; married; at least		the control group at 3 and 12 months, respectively; thus, actual
1 pre-school-aged child		weight loss achieved was significantly larger than the net values
$N = 168$		presented above.
% Minorities: 100% Mexican		**Retention:** analysis includes only the 51% (86 participants) who
American		provided data at all four measurement points (baseline, 3, 6, and
Controlled: yes		12 months).
		Comment: both treatment groups lost significantly more than the
Source: Cousins et al. (1992)		control. Though the family-oriented group achieved greater
		weight loss than those in the individually-oriented arm,
		differences were not statistically significant.

Table 5
(Continued)

Study (duration)	Cultural adaptations	Findings
Avila, 1994 (10 weeks) **Participants** **Age (year):** 18+ **Weight:** ≥ 20% overweight (MetLife) **Sex:** female $N = 44$ **% Minorities:** 100% Hisp. **Controlled:** yes Source: Avila and Hovell (1994)	• Bilingual • Instructed by a bi-cultural Spanish speaking doctor • Buddy system	**Net weight loss:** **Short-term (10 weeks):** **End of study (3 months post-training):** Hisp(f): −3.2 kg Hisp(f): −5.7 kg **Other:** exercise rate increased in intervention group from 0.049 to 0.076 miles/minute while control group rates remained constant at 0.048. **Retention:** only 45% returned for follow-up at 3 months post-training. **Comment:** with a net change in BMI of −3.7, study authors cite this as one of few published interventions to demonstrate "therapeutic effectiveness" of diet/exercise programs in US Latinas.

Table 5
(Continued)

Study (duration)	Cultural adaptations	Findings
	Asian Pacific Islanders/Native Hawaiians	
Waianae Diet Program (34 month average) **Participants** **Age (year):** 24–64 **Weight:** obese, BMI ≥ 27 (120 kg) **Sex:** Both **Other:** $N = 173$ **% Minorities:** 100% Native Hawaiians **Controlled:** No Sources: Shintani et al. (1991); Shintani et al. (1999)	• Traditional foods (pre-Western contact Hawaiian diet) • Community wide fed meals and pot-lucks	**Net weight loss:** **Short-term (21 days):** **End of study (34 months average):** Native Hawaiian: −6.3 kg Native Hawaiian: −6.9 kg **Other:** short-term (21 day) weight loss reported is that of those who provided long-term follow-up data; however it is similar to or less than short-term weight losses reported for entire cohorts (e.g., −7.8 kg). **Retention:** 47.4% of eligible participants provided long-term follow-up data. **Comment:** this intervention achieved statistically significant and clinically meaningful weight loss (6–8 kg or 6–7% baseline weight) which appears well maintained or even increased over several years in those providing long-term follow-up. Weight loss was generally achieved by reducing average daily energy intake by about 41% while participants continued to report high levels of satiety.

Table 5
(Continued)

Study (duration)	Cultural adaptations	Findings
Samoan Church, NZ (2 years) **Participants** **Age (year):** 20+ (20–77) **Weight:** no restrictions (average = 94 kg) **Sex:** both **Other:** member of selected churches $N = 471$ **% Minorities:** 100% Samoan (API) **Controlled:** yes Source: Bell et al. (2001)	• Bilingual • Church based • Inclusion of "culturally appropriate" and traditional foods • Whole family and community sessions • Church wide meals	**Weight loss: actual (net)** **Short-term (1 year):** **End of study (2 years):** Samoan: −0.4 kg (-1.7 kg) Samoan: −0.2 kg **Other:** Actual 1-year weight loss achieved by those providing 2-year follow-up data was larger than average at 1.0 kg. **Retention:** 66% of participants provided post-intervention 1-year follow-up data; 25% provided post-maintenance 2-year follow-up data. Participants lost to follow-up were younger, less obese, and better educated. **Comment:** study limitations include a "quasi-experimental," non-blinded, and non-randomized design. The minimal weight-loss initially achieved was largely regained by the end of the maintenance year and accompanied a shift toward less healthy lifestyle choices regarding dietary fat and exercise.

Table 5
(Continued)

Study (duration)	Cultural adaptations	Findings

W. Samoan Church, NZ-pilot (2 years)
Participants
Age (year): (14–102)
Weight: (average:
  control = 87.7 kg,
  intervention = 83.6 kg)
Sex: both
Other: member of selected
  churches
N = 182
% Minorities: 100% Western
  Samoan
Controlled: yes
 	
Source: Simmons et al. (1998)
	• Samoan interventionists
	• Bilingual
	• Materials made specifically for
	  Pacific Islanders
	• Church based
		Net weight loss:
		End of study (2 years):
		Samoan: −3.1 kg
		Other: no actual weight loss was achieved; however, intervention participants increased physical activity and significantly reduced reported fat intake.
		Retention: 75% of intervention members and 80% of controls provided 2 year follow-up data.
		Comment: study limitations include a "quasi-experimental," non-blinded, and non-randomized design. Though no actual weight loss was achieved, intervention participants maintained a steady weight while their control counterparts gained roughly 3 kg. Intervention members also improved diet and exercise behaviors.

* Information presented is estimated from available data.

albeit limited, suggests that certain Asian/Pacific Islander groups (such as Samoans in New Zealand) and Native Hawaiians have an extremely high prevalence of overweight and obesity *(66)*. Data from the Diabetes Prevention Program suggest that Asian/Pacific Islanders experience less weight loss success than whites *(63)* (see Fig. 9). A few non-randomized intervention studies in Samoans had limited success (Table 5) *(67,68)*.

In contrast, the Waianae Diet Program *(69,70)* reported high levels of success at achieving and maintaining weight loss long term in Native Hawaiians. The program encouraged participants to eat to satiety while maintaining a diet of ethnic whole foods with limited amounts of chicken and fish.

6.3. Native Americans/American Indians

Despite the high prevalence of overweight and obesity in Native Americans *(9,10)*, remarkably few trials have been conducted in these populations. Data from the Diabetes Prevention Program suggest that despite being more likely to meet physical activity targets, Native Americans were less successful in achieving weight loss goals than whites (Fig. 9). A few trials developed and tested targeted interventions for Native American populations. The Zuni Diabetes Project is one such study; however, the presentation of data hinders interpretation of trial results *(71,72)*.

Some school-based, culturally adapted interventions among Native American children and adolescents have also been conducted but with limited success. Pathways, the most recent and largest of these studies, was a controlled trial that followed nearly 2000 second graders over 3 years *(73)*. Though intervention participants successfully reduced fat intake and increased health knowledge relative to members of the control group, the intervention had no effect on anthropomorphic measurements. Members of both the intervention and the control groups experienced a 7% increase in percent body fat over the 3-year study period.

"Growing Healthy" *(9)*, a year-long school-based initiative among Native Americans aged 4–13 years old, provided slightly more promising results. Compared to 176 non-participants, the 130 program participants "gained weight more slowly", that is, their BMI increased only $0.42 \, \text{kg/m}^2$ during the school year, while their non-participant peers experienced a $0.97 \, \text{kg/m}^2$ gain. However, the difference was somewhat attenuated because during the summer months, BMI rose by $0.94 \, \text{kg/m}^2$ among program participants compared to only $0.70 \, \text{kg/m}^2$ among non-participants.

7. CONCLUSIONS

The problem of excess weight in minority populations is a public health crisis. In clinical trials, African-Americans, particularly women, achieve less weight loss than Caucasians. Despite their conceptual appeal, culturally adapted intervention programs that target African-Americans have likewise had mixed results. Explanations for the limited success of weight loss programs in African-Americans include social–cultural–environmental factors as well as physiologic factors; indeed, a rather consistent body of evidence suggests that African-American women have lower resting energy expenditure than Caucasian women. The dearth of weight loss studies in Hispanic Americans, Native Americans, and Native Hawaiian/Pacific Islander populations is striking. The magnitude of the obesity epidemic in combination with the lack of effective interventions in minority populations argues strongly for additional research.

REFERENCES

1. Wang Y, Wang QJ. The prevalence of prehypertension and hypertension among US adults according to the new joint national committee guidelines: New challenges of the old problem. *Arch Intern Med* 2004; 164:2126–2134.
2. Appel LJ. At the tipping point: accomplishing population-wide sodium reduction in the United States. *J Clin Hypertens (Greenwich)* 2008; 10:7–11.
3. Vasan RS, Beiser A, Seshadri S, et al. Residual lifetime risk for developing hypertension in middle-aged women and men: The Framingham Heart Study. *JAMA* 2002; 287: 1003–1010.
4. Appel LJ, Brands MW, Daniels SR, et al. Dietary approaches to prevent and treat hypertension: a scientific statement from the American Heart Association. *Hypertension* 2006; 47:296–308.
5. Dietary Guidelines Advisory Committee. 2005 Report of the Dietary Guidelines Advisory Committee on the Dietary Guidelines for Americans. US Department of Agriculture, Agricultural Research Service; 2005.
6. Ogden CL, Carroll MD, Curtin LR, McDowell MA, Tabak CJ, Flegal KM. Prevalence of overweight and obesity in the united states, 1999-2004. *JAMA* 2006; 295:1549–1555.
7. Allison DB, Fontaine KR, Manson JE, Stevens J, VanItallie TB. Annual deaths attributable to obesity in the United States. *JAMA* 1999; 282:1530–1538.
8. Hedley AA, Ogden CL, Johnson CL, Carroll MD, Curtin LR, Flegal KM. Prevalence of overweight and obesity among US children, adolescents, and adults, 1999-2002. *JAMA* 2004; 291:2847–2850.
9. Broussard BA, Sugarman JR, Bachman-Carter K, et al. Toward comprehensive obesity prevention programs in native American communities. *Obes Res* 1995; 3(Suppl 2): 289s–297s.
10. Wang Y, Beydoun MA. The obesity epidemic in the United States–gender, age, socioeconomic, racial/ethnic, and geographic characteristics: a systematic review and meta-regression analysis. *Epidemiol Rev* 2007; 29:6–28.
11. Kannel WB, Brand N, Skinner JJ, Jr, Dawber TR, McNamara PM. The relation of adiposity to blood pressure and development of hypertension. The Framingham Study. *Ann Intern Med* 1967; 67:48–59.
12. Field AE, Coakley EH, Must A, et al. Impact of overweight on the risk of developing common chronic diseases during a 10-year period. *Arch Intern Med* 2001; 161: 1581–1586.
13. Juhaeri J, Stevens J, Chambless LE, et al. Associations of weight loss and changes in fat distribution with the remission of hypertension in a bi-ethnic cohort: Atherosclerosis Risk in Communities. *Prev Med* 2003; 36:330–339.

14. Wadden TA, Butryn ML, Wilson C. Lifestyle modification for the management of obesity. *Gastroenterology* 2007; 132:2226–2238.
15. Ledikwe JH, Rolls BJ, Smiciklas-Wright H, et al. Reductions in dietary energy density are associated with weight loss in overweight and obese participants in the PREMIER trial. *Am J Clin Nutr* 2007; 85:1212–1221.
16. Hill JO, Wyatt H, Phelan S, Wing R. The national weight control registry: is it useful in helping deal with our obesity epidemic? *J Nutr Educ Behav* 2005; 37:206–210.
17. Raynor DA, Phelan S, Hill JO, Wing RR. Television viewing and long-term weight maintenance: results from the national weight control registry. *Obesity (Silver Spring)* 2006; 14:1816–1824.
18. Neter JE, Stam BE, Kok FJ, Grobbee DE, Geleijnse JM. Influence of weight reduction on blood pressure: a meta-analysis of randomized controlled trials. *Hypertension* 2003; 42:878–884.
19. Stevens VJ, Corrigan SA, Obarzanek E, et al. Weight loss intervention in phase 1 of the trials of hypertension prevention. The TOHP Collaborative Research Group. *Arch Intern Med* 1993; 153:849–858.
20. Whelton PK, Appel LJ, Espeland MA, et al. Sodium reduction and weight loss in the treatment of hypertension in older persons: a randomized controlled trial of nonpharmacologic interventions in the elderly (TONE). TONE Collaborative Research Group. *JAMA* 1998; 279:839–846. Available from: PM: 9515998.
21. Kumanyika S. Obesity treatment in minorities. In: Wadden TA, Stunkard AJ, ed. Handbook of Obesity Treatment. New York: The Guilford Press; 2002:416–446.
22. Knowler WC, Barrett-Connor E, Fowler SE, et al. Reduction in the incidence of type 2 diabetes with lifestyle intervention or metformin. *N Engl J Med* 2002; 346:393–403.
23. Effects of weight loss and sodium reduction intervention on blood pressure and hypertension incidence in overweight people with high-normal blood pressure. the trials of hypertension prevention, phase II. The trials of hypertension prevention collaborative research group. *Arch Intern Med* 1997; 157:657–667.
24. National Institutes of Health. NHLBI clinical guidelines on the identification, evaluation, and treatment of overweight and obesity in adults, executive summary. U.S. Department of Health and Human Services; 1998.
25. Stevens VJ, Obarzanek E, Cook NR, et al. Long-term weight loss and changes in blood pressure: results of the trials of hypertension prevention, phase II. *Ann Intern Med* 2001; 134:1–11.
26. Stamler R. Implications of the INTERSALT study. *Hypertension* 1991; 17:I16–I20.
27. Cook NR, Cohen J, Hebert PR, Taylor JO, Hennekens CH. Implications of small reductions in diastolic blood pressure for primary prevention. *Arch Intern Med* 1995; 155:701–709.
28. Trails of Hypertension Prevention Collaborative Research Group. The effects of nonpharmacologic interventions on blood pressure of persons with high normal levels. Results of the trials of hypertension prevention, phase I. *JAMA* 1992; 267:1213–1220.
29. Jeffery RW, Drewnowski A, Epstein LH, et al. Long-term maintenance of weight loss: current status. *Health Psychol* 2000; 19:5–16.
30. Hamm P, Shekelle RB, Stamler J. Large fluctuations in body weight during young adulthood and twenty-five-year risk of coronary death in men. *Am J Epidemiol* 1989; 129:312–318.
31. Blair SN, Shaten J, Brownell K, Collins G, Lissner L. Body weight change, all-cause mortality, and cause-specific mortality in the multiple risk factor intervention trial. *Ann Intern Med* 1993; 119:749–757.
32. Field AE, Byers T, Hunter DJ, et al. Weight cycling, weight gain, and risk of hypertension in women. *Am J Epidemiol* 1999; 150:573–579.

33. Wing RR, Jeffery RW, Hellerstedt WL. A prospective study of effects of weight cycling on cardiovascular risk factors. *Arch Intern Med* 1995; 155:1416–1422.

34. Vollmer WM, Sacks FM, Ard J, et al. Effects of diet and sodium intake on blood pressure: subgroup analysis of the DASH-sodium trial. *Ann Intern Med* 2001; 135:1019–1028.

35. Kumanyika SK, Obarzanek E, Stevens VJ, Hebert PR, Whelton PK. Weight-loss experience of black and white participants in NHLBI-sponsored clinical trials. *Am J Clin Nutr* 1991; 53:1631S–1638S.

36. Svetkey LP, Erlinger TP, Vollmer WM, et al. Effect of lifestyle modifications on blood pressure by race, sex, hypertension status, and age. *J Hum Hypertens* 2005; 19:21–31.

37. Whelton PK, Babnson J, Appel LJ, et al. Recruitment in the trial of nonpharmacologic intervention in the elderly (TONE). *J Am Geriatr Soc* 1997; 45:185–193.

38. Kumanyika SK, Espeland MA, Bahnson JL, et al. Ethnic comparison of weight loss in the trial of nonpharmacologic interventions in the elderly. *Obes Res* 2002; 10:96–106.

39. Wing RR, Hamman RF, Bray GA, et al. Achieving weight and activity goals among diabetes prevention program lifestyle participants. *Obes Res* 2004; 12:1426–1434.

40. Kumanyika SK, Shults J, Fassbender J, et al. Outpatient weight management in African-Americans: The Healthy Eating and Lifestyle Program (HELP) Study. *Prev Med* 2005; 41:488–502.

41. Karanja N, Stevens VJ, Hollis JF, Kumanyika SK. Steps to soulful living (steps): a weight loss program for African-American women. *Ethn Dis* 2002; 12:363–371.

42. Kanders BS, Ullmann-Joy P, Foreyt JP, et al. The black American lifestyle intervention (BALI): the design of a weight loss program for working-class African-American women. *J Am Diet Assoc* 1994; 94:310–312.

43. Kumanyika SK, Charleston JB. Lose weight and win: a church-based weight loss program for blood pressure control among black women. *Patient Educ Couns* 1992; 19:19–32.

44. McNabb W, Quinn M, Kerver J, Cook S, Karrison T. The PATHWAYS church based weight loss program for urban African-American women at risk for diabetes. *Diabetes Care* 1997; 20:1518–1523.

45. Fitzgibbon ML, Stolley MR, Ganschow P, et al. Results of a faith-based weight loss intervention for black women. *J Natl Med Assoc* 2005; 97:1393–1402.

46. Kennedy BM, Paeratakul S, Champagne CM, et al. A pilot church-based weight loss program for African-American adults using church members as health educators: a comparison of individual and group intervention. *Ethn Dis* 2005; 15:373–378.

47. Schmidt M, Affenito SG, Striegel Moore R, et al. Fast food intake and diet quality in black and white girls: The National Heart, Lung, and Blood Institute Growth and Health Study. *Arch Pediatr Adolesc Med* 2005; 159:626–631.

48. Lovejoy JC, Champagne CM, Smith SR, de Jonge L, Xie H. Ethnic differences in dietary intakes, physical activity, and energy expenditure in middle-aged, premenopausal women: The Healthy Transitions Study. *Am J Clin Nutr* 2001; 74:90–95.

49. Crespo CJ, Smit E, Andersen RE, Carter-Pokras O, Ainsworth BE. Race/ethnicity, social class and their relation to physical inactivity during leisure time: Results from the third national health and nutrition examination survey, 1988-1994. *Am J Prev Med* 2000; 18:46–53.

50. Marshall SJ, Jones DA, Ainsworth BE, Reis JP, Levy SS, Macera CA. Race/ethnicity, social class, and leisure-time physical inactivity. *Med Sci Sports Exerc* 2007; 39:44–51.

51. Tuten C, Petosa R, Sargent R, Weston A. Biracial differences in physical activity and body composition among women. *Obes Res* 1995; 3:313–318.

52. Lewis TT, Everson-Rose SA, Sternfeld B, Karavolos K, Wesley D, Powell LH. Race, education, and weight change in a biracial sample of women at midlife. *Arch Intern Med* 2005; 165:545–551.
53. Kumanyika S, Adams-Campbell LL. Obesity, diet, and psychosocial factors contributing to cardiovascular disease in blacks. *Cardiovasc Clin* 1991; 21:47–73.
54. Baturka N, Hornsby PP, Schorling JB. Clinical implications of body image among rural African-American women. *J Gen Intern Med* 2000; 15:235–241.
55. Padgett J, Biro FM. Different shapes in different cultures: body dissatisfaction, overweight, and obesity in African-American and Caucasian females. *J Pediatr Adolesc Gynecol* 2003; 16:349–354.
56. Caldwell MB, Brownell KD, Wilfley DE. Relationship of weight, body dissatisfaction, and self-esteem in African American and white female dieters. *Int J Eat Disord* 1997; 22:127–130.
57. Annesi JJ. Relations of changes in exercise self-efficacy, physical self-concept, and body satisfaction with weight changes in obese white and African American women initiating a physical activity program. *Ethn Dis* 2007; 17:19–22.
58. Jakicic JM, Wing RR. Differences in resting energy expenditure in African-American vs Caucasian overweight females. *Int J Obes Relat Metab Disord* 1998; 22: 236–242.
59. Jakicic JM, Lang W, Wing RR. Do African-American and Caucasian overweight women differ in oxygen consumption during fixed periods of exercise? *Int J Obes Relat Metab Disord* 2001; 25:949–953.
60. Weinsier RL, Hunter GR, Zuckerman PA, et al. Energy expenditure and free-living physical activity in black and white women: comparison before and after weight loss. *Am J Clin Nutr* 2000; 71:1138–1146.
61. Gannon B, DiPietro L, Poehlman ET. Do African Americans have lower energy expenditure than Caucasians? *Int J Obes Relat Metab Disord* 2000; 24:4–13.
62. Hong K, Li Z, Wang HJ, Elashoff R, Heber D. Analysis of weight loss outcomes using VLCD in black and white overweight and obese women with and without metabolic syndrome. *Int J Obes (Lond)* 2005; 29:436–442.
63. Wing RR. Behavioral weight control. In: Wadden TA, Stunkard AJ, ed. Handbook of Obesity Treatment. New York: Guilford Press; 2002:301–16.
64. Cousins JH, Rubovits DS, Dunn JK, Reeves RS, Ramirez AG, Foreyt JP. Family versus individually oriented intervention for weight loss in Mexican American women. *Public Health Rep* 1992; 107:549–555.
65. Avila P, Hovell MF. Physical activity training for weight loss in Latinas: a controlled trial. *Int J Obes Relat Metab Disord* 1994;18:476–482.
66. Davis J, Busch J, Hammatt Z, et al. The relationship between ethnicity and obesity in Asian and Pacific Islander populations: a literature review. *Ethn Dis* 2004; 14: 111–118.
67. Simmons D, Fleming C, Voyle J, Fou F, Feo S, Gatland B. A pilot urban church-based programme to reduce risk factors for diabetes among western Samoans in New Zealand. *Diabet Med* 1998;15:136–142.
68. Bell AC, Swinburn BA, Amosa H, Scragg RK. A nutrition and exercise intervention program for controlling weight in Samoan communities in New Zealand. *Int J Obes Relat Metab Disord* 2001; 25:920–927.
69. Shintani TT, Hughes CK, Beckham S, O'Connor HK. Obesity and cardiovascular risk intervention through the ad libitum feeding of traditional Hawaiian diet. *Am J Clin Nutr* 1991; 53:1647S–1651S.
70. Shintani T, Beckham S, Tang J, O'Connor HK, Hughes C. Waianae diet program: long-term follow-up. *Hawaii Med J* 1999; 58:117–122.

71. Heath GW, Leonard BE, Wilson RH, Kendrick JS, Powell KE. Community-based exercise intervention: Zuni diabetes project. *Diabet Care* 1987; 10:579–583.
72. Heath GW, Wilson RH, Smith J, Leonard BE. Community-based exercise and weight control: diabetes risk reduction and glycemic control in Zuni Indians. *Am J Clin Nutr* 1991; 53:1642S–1646S.
73. Caballero B, Clay T, Davis SM, et al. Pathways: a school-based, randomized controlled trial for the prevention of obesity in American Indian schoolchildren. *Am J Clin Nutr* 2003; 78:1030–1038.

10 Obesity and the Cardiometabolic Syndrome: Impact on Chronic Kidney Disease and CVD

Abrar Ahmed, MD,
Guido Lastra, MD,
Camila Manrique, MD, *and*
James R. Sowers, MD

CONTENTS

From: *Contemporary Cardiology: Cardiovascular Disease in Racial and Ethnic Minorities*
Edited by: K.C. Ferdinand and A. Armani, DOI 10.1007/978-1-59745-410-0_10
© Humana Press, a part of Springer Science+Business Media, LLC 2009

Abstract

The prevalence of the cardiometabolic syndrome (CMS), a cluster of car-diovascular disease (CVD) risk factors which include central obesity, dysg-lycemia, atherogenic dyslipidemia, hypertension (hypertension), and microal-buminuria (MAU), has increased. Obesity largely drives the dramatic increase in the incidence and prevalence of the CMS worldwide. Recently there has been increasing interest in the association between CMS, obesity, and chronic kidney disease (CKD), which is multifactorial and includes genetic as well as environ-mental factors. Obesity, hypertension, and dysglycemia are strongly associated with a systemic chronic low-grade inflammation, inappropriate activation of the renin–angiotensin–aldosterone system (RAAS), and increased oxidative stress. The link between RAAS activation and oxidative stress has been a subject of great interest over the past several years.

African-Americans have a greater prevalence of other cardiovascular risk fac-tors, especially obesity and hypertension. There is a question as to whether race or ethnicity should be a significant consideration in the choice of individual antihypertensive drugs, specifically for monotherapy or the use of combination antihypertensive drug therapy. Microalbuminuria is currently recognized as an independent risk factor for progressive CKD and CVD in individuals with type 2 diabetes. Visceral obesity, which by definition is the excess fat tissue in parain-testinal and omental areas, is a feature strongly associated with the CMS and increased risk of CVD. Patients with hypertension have higher fasting and post-prandial insulin levels and evidence of insulin resistance, independent of body mass index or body fat distribution. Both insulin resistance and hypertension predispose to atherosclerosis. Hypertension is a pathophysiologic stimulus for NADPH oxidase complex activation.

Key Words: Cardiometabolic syndrome; Chronic kidney disease; Obesity; Adipokines; Dysglycemia; Oxidative stress; Microalbuminuria; Visceral obesity; Hypercoagulability.

1. INTRODUCTION

In the United States currently, the prevalence of obesity has increased by 110%, when compared to the 1970s (1). More than 65% of the total US population is overweight or obese, and excess-associated metabolic complications affect more than half US adults *(2)*. Overweight is defined by the World Health Organization (WHO) as body mass index (BMI) between 25 and 29.9, while obesity is defined as BMI above 30. The definition of obesity must, however, also consider other anthropometric measurements, such as waist circumference (WC) and waist to hip ratio (WHR), factors influenced by race or ethnicity.

2. CARDIOMETABOLIC SYNDROME: A CLUSTER OF CVD RISK FACTORS

The prevalence of the cardiometabolic syndrome (CMS), a cluster of cardiovascular disease (CVD) risk factors which include central obesity, dysglycemia, atherogenic dyslipidemia, hypertension (HTN), and microalbuminuria (MAU) (Table 1), has also increased, and obesity is considered the main culprit. According to recent analysis from the Third National Health and Nutrition Examination Survey (NHANES III) *(3)*, the prevalence of CMS could exceed 34% of the US population. Importantly, obesity in children and adolescent populations is dramatically rising and has also been linked to a higher prevalence of the CMS, according to the NHANES III survey *(4)*.

In both adult and pediatric populations, minorities appear to be at increased risk of excess adiposity and associated comorbidities. Indeed, it has been demonstrated that Hispanic and non-Hispanic African-Americans are at higher risk *(5)*. The National Cholesterol Education Panel (NCEP-ATP III) has acknowledged these considerations and has tracked the causes of the CMS to genetic/ethnic factors and physical inactivity *(5)*. For instance, within the United States, the Hispanic population is rapidly growing, and it is estimated that it will comprise approximately one quarter of the total US population by the year 2050, according to the US Census Bureau in 2005 (available online at www.census.gov). A recent analysis of 1438 Mexican-American adults included in the San Antonio Heart Study followed-up during an average period of 14.5 years found a similar risk for all-cause mortality, CVD, and coronary heart disease (CHD) in non-diabetics as well as in diabetics treated with insulin, when compared to non-Hispanic whites *(6)*. Moreover, in this study the risk of mortality was significantly higher in the Hispanic diabetic group not treated with insulin.

As previously stated, obesity largely drives the dramatic increase in the incidence and prevalence of the CMS worldwide *(7)*. Ethnicity, which has been taken into account in the newer IDF definition criteria (according to which the WC cut-off in Hispanic men is 90 cm and 80 cm in women), also plays a key role in the CMS features, as is exemplified by a significantly higher prevalence of CMS in Mexican-Americans (50.6%), compared to non-Hispanics Whites *(3)* (Table 1).

Table 1
Classification Criteria of the Cardiometabolic Syndrome

WHO 1998	EGIR 1999	ATP III 2001
Dysglycemia: Fasting glycemia ≥110 mg/dl or impaired glucose tolerance (>140 mg/dl or insulin resistance) and Two or more of the following: Dyslipidemia: TG ≥150 and/or HDL <35 M, <40 W BP: >140/90 mmHg Microalbuminuria >20 μg/min	Insulin resistance – Hyperinsulinemia >25% and Two or more of the following: Central obesity: waist circumference ≥94 men, ≥80 women Dyslipidemia: TG >170 or HDL <40 Hypertension: BP ≥140/90 mmHg and/or on medication Dysglycemia ≥110 mg/dl	Three or more of the following: Central obesity: waist circumference ≥102 cm in men, ≥88 women Dyslipidemia: TG ≥150 mg/dl, HDL <40 men, HDL, 50 women Hypertension: BP ≥135/85 mmHg or on medication Fasting glucose >110 (100) MG/DL

IDF 2005	AACE 2003	
Central obesity plus two other factors Central obesity: waist circumference ≥94 cm men, ≥80 women (euripoids) Hispanics: men: 90 cm, women: 80 cm Dysglycemia: fasting glycemia ≥100 mg/dl Dyslipidemia: triglycerides ≥150 mg/dl or on medication	Risk factors Overweight: a body mass index (BMI) >25 or a waist circumference of >40 in. for men, >35 in. for women (10–15% lower for non-Caucasians) Sedentary lifestyle Age >40 years Non-Caucasian ethnicity	

Table 1
(Continued)

IDF 2005	AACE 2003
HDL <40 men, <50 women mg/dl or on medication	Family history of type 2 diabetes, hypertension, or cardiovascular disease
Hypertension: SBP ≥130 or DBP ≥85 mmHg or on medication	History of glucose intolerance or gestational diabetes
	Acanthosis nigricans
	Polycystic ovary syndrome
	Non-alcoholic fatty liver disease
	Characteristic abnormalities of Insulin Resistance syndrome
	Dyslipidemia: TG ≥150 mg/dl, HDL <40 men, HDL, 50 women
	Hypertension: BP ≥135/85 mmHg or on medication
	Fasting glucose >110 (100) MG/DL
	Diagnosis is made by the presence of one risk factor and two or more characteristic abnormalities

2.1. CMS and Inflammatory Markers

Adiponectin levels, a cytokine produced in adipose tissue, may vary according to race and ethnicity and are negatively related to insulin resistance, fat mass (particular visceral fat), dyslipidemia, and type 2 diabetes mellitus (T2DM). The mechanism of action of adiponectin has not been fully elucidated, however, this adipokine seems to induce a rise in fatty acids (FA) oxidation in skeletal muscle, which otherwise would act as potent inducers of lipotoxicity (8). A recent study by Hanley et al. found ethnic differences (9) in adiponectin related to the CMS. A cross-sectional analysis derived from the Insulin Resistance and Atherosclerosis Family study (IRAS Family) studied adiponectin in 1636 non-diabetic Hispanic and African-American participants, relative to indices of insulin sensitivity, lipid profile, CRP, visceral, and subcutaneous adiposity. Adiponectin levels were positively correlated with age, gender (female), high density lipoproteins (HDL), subcutaneous fat, and insulin sensitivity, while CRP, visceral fat, and basal glycemia were negatively correlated to adiponectin. The association between adiponectin, insulin sensitivity, and both visceral and subcutaneous-type adiposity was independent of the other components of the CMS. There was a significantly lower association between visceral adiposity and adiponectin in Hispanics compared to African-Americans, again suggesting ethnicity-related variation in the role of adiponectin in the development of the CMS. Indeed, available studies suggest different patterns of adiponectin association with the CMS in Hispanics and other ethnic minorities, which will need to be taken into account when designing therapeutic interventions directed at preventing and/or controlling the development of CMS in these populations.

2.2. The Link Between CMS, T2DM, and ESRD

On the other hand, the link between the CMS and the future development of T2DM and CVD is well recognized, and there is also emerging evidence of an important relationship among CMS, obesity, and both MAU and chronic kidney disease (CKD). This relationship has been confirmed in large population-based studies, as shown by the relationship between body mass index (BMI) and End-Stage Renal Disease (ESRD) in a Japanese population of over 100,000 people followed for 17 years. The cumulative incidence of ESRD increased significantly with rising BMI; after adjustment for age, systolic blood pressure, and proteinuria, the odds ratio of BMI for developing ESRD was 1.273 in men. Likewise, in 10,096 non-diabetic participants in the Atherosclerosis Risk In Communities Study (ARIC), the odds ratio for developing CKD in those with CMS, compared with those without the syndrome, reached a significant 1.436 value. These data support the original observation that CMS is related to accelerated progression to ESRD.

A retrospective study in 320,252 American adults showed similar results, with the rate of ESRD increased in a proportional manner to rising BMI. The association between the CMS and the risk for CKD and MAU was also analyzed in patients participating in the NHANES III using the NCEP-ATP III diagnostic criteria. A significant association was found in multivariate-adjusted analysis. The risk of CKD and MAU was proportional to the number of components of CMS documented. These findings were reproduced in a Japanese population, in which a significant influence of CMS on the development of CKD was documented in men younger than 60 years *(10)*.

3. IMPACT OF OBESITY AND THE CMS ON DEVELOPMENT OF CKD

Recently there has been increasing interest in the association between CMS, obesity, and CKD. There is evidence implicating obesity and its related pathophysiologic conditions, in particular insulin resistance with compensatory hyperinsulinemia, as important players in the emergence of CKD. CKD has been defined either as the presence of kidney injury, demonstrated by pathologic abnormalities or by other markers of kidney damage, or as the presence of a glomerular filtration rate (GFR) less than 60 mL/min/1 73 m^2 for a period longer than 3 months *(11)*. CKD is a major health-care problem, as approximately 8 million adults in the United States meet GFR criteria for CKD. A recent study, based on data from the NHANES III Survey, demonstrated a strong association between hyperinsulinemia, insulin resistance measured by homeostasis model assessment (HOMA-IR), and the prevalence of CKD in 6453 non-diabetic participants in the United States, after adjustment for age, gender, ethnicity, blood pressure, total cholesterol, physical activity, and tobacco use. Dyslipidemia, intimately connected to obesity and a key feature of CMS, is also related to CKD. A recent prospective study in patients with mild to moderate renal dysfunction followed for up to 7 years demonstrated kidney disease progression (defined as the doubling time of baseline creatinine or terminal kidney failure requiring renal-replacement therapy) in those patients who had a significantly higher baseline serum apolipoprotein IV and triglyceride concentrations and low high density lipoproteins (IIDL) cholesterol. In addition, analysis showed that baseline GFR and apolipoprotein IV were strong predictors of CKD worsening *(12)*.

4. ROLE OF OBESITY, INSULIN RESISTANCE, AND COMPENSATORY HYPERINSULINEMIA

Obesity, in particular visceral-type, is characterized by dysfunctional adipose tissue and is a known source of proinflammatory adipokines which include TNF-alpha, IL-1, IL-6, leptin, and resistin, all of which have been implicated in the development of insulin resistance *(13)*. The combination of decreased insulin sensitivity and hyperinsulinemia results in glomerular changes that include expansion and thickening of the glomerular basement membranes. The relation between obesity, CMS, and CKD is multifactorial and includes genetic as well as environmental factors. Genetic mutations involved in lipolysis, insulin production, adipose-tissue distribution, and appetite have been identified in individuals with CMS *(14,15)*. These factors interact with environmental influences, especially dietary and physical activity to further enhance kidney damage. Chronic hyperinsulinemia induced by insulin resistance in obesity and CMS impairs renal hemodynamics *(16)*. Reduced-pressure natriuresis, vascular sodium retention, and salt sensitivity are all increased by hyperinsulinemia, contributing to increased glomerular pressure, hyperfiltration, and increased urinary albumin excretion in CMS and diabetic patients *(17)* (Fig. 1). Insulin resistance and compensatory

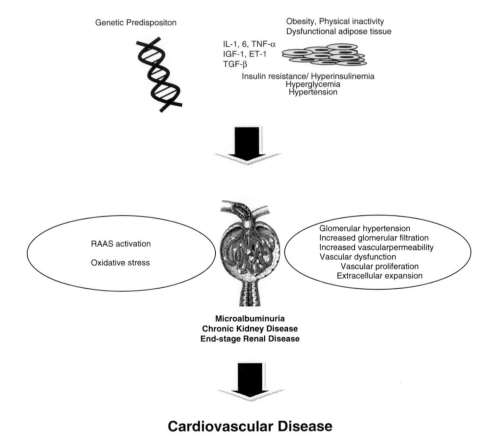

Fig. 1. Multifactorial pathophysiological events implicated in the relationship between features of the Cardiometabolic Syndrome and the development of Chronic Kidney Disease, end-stage renal disease and cardiovascular disease, involving genetic, environmental factors, and renal hemodynamics impairment.

hyperinsulinemia also cause proliferation of the mesangial vascular cells and expansion of the extracellular matrix *(18)*. This and the production of growth factors like Transforming Growth Factor 1 (TGF-1) contribute to interstitial fibrosis. Endothelin 1 (ET-1), a potent vasoconstrictor produced by endothelial cells and upregulated in hyperinsulinemic conditions, has also been shown to induce mesangial cell proliferation *(19)*. Furthermore, plasminogen activator inhibitor -1 (PAI-1) levels are elevated in conditions of obesity and hyperinsulinemia *(20)*. These increased levels of PAI-1 in experimental conditions have been shown to inhibit matrix metalloproteinases leading to impaired extracellular matrix degradation and subsequent expansion and fibrosis *(12)*.

On the other hand, MAU, defined as the albumin excretion of 30–300 or 30–300 mg/gm of creatinine in a spot collection, is a known cardiovascular risk factor and is one of the diagnostic features in the CMS definition of the WHO. The presence of MAU is a marker of increased vascular permeability, systemic low grade inflammation, and increased risk of CVD *(22,23)*. There is increasing evidence demonstrating that the kidney is a target for insulin actions, and insulin resistance at the podocyte level has been shown to be a potentially key factor in the development of MAU and ongoing kidney damage *(24)*.

5. ROLE OF RENIN–ANGIOTENSIN–ALDOSTERONE SYSTEM IN THE PATHOGENESIS OF CKD IN THE CONTEXT OF THE CMS

Obesity, hypertension, and dysglycemia are strongly associated with a systemic chronic low-grade inflammation, inappropriate activation of the renin-angiotensin-aldosterone system (RAAS), and increased oxidative stress *(25)*. The deleterious effects of the intrarenal RAAS activation are mediated at least in part by the interaction of angiotensin II (Ang II) with its specific receptors AT_1R and AT_2R. Upon interaction with AT_1R and its subsequent activation, Ang II promotes the production of ROS by upregulating the activity of the NADPH oxidase enzymatic complex *(26)*. In addition, intrarenal fibrosis is induced through the production of the profibrotic growth factors such as TGF-b1 and connective tissue growth factor (CTGF). These profibrotic growth factors are implicated in mesangial cell hypertrophy, matrix expansion, and fibroblast proliferation, events that collectively lead to relentless progression of CKD.

6. THE ROLE OF OXIDATIVE STRESS

The link between RAS activation and oxidative stress has been a subject of great interest over the past several years. Ang II promotes the production of ROS in adipose tissue, skeletal muscle, and cardiovascular tissue *(27)*. In turn, ROS induces a shift toward proinflammatory and proatherogenic patterns and mitogenic actions in vascular smooth muscle cells (VSMC) *(28)*. In mammalian cells, NADPH oxidase, nitric oxide synthase, cytochrome p450 enzymatic complex, the mitochondrial electron transport system, and xanthine oxidase systems are all capable of ROS production. However, the NADPH oxidase complex is probably the most important system implicated in excessive oxidative stress leading to vascular dysfunction in cardiovascular tissue *(29)*.

The NADPH oxidase enzymatic complex is composed of cytosolic proteins (small GTPase Rac1, p47^{phox}, p67^{phox}) and membrane catalytic proteins Nox 2 (gp 91) and p22^{phox}. Ang II, via AT$_1$R, stimulates intracellular pathways that result in translocation of all subunits to the plasma membrane, a key step in NADPH oxidase activation and production of superoxide (O$_2^-$) (Fig. 2). Experimental studies suggest that Ang II-mediated NADPH activation and production of ROS involve transcriptional as well as non-transcriptional mechanisms *(30)*. The experimental demonstration of the abrogation of NADPH-induced oxidative stress through AT$_1$R antagonist

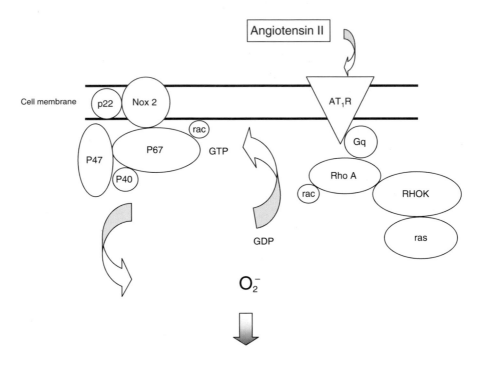

Fig. 2. Simplified version of the interplay between Ang-II-mediated activation of AT$_1$R and translocation of cytosolic units (rac, p47phox, p67phox) to the cell membrane and subsequent activation of the NADPH oxidase enzymatic complex, which in turn triggers production of superoxide anion and increased oxidative stress.

therapy in experimental models supports the role of RAS as an important player in ROS formation *(31)*.

ROS activity has been linked to multiple intracellular signaling pathways regulating vascular cell growth and differentiation. AT_1R-mediated activation of ROS production can induce the inflammatory NF-κB pathway and can lead to increased expression of vascular adhesion molecule 1 (VCAM-1), as demonstrated by Pueyo and coworkers in rat endothelial cells *(32)*. In addition, Ang II can activate through a ROS-dependent mechanism different intracellular tyrosine kinase pathways such as extracellular signal-regulated kinase 1 and 2 (ERK1 and ERK2), thus influencing vascular cells growth and proliferation. Furthermore, ROS can also act as second messengers in the transactivation of other growth factor receptors such as EGFR, and in the triggering of the Jak-STAT pathway, which leads to increased production of IL-6, leading to further inflammation *(33)*.

7. IMPACT OF OBESITY AND THE CMS ON DEVELOPMENT OF CARDIOVASCULAR DISEASE (CVD)

The CMS and its individual components lead to an increase the risk of CVD end points, such as stroke, congestive heart failure, chronic kidney disease, and overall mortality. The association of this syndrome with all cause and cardiovascular mortality from all causes was assessed during an 11-year follow up in a population-based cohort of middle-aged Finnish men who did not have CVD or diabetes at baseline. In this study, there was a significantly increased incidence of CVD, and overall mortality, in patients with the CMS. Similarly, in another population-based study in Finland and Sweden, in which 3606 subjects were followed over an average period of 6.9 years, it was observed that the risk of coronary heart disease (CHD) and stroke was increased three-fold in subjects with the CMS. Among the individual components of the CMS, MAU conferred the strongest risk for CVD-related death.

8. MICROALBUMINURIA

MAU is currently recognized as an independent risk factor for progressive CKD and CVD in individuals with DM2. The pathophysiologic alterations that characterize diabetic glomerulosclerosis parallel those of vascular atherosclerosis. MAU is associated with insulin resistance/compensatory hyperinsulinemia, central obesity, dyslipidemia, salt sensitivity, systolic hypertension, loss of nocturnal decreases in blood pressure and heart rate, left ventricular hypertrophy, hyperuricemia, and increased markers of cardiovascular inflammation.

These findings and the ongoing research in this field indicate that the presence of CMS is associated with increased risk of developing CVD and diabetes. Patients with the CMS have at least a two-fold increased risk of CVD compared with those without. How various components of the CMS translate into increased risk of CVD will be discussed below.

9. VISCERAL OBESITY

Visceral obesity, which by definition is the excess fat tissue in paraintestinal and omental areas, is a feature strongly associated with the CMS and increased risk of CVD. Relative to the peripheral fat tissue, visceral fat is characterized by enlarged and dysfunctional adipocytes, and is more resistant to the metabolic effects of insulin. In addition, this tissue appears to be more sensitive to the metabolic effects of lipolytic hormones such as glucocorticoids and catecholamines *(34,35)*. As a result, there is increased release of fatty acids (FA) into the portal system providing increased substrate for hepatic production of triglycerides and impairing first pass metabolism of insulin which leads to atherogenic dyslipidemia and hyperinsulinemia *(35)*.

The dyslipidemia associated with visceral obesity typically consists of increased apolipoprotein B (Apo B) particles, elevated proportion of small, dense lipoprotein particles; decreased HDL cholesterol; and elevated triglyceride levels. Several large prospective studies have shown that hyperinsulinemia is a predictor of CVD and stroke. Collectively, all factors associated with visceral obesity and hyperinsulinemia predispose patients to atherosclerosis and premature CVD *(36)*.

10. HYPERTENSION

Hypertension is a powerful and highly prevalent risk factor, especially in African-Americans. Approximately 25–47% of subjects with hypertension have insulin resistance or impaired glucose tolerance, or both, supporting the evidence that HTN, insulin resistance, and compensatory hyperinsulinemia may be causally related. Patients with HTN have higher fasting and postprandial insulin levels and evidence of insulin resistance, independent of body mass index or body fat distribution. In spite of still unclear understanding of the mechanisms by which insulin resistance relates to HTN, studies have shown that improvement in insulin resistance have a positive effect on blood pressure control *(37)*. Both insulin resistance and HTN per se predispose to atherosclerosis. HTN is a pathophysiologic stimulus for NADPH oxidase complex activation and production of reactive oxygen species (ROS) *(27,38)*, which in turn lead to loss of endothelium-dependant vasodilatation, gene expression, inflammatory responses, and finally a vicious cycle of worsening hypertension, all leading to atherosclerosis and premature CVD.

11. ATHEROGENIC DYSLIPIDEMIA

Regardless of race/ethnicity, dyslipidemia remains an important predictor of atherosclerosis. Atherogenic dyslipidemia is characterized by increased triglyceride-rich lipoproteins; low–HDL cholesterol; small, dense LDL particles; increased post-prandial lipemia; and abnormal ApoA1 and Apo B metabolism that accelerate atherosclerosis. CMS is characterized by increased FA flux to liver as a result of increased lipolysis from the underlying insulin-resistant condition. This increases the triglyceride content of the liver and with the insulin-resistant state that accompanies these changes results in gluconeogenesis and elevated levels of VLDL cholesterol. High levels of VLDL result in increased triglycerides, ApoB, and small dense LDL, which are easily oxidized and pro-atherogenic. Measurement of Apo-B level, which is present in VLDL and LDL, can be used as a measure of atherogenic dyslipidemia *(39)*. Elevated triglycerides impair endothelium-dependent vasodilatation in hypercholesterolemic patients without diabetes, as a surrogate of endothelial dysfunction *(38)*.

12. HYPERCOAGULABILITY

The delicate balance between coagulation and fibrinolysis/thrombolysis that modulates hemostasis is tilted toward clot formation in insulin-resistant/hyperinsulinemic patients *(40)*. Increased levels of plasminogen activator inhibitor 1 (PAI-I) are seen in patients with CMS. Both visceral obesity and insulin resistance contribute to elevated levels of PAI-I. In turn, PAI-I combines with tissue-type plasminogen activator and results in blunting of fibrinolytic activity. High levels of PAI-I relative to plasminogen activator predispose patients to increased incidence of thrombosis and CVD. Other CVD risk factors that are increased in insulin-resistant states are increased levels of fibrinogen and CRP as well as blood viscosity *(40)*. In addition with CMS, deficiencies have been noted in endogenous antithrombogenic substances like factor C and S and antithrombin III *(35,40,41)*. Collectively, these changes result in hypercoagulability, which in turns also increases endothelial dysfunction, atherogenesis and hence the likelihood of CVD *(42)*.

13. THERAPY: INFLUENCE OF ETHNICITY AND PERSPECTIVES

The prevalence, impact, and control of hypertension differ across racial and ethnic subgroups of the US population. In African-Americans, HTN is more common, more severe, develops at an earlier age, and leads to more clinical morbidity than in age-matched non-Hispanic whites *(43,44)*. Mexican-Americans and Native American have lower control rates than non-Hispanic whites and African-Americans *(45,46)*.

The pathogenesis of HTN in different racial subgroups may differ with respect to the contributions of factors such as salt and potassium homeostasis, stress, cardiovascular reactivity, body weight, nephron number, sodium handling, or hormonal systems, but in all subgroups the pathogenesis is multifactorial *(44,47)*.

African-Americans have a greater prevalence of other cardiovascular risk factors, especially obesity and HTN *(44,47)*. Weight reduction and sodium reduction are recommended for all prehypertensive (defined as SBP 120–139 mmHg or DBP of 80–89 mmHg) and hypertensive patients but may be particularly effective in minorities. The low-sodium DASH (for "Dietary Approaches to Stop Hypertension") eating plan was associated with greater reductions in blood pressure in African-Americans than other demographic subgroups *(48)*. In clinical trials, lowering blood pressure prevents hypertensive complications in all racial or ethnic groups *(44,47)*.

However, there are no clinical trial data at the present time to suggest that lower-than-usual blood pressure targets should be set for high-risk demographic groups, including African-Americans, Hispanics, and certain other racial/ethnic minorities. Large randomized clinical trials *(49–54)* have demonstrated that 2–4 antihypertensive agents are required to achieve diastolic blood pressure (DBP) and systolic blood pressure (SBP) goals in adults with uncomplicated HTN. Patients with diabetes or renal disease require an average of 2.6–4.3 different antihypertensive medications to achieve a blood pressure goal of lower than 130/80 mmHg *(55)*. This was exemplified in the AASK *(47)*, where 2–3 drugs were needed, on an average, to reduce mean arterial blood pressure to lower than 92–107 mmHg in African-Americans with HTN and mild-to-moderate renal dysfunction.

Until recently, DBP was generally preferred as an outcome measure for efficacy when evaluating the blood pressure-lowering effects of antihypertensive agents. However, large observational epidemiologic studies such as the Framingham Heart Study *(56)* have consistently indicated that SBP is a better predictor of cardiovascular events than DBP. Randomized, controlled trials have demonstrated that the association between the SBP and the risk of CHD, stroke, increased left ventricular mass, and ESRD is continuous, graded, and independent *(57)* and is typically stronger than the association of DBP with these same outcomes *(58)*.

When combination therapy using agents from two major drug classes is required to achieve blood pressure goals, based on data from randomized controlled clinical trials, the following combinations may be considered effective: beta-blocker/diuretic, angiotensin-converting enzyme (ACE) inhibitor/diuretic, ACE inhibitor/calcium channel blocker (CCB), or angiotensin II receptor blocker (ARB)/diuretic. All antihypertensive drug classes are associated with blood pressure-lowering efficacy in African-Americans *(59,60)*. Thus, in terms of efficacy, there would be no rationale for using race as a reason to avoid certain classes of agents in African-American patients with high blood pressure *(61,62)*. Patients whose blood pressure target is lower than 140/90 mmHg and who have untreated blood pressure that is lower than 155/100 mmHg may receive the recommended starting dose of an antihypertensive agent from any of the following major antihypertensive classes: diuretics, β-blockers, CCBs (dihydropyridine or non-dihydropyridine), and ACE inhibitors. The blood pressure-lowering efficacy of either chlorthalidone (a diuretic) or amlodipine (a dihydropyridine CCB) was recently confirmed to be superior to that of the ACE inhibitor lisinopril in African-Americans *(49)*. In many cases, a single drug will not achieve the desired blood pressure-lowering effect of 15 mmHg for SBP and 10 mmHg for DBP.

Centrally acting agents and direct vasodilators are not well suited for initial monotherapy because they produce annoying adverse effects in many patients *(63,64)*. Based on data reported from ALLHAT, [alpha]-adrenergic blockers should not be used as first-line agents in patients at high risk for hypertension.

It has been well documented that, as monotherapy or in the absence of a diuretic, beta-blockers, ACE inhibitors, and ARBs do not lower blood pressure to the same extent in African-American patients that they do in white patients with hypertension *(49,58,59,65,67)*. It has also been reported that, as monotherapy, thiazide diuretics and CCBs have greater blood pressure-lowering efficacy than do other drug classes in African-Americans. In the ALLHAT trial, which included more than 15,000 African-Americans, the ACEIs were less effective in lowering blood pressure than either the thiazide-type diuretic or the CCBs. This was associated with a 40% greater risk of stroke, 32% greater risk of HF, and 19% greater risk of CVD in those randomized to the ACEI versus the diuretic *(49)*. The interracial differences in BP-lowering efficacy observed with these drugs were abolished when they were combined with a diuretic. Furthermore, high-dose diuretic therapy, frequently used in the past, is no longer routinely recommended *(47,49)*.

When indications arise for target organ protection, RAAS-blocking agents (either ACE inhibitors or ARBs) or β-blockers should be used in the same manner in African-American patients as in any other ethnic subgroup. While lowering blood pressure to the target goal is the primary clinical approach to reduce the risk of adverse cardiovascular and renal events, some data also indicate greater benefits with specific classes of agents in high-risk patients. ALLHAT compared four antihypertensive agents as initial therapy in approximately 42,400 North American patients 55 years or older with hypertension and at least one other CHD risk factor; approximately 35% of subjects were African-American and approximately 36% had type 2 diabetes mellitus. In this trial, patients were randomly assigned to initial therapy with a diuretic (chlorthalidone), an ACE inhibitor (lisinopril), an alpha blocker (doxazosin), or a dihydropyridine CCB (amlodipine). An interim review by the data and safety monitoring board and an independent review panel determined that doxazosin-treated patients developed congestive heart failure at a greater rate than did diuretic-treated patients, and thus, the doxazosin arm was discontinued in 2000. Based on these data, it appears that alpha adrenergic blockers should not be used as first-line agents in high-risk patients. Chlorthalidone, lisinopril, and amlodipine did not differ in preventing major coronary events, the primary outcome of the trial, or in their effect on overall survival. However, chlorthalidone was associated with significantly fewer combined cardiovascular disease events, including fewer strokes and less heart failure, and better blood pressure control as than lisinopril, and the difference was greater in the African-American and other black ALLHAT participants. Amlodipine and chlorthalidone had similar results in terms of these secondary outcomes, with the exception of a higher rate of heart failure with amlodipine. By the completion of the trial, after approximately 5 years of treatment, patients received an average of two antihypertensive medications to achieve blood pressures lower than 140/90 mmHg.

As far as RAAS-blocking agents are concerned, data are clear on use of these agents in African-Americans with renal disease *(50)*. There is also a strong rationale for their use in patients with left ventricular hypertrophy (LVH) in the presence or absence of diabetes *(67,68)* in diabetic nephropathy *(69,70)*. The AASK trial *(50,71)* evaluated the impact of treatment with an ACE inhibitor (ramipril), a beta-blocker (metoprolol), and a CCB (amlodipine) on the progression of hypertensive kidney disease in African-Americans with mild to moderate renal insufficiency. It was seen that ramipril had greater renoprotective effects than amlodipine and hence the amlodipine arm was prematurely terminated. The final results of AASK showed that ramipril reduced the decline in kidney function to a significantly greater extent than did metoprolol or amlodipine. Also, ramipril reduced glomelular filtration rate, ESRD, or death in patients with renal dysfunction and high levels of proteinuria by 46% *(P = 0.004)* compared with amlodipine. Differences in blood pressure level did not account for the protective effects on renal function. These data provide strong evidence for including an ACE inhibitor in the antihypertensive regimen for African-American patients with renal disease.

ARBs have demonstrated blood pressure-lowering efficacy in African-American patients, particularly when combined with hydrochlorothiazide *(72–74)*. Recent trial evidence has shown that in patients with diabetic nephropathy, ARBs slow the rate of progression of nephropathy and proteinuria *(69,70)* and also blunt an increase in microalbuminuria in patients with early diabetic nephropathy *(75)*. Hence, it is assumed that an ARB may be considered at least as effective as an ACE inhibitor in the treatment of all patients with diabetic nephropathy who cannot reach the target blood pressure *(76)*. The Losartan Intervention for Endpoint Reduction in Hypertension (LIFE) study *(77,78)* included 9193 patients with high blood pressure and LVH (6% were African-American) who were randomized to receive either the ARB losartan or the beta-blocker atenolol for a mean of 4.8 years. Patients with LVH were selected because they had evidence of target-organ damage. There was little difference between the two groups in the degree of blood pressure reduction; however, losartan reduced the incidence of stroke by 25% more than did atenolol, and 25% fewer losartan-treated patients were diagnosed with new-onset diabetes during the course of the study. Losartan was also more effective than atenolol in reducing cardiovascular morbidity and mortality and all-cause mortality in the subpopulation of patients with high blood pressure, LVH, and diabetes. However, the benefit found in the above studies may not extend to the very small groups of African-Americans included in these trials.

When prescribing ACE inhibitors, it is important to note that compared with whites, African-Americans appear to be at increased risk for ACE inhibitor-associated angioedema, cough (reference), or both (46). If the ACE inhibitor-associated cough is intolerable, an ARB would be a reasonable alternative. Unfortunately, sufficient numbers of Mexican-Americans, other Hispanic Americans, Native Americans, or Asian/Pacific Islanders have not been included in most of the major clinical trials to allow strong conclusions about their responses to individual antihypertensive therapies.

Irrespective of the question as to whether race or ethnicity should be a significant consideration in the choice of individual antihypertensive drugs, specifically for monotherapy, the use of combination or multiple antihypertensive drug therapy, which usually includes a thiazide-type diuretic, in all patients including minority groups will lower BP and reduce hypertension-related cardiovascular and renal disease.

14. CONCLUSION

The increased rates of CKD in patients with obesity, especially in African-Americans and Hispanics indicate the need to calculate GFR and consider the use of ACEI and alternatively ARBs as part of an anti-hypertensive cardiovascular and renal protective program. As the wider burden of obesity grows with concomitant increase in CMS, it is expected there will be a significantly wider prevalence in cardiovascular and renal complications.

REFERENCES

1. Stein CJ, Colditz GA. The epidemic of obesity. *J Clin Endocrinol Metab* 2004; 89: 2522–2525.
2. King H, Aubert RE, Herman WH. Global Burden of diabetes, 1995–2025: prevalence, numerical estimates and projections. *Diabet Care* 1998; 21:1414–1431.
3. Ford ES. Prevalence of the metabolic syndrome defined by International Diabetes Federation among adults in the U.S. *Diabet Care* 2005; 28:2745–2749.
4. De Ferranti SD, Gauvreau K, Ludwig DS, et al. Prevalence of the metabolic syndrome in American adolescents: findings from the Third National Health and Nutrition Examination Survey. *Circulation* 2004; 110:2494–2497.
5. National Cholesterol Education Program (NCEP) Expert Panel on Detection, Evaluation, and Treatment of high blood cholesterol in adults (Adult Treatment Panel III) final report. *Circulation* 2002; 106:3143–3421.

6. Hunt KJ, Rsendez RG, Williams, et al. All-cause and cardiovascular mortality among Mexican-American and Non-Hispanic white older participants in the San Antonio Heart Study-Evidence against the "Hispanic Paradox". *Am J Epidemiol* 2003; 158:1048–1057.
7. Manrique C, Lastra G, Whaley-Connell A, et al. Hypertension and the cardiometabolic syndrome. *J Clin Hypertens* 2003; 7:471–476.
8. Boden G, Shulman GI. Free fatty acids in obesity and type 2 diabetes: defining their role in the development of insulin resistance and β-cell dysfunction. *Eur J Clin Invest* 2002; 32:14–23.
9. Hanley AJG, Bowden D, Wagenknecht LE, et al. Associations of adiponectin with body fat distribution and insulin sensitivity in non-diabetic Hispanic and African Americans. *J Clin Endocrinol Metab* 2007; 10:2006–2614.
10. Tanaka H, Shiohira Y, Uezu Y, et al. Metabolic syndrome and chronic kidney disease in Okinawa, Japan. *Kidney Int* 2006; 69:369–374.
11. Kidney Disease Outcome Quality Initiative. K/DOQI clinical practice guidelines for chronic kidney disease: evaluation, classification and stratification. *Am J Kidney Dis* 2002; 39(Suppl.):S1–S246.
12. Boes E, Fliser D, Ritz E, et al. Apolipoprotein A-IV predicts progression of chronic kidney disease: The Mild to Moderate Kidney Disease Study. *J Am Soc Nephrol* 2006; 17:528–536.
13. Wisse BE: The inflammatory syndrome. The role of adipose tissue cytokines in metabolic disorders linked to obesity. *J Am Soc Nephrol* 2004; 15:2792–2800.
14. El-Atat F, Aneja A, McFarlane S, et al. Obesity and hypertension. *Endocrinol Metab Clin North Am* 2003; 32:823–854.
15. Cheng LS, Davis RC, Raffel LJ, et al. Coincident linkage of fasting plasma insulin and blood pressure to chromosome 7q in hypertensive Hispanic families. *Circulation* 2001; 104:1255–1260.
16. Cohen AJ, McCarthy DM, Stoff JS. Direct homodynamic effect of insulin in the isolated perfused kidney. *Am J Physiol* 1989; 257:580–585.
17. Catalano C, Muscelli E, Quinones, et al. Effect of insulin on systemic and renal handling of albumin in nondiabetic and NIDDM subjects. *Diabetes* 1997; 46:868–875.
18. Young BA, Johnson RJ, Alpers CE, et al. Cellular events in the evolution of diabetic nephropathy. *Kidney Int* 1995; 47:935–944.
19. Simnonson MS, Herman WH. Protein kinase C and protein tyrosine kinase activity contribute to mitogenic signaling by endothelin-1: cross-talk between G-protein coupled receptors and pp60c-src. *J Biol Chem* 1993; 268:9347–9357.
20. Juhan-Vague I, Alessi MC. PAI-1, obesity, insulin resistance and risk of cardiovascular events. *Thromb Haemost* 1997; 78:656–660.
21. Rerolle JP, Hertig A, Nguyen G, et al. Plasminogen activator inhibitor type 1 is a potential target in renal fibrogenesis. *Kidney Int* 2000; 58:1841–1850.
22. Steinke JM, Sinaiko AR, Kramer MS, et al. The early natural history of nephropathy in type 1 diabetes. III. Predictors of 5-year urinary albumin excretion rate patterns in initially normoalbuminuric patients. *Diabetes* 2005; 54:2164–2171.
23. Bakris GL. Clinical importance of microalbuminuria in diabetes and hypertension. *Curr Hypertens Rep* 2004; 6:352–356.
24. Coward RJM, Welsh GI, Yang J, et al. The human glomerular podocyte is a novel target for insulin action. *Diabetes* 2005; 54:3095–3102.
25. Campbell RC. The rennin-angiotensin system: a 21st century perspective. *J Am Soc Nephrol* 2004; 15:1963–1964.
26. Rodriguez-Vita J, Sanchez-Lopez E, Esteban V, et al. Angiotensin II activates the Smad pathway in vascular smooth muscle cells by a transforming growth factor-beta independent mechanism. *Circulation* 2005; 111:2509–2517.

27. Sowers JR. Hypertension, angiotensin II and oxidative stress. *N Engl J Med* 2002; 346:1999–2001.
28. Nickenig G, Harrison DG. The AT1-type angiotensin receptor in oxidative stress and atherogenesis. Part I: oxidative stress and atherogenesis. *Circulation* 2002; 105: 393–396.
29. Ushio-Fukai M, Tabg Y, Fukai T, et al. Novel role of gp91phox containing NADPH oxidase in vascular endothelial growth factor induced signaling and angiogenesis. *Circ Res* 2002; 91:1160–1167.
30. Pagano PJ, Chanock SJ, Siwik DA, Colucci WS, Clark JK. Angiotensin II induces p67phox mRNA expression and NADPH oxidase superoxide generation in rabbit aortic adventitial fibroblasts. *Hypertension* 1998; 32:331–337
31. Wang HD, Hope SK, Du Y, Quinn MT, Cayatte AJ, Cohen RA. Paracrine role of adventitial superoxide anion in spontaneous tone in the isolated rat aorta in angiotensin II-induced hypertension. *Hypertension* 1999; 33:1225–1232.
32. Pueyo ME, Gonzalez W, Nicoletti A, Savoie F, Arnal J, Michel J. Angiotensin II stimulates endothelial vascular cell adhesion molecule – 1 via nuclear factor_B activation induced by intracellular oxidative stress. *Arterioscler Thromb Vasc Biol* 2000; 20: 645–654.
33. Berry C, Touyz R, Dominiczak AF, Webb RC, Johns DG. Angiotensin receptors: signaling, vascular pathophysiology, and interactions with ceramide. *Am J Physiol Heart Circ Physiol* 2001; 281:H2337–H2365.
34. Tchernof A, Lamarche B, Prud'Homme D, et al. The dense LDL phenotype: association with plasma lipoprotein levels, visceral obesity, and hyperinsulinemia in men. *Diabet Care* 1996; 19:629–637.
35. Banerji MA, Lebowitz J, Chaiken RI, et al. Relationship of visceral adipose tissue and glucose disposal is independent of sex in black NIDDM subjects. *Am J Physiol* 1997; 273:E425–32.
36. Despres JP, Lamarche B, Mauriege P, et al. Hyperinsulinemia as an independent risk factor for ischemic heart disease. *N Engl J Med* 1996; 334:952–957.
37. Shen DC, Sheih SM, Fuh MM, et al. Resistance to insulin stimulated glucose uptake in patients with hypertension. *J Clin Endocrinol Metab* 1988; 66:580–583.
38. Schneider MP, Delles C, Fleischmann E, et al. Effect of elevated triglyceride levels on endothelium-dependant vasodilation in patients with hypercholesterolemia. *Am J Cardiol* 2003; 91:482–484.
39. Sniderman AD. How, when and why to use apolipoprotein B in clinical practice. *Am J Cardiol* 2002; 90:48i–54i.
40. McFarlane SI, Banerji M, Sowers JR. Insulin resistance and cardiovascular disease. *J Clin Endocrinol Metab* 2001; 86:713–718.
41. Chen YQ, Su M, Walia RR, et al. Sp1 sites mediate activation of the plasminogen activator inhibitor-1 promoter by glucose in vascular smooth muscle cells. *J Biol Chem* 1998; 273:8225–8231.
42. Laine H, Yki-Jarvinen H, Kirvela O, et al. Insulin resistance of glucose uptake in skeletal muscles cannot be ameliorated by enhancing endothelium-dependant blood flow in obesity. *J Clin Invest* 1998; 101:1156–1162.
43. Chobanian AV, Bakris GL, Black HR, et al. Seventh report of the Joint National Committee on Prevention, Detection, Evaluation, and Treatment of High Blood Pressure. *Hypertension* 2003; 42:1206–1252.
44. Cooper R, Rotimi C. Hypertension in blacks. *Am J Hypertens* 1997; 10:804–812.
45. National Heart, Lung, and Blood Institute. Strong Heart Study Data Book: a report to American Indians communities. Bethesda, MD: National Institutes of Health, National Heart, Lung, and Blood Institute. NIH Publication No. 01–3285; 2001.

46. Crespo CJ, Loria CM, Burt VL. Hypertension and other cardiovascular disease risk factors among Mexican Americans, Cuban Americans, and Puerto Ricans from the Hispanic Health and Nutrition Examination Survey. *Public Health Rep* 1996; 111:7–10.

47. Douglas JG, Bakris GL, Epstein M, Ferdinand KC, Ferrario C, Flack JM, et al. Management of high blood pressure in African Americans: consensus statement of the Hypertension in African Americans Working Group of the International Society on Hypertension in Blacks. *Arch Intern Med* 2003; 163:525–541.

48. Sacks FM, Svetkey LP, Vollmer WM, Appel LJ, Bray GA, Harsha D, et al. Effects on blood pressure of reduced dietary sodium and the Dietary Approaches to Stop Hypertension (DASH) diet. DASH-Sodium Collaborative Research Group. *N Engl J Med* 2001; 344:3–10.

49. The ALLHAT Officers and Coordinators, for the ALLHAT Collaborative Research Group. Major outcomes in high-risk hypertensive patients randomized to angiotensin-converting inhibitor or calcium channel blocker vs diuretic: the Antihypertensive and Lipid-Lowering Treatment to Prevent Heart Attack Trial (ALLHAT). *JAMA* 2002; 288:2981–2197.

50. Wright Jr JT, Bakris G, Greene T, et al. Effect of blood pressure lowering and antihypertensive drug class on progression of hypertensive kidney disease: results from the AASK trial. *JAMA* 2002; 288:2421–2431.

51. Hansson L, Zanchetti A, Carruthers SG, et al. Effects of intensive blood-pressure lowering and low-dose aspirin in patients with hypertension: principal results of the Hypertension Optimal Treatment (HOT) randomised trial. *Lancet* 1998; 351:1755–1762.

52. Hansson L, Lindholm LH, Ekbom T, et al. Randomised trial of old and new antihypertensive drugs in elderly patients: cardiovascular mortality and morbidity: the Swedish Trial in Old Patients With Hypertension-2 study. *Lancet* 1999; 354:1751–1756.

53. SHEP Cooperative Research Group. Prevention of stroke by antihypertensive drug treatment in older persons with isolated systolic hypertension: final results of the Systolic Hypertension in the Elderly Program (SHEP). *JAMA* 1991; 265:3255–3264.

54. Staessen JA, Fagard R, Thijs L, et al, for the Systolic Hypertension in Europe (SYST-EUR) Trial Investigators. Randomised double-blind comparison of placebo and active treatment for older patients with isolated systolic hypertension. *Lancet* 1997; 350:757–764.

55. Bakris GL. Maximizing cardiorenal benefit in the management of hypertension: achieve blood pressure goals. *J Clin Hypertens (Greenwich)* 1999; 1:141–147.

56. Kannel WB. Elevated systolic blood pressure as a cardiovascular risk factor. *Am J Cardiol* 2000; 85:251–255.

57. He J, Whelton PK. Elevated systolic blood pressure as a risk factor for cardiovascular and renal disease. *J Hypertens Suppl* 1999; 17:S7–S13.

58. He J, Whelton PK. Elevated systolic blood pressure and risk of cardiovascular and renal disease: overview of evidence from observational epidemiologic studies and randomized controlled trials. *Am Heart J* 1999; 138(3, pt 2):211–219.

59. Saunders E, Weir MR, Kong BW, et al. A comparison of the efficacy and safety of a [beta]-blocker, a calcium channel blocker, and a converting enzyme inhibitor in hypertensive blacks. *Arch Intern Med* 1990; 150:1707–1713.

60. Materson BJ, Reda DJ, Williams D, for the Department of Veterans Affairs Cooperative Study Group on Antihypertensive Agents. Lessons from combination therapy in veterans affairs studies. *Am J Hypertens* 1996; 9:187S–191S.

61. Schwartz RS. Racial profiling in medical research. *N Engl J Med* 2001; 344:1392–1393.

62. Flack JM, Mensah GA, Ferrario CM. Using angiotensin converting enzyme inhibitors in African American hypertensives: a new approach to treating hypertension and preventing target-organ damage. *Curr Med Res Opin* 2000; 16:66–79.

63. Joint National Committee on Prevention, Detection, Evaluation, and Treatment of High Blood Pressure. The sixth report of the Joint National Committee on Prevention, Detection, Evaluation, and Treatment of High Blood Pressure (JNC VI). *Arch Intern Med* 1997; 157:2413–2466.

64. Guidelines Subcommittee of the World Health Organization–International Society of Hypertension (WHO-ISH) Mild Hypertension Liaison Committee. World Health Organization–International Society of Hypertension guidelines for the management of hypertension. *J Hypertens* 1999; 17:151–183.

65. Richardson AD, Piepho RW. Effect of race on hypertension and antihypertensive therapy. *Int J Clin Pharmacol Ther* 2000; 38:75–79.

66. Cushman WC, Reda DJ, Perry HM, Williams D, Abdellatif M, Materson BJ, for the Department of Veterans Affairs Cooperative Study Group on Antihypertensive Agents. Regional and racial differences in response to antihypertensive medication use in a randomized controlled trial of men with hypertension in the United States. *Arch Intern Med* 2000; 160:825–831.

67. Dahlöf B, Devereux RB, Kjeldsen SE, et al. Cardiovascular morbidity and mortality in the Losartan Intervention For Endpoint reduction in hypertension study (LIFE): a randomised trial against atenolol. *Lancet* 2002; 359:995–1003.

68. Lindholm LH, Ibsen H, Dahlöf B, et al. Cardiovascular morbidity and mortality in patients with diabetes in the Losartan Intervention For Endpoint reduction in hypertension study (LIFE): a randomised trial against atenolol. *Lancet* 2002; 359:1004–1010.

69. Lewis EJ, Hunsicker LG, Clarke WR, et al. Renoprotective effect of the angiotensin-receptor antagonist irbesartan in patients with nephropathy due to type 2 diabetes. *N Engl J Med* 2001; 345:851–860.

70. Brenner BM, Cooper ME, De Zeeuw D, et al. Effects of losartan on renal and cardiovascular outcomes in patients with type 2 diabetes and nephropathy. *N Engl J Med* 2001; 345:861–869.

71. Agodoa LY, Appel L, Bakris GL, et al. Effect of ramipril vs amlodipine on renal outcomes in hypertensive nephrosclerosis: a randomized controlled trial. *JAMA* 2001; 285:2719–2728.

72. Flack JM, Saunders E, Gradman A, et al. Antihypertensive efficacy and safety of losartan alone and in combination with hydrochlorothiazide in adult African Americans with mild to moderate hypertension. *Clin Ther* 2001; 23:1193–1208.

73. McGill JB, Reilly PA. Telmisartan plus hydrochlorothiazide versus telmisartan or hydrochlorothiazide monotherapy in patients with mild to moderate hypertension: a multicenter, randomized, double-blind, placebo-controlled, parallel-group trial. *Clin Ther* 2001; 23:833–850.

74. Weir MR, Smith DHG, Neutel JM, Bedigian MP. Valsartan alone or with a diuretic or ACE inhibitor as treatment for African American hypertensives: relation to salt intake. *Am J Hypertens* 2001; 14:665–671.

75. Parving HH, Lehnert H, Bröchner-Mortensen J, Gomis R, Anderson S, Arner P; for the Irbersartan in Patients with Type 2 Diabetes and Microalbuminuria Study Group. The effect of irbesartan on the development of diabetic nephropathy in patients with type 2 diabetes. *N Engl J Med* 2001; 345:870–878.

76. Sica DA, Bakris GL. Type 2 diabetes: RENAAL and IDNT—the emergence of new treatment options. *J Clin Hypertens (Greenwich)* 2002; 4:52–57.

77. Dahlöf B, Devereux RB, Kjeldsen SE, et al. Cardiovascular morbidity and mortality in the Losartan Intervention For Endpoint reduction in hypertension study (LIFE): a randomised trial against atenolol. *Lancet* 2002; 359:995–1003.

78. Lindholm LH, Ibsen H, Dahlöf B, et al. Cardiovascular morbidity and mortality in patients with diabetes in the Losartan Intervention For Endpoint reduction in hypertension study (LIFE): a randomised trial against atenolol. *Lancet* 2002; 359:1004–1010.

11 Risk Calculation and Clustering Within Racial/Ethnic Groups

P.W.F. Wilson, MD

Abstract

Several methods have been suggested to estimate the risk for initial coronary heart disease (CHD) events. Prior to the availability of modern computer methods, there was no easy way to adapt risk estimates to clinical practice. In 1998, the Framingham CHD risk approach was simplified, leading to greater interest in using risk prediction algorithms for clinical care. This formulation used categories of blood pressure, total cholesterol, HDL cholesterol, and simple groupings for smokers and diabetes mellitus to assess CHD risk. In 1999, the National Heart, Lung, and Blood Institute convened a CHD Prediction Workshop to

From: *Contemporary Cardiology: Cardiovascular Disease in Racial and Ethnic Minorities*
Edited by: K.C. Ferdinand and A. Armani, DOI 10.1007/978-1-59745-410-0_11
© Humana Press, a part of Springer Science+Business Media, LLC 2009

address the use of Framingham CHD risk functions to varied populations. Validation of the Framingham CHD prediction scores was achieved with data from a large number of observational data sources, representing multiple ethnic groups. As part of the proceedings of the CHD workshop, D'Agostino demonstrated the relative effects of most CHD risk factors. The equations derived in Framingham were tested in each site and showed good predictive capabilities in outcomes for the various ethnic groups and ages represented, with some exceptions. In regions where CHD risk was low, such as in the Honolulu Heart Program, the Framingham risk algorithms overestimated the CHD experience of the participants.

By the late 1990s, concern had risen among European scientists as to how well Framingham algorithms predicted CHD risk in their region. A large-scale, multinational European study was undertaken to address this issue – the Systematic Coronary Risk Estimation (SCORE) project – assembling data from 12 primarily Caucasian, European countries. A variety of issues relating to CHD risk estimation are of particular importance to high-risk population groups such as African-Americans. Blood pressure elevation has been consistently shown to be an important CHD risk predictor and levels are typically higher in black American populations. A variety of cardiovascular techniques are now available to assess subclinical arteriosclerosis. Estimation of risk for cardiovascular events is a dynamic field and it is expected that the approaches will undergo modification, as better information is obtained and more contemporary data become available.

Key Words: Risk clustering; Risk calculation; Framingham; Left ventricular hypertrophy; Racial/ethnic minorities; Risk validation.

1. BACKGROUND

Several methods have been suggested to estimate the risk for initial coronary heart disease (CHD) events. This approach originated in the late 1940s, when observational studies initiated long-term CHD studies over intervals that typically spanned 5–15 years. The earliest reports noted that combinations of high cholesterol, high blood pressure, and cigarette smoking led to a greater risk of CHD events. Risks were generally higher in men than in women and age was a critical factor for both sexes.

Prior to the availability of modern computer methods, there was no easy way to adapt risk estimates to clinical practice. The typical assessment tool was simple risk factor counting, utilizing persons with no risk factors as the referent group and universally relating age, sex, blood pressure, cholesterol, cigarette smoking, and diabetes mellitus history to risk for initial CHD events. Then, in the early 1980s, the advent of testing for different lipoprotein particles and general use of high-density lipoprotein (HDL) cholesterol screening on a population basis provided yet another important variable.

In the office setting, physicians tended to emphasize relative risk for CHD, which allowed comparison of risks for individuals of the same age and sex versus others with different combinations of factors. Longitudinal studies, however, eventually led to the development of risk equations that provided absolute risk estimates, leading to the adaptation of pocket calculators with special programming to put this approach into use. In the early 1990s, this approach was adapted to score sheets as described by Anderson *(1)* and adopted by experts in preventive cardiology across Europe, recognizing that no single algorithm was optimal. The Framingham experience served as a reasonable source for estimates, and various modifications were used to guide prevention programs.

In 1998, the Framingham CHD risk approach was simplified, leading to greater interest in using risk prediction algorithms for clinical care. This formulation used categories of blood pressure, total cholesterol, HDL cholesterol, and simple groupings for smokers and diabetes mellitus to assess CHD risk. The categories followed the blood pressure levels determined by, and currently followed by, the Seventh Report of the Joint National Committee on Prevention, Detection, Evaluation, and Treatment of High Blood Pressure (JNC 7), as well as the cholesterol and HDL cholesterol cutpoints for lipoprotein levels created by the National Cholesterol Education Program (NCEP) *(2,3)*

Examples of absolute and relative risk estimates from the Framingham CHD experience are shown in Fig. 1. The left bar in the figure represents the estimated 10-year hard CHD risk for a 55-year-old man. For the risk

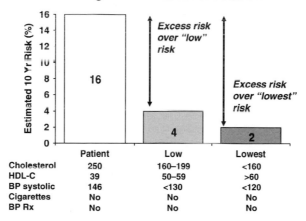

Fig. 1. Estimated 10-year hard CHD risk in a 55-year-old man according to levels of various risk factors. Estimates are shown for a representative patient, a low risk individual, and a lowest risk individual for comparisons.

factors displayed, the individual has a 16% risk of developing a first hard CHD event (myocardial infarction or CHD death) over a 10-year interval. For comparison purposes, a low-risk 55-year-old man, shown in the middle bar, would be expected to have a 4% risk over 10 years. The bar at the right shows the risk estimate of 2% over a ten years for a 55-year-old man with optimal risk factor levels, with excess risks shown as the difference between the risk estimates. On the other hand, relative risks are derived from the ratio of the absolute estimates. For example, 16%/4% ratio implies a relative risk of four when comparing the test subject to a low-risk individual, and a 16%/2% ratio implies a relative risk of eight when comparing the test subject to an individual at the lowest risk.

In 1999, the National Heart, Lung, and Blood Institute convened a CHD Prediction Workshop to address the use of Framingham CHD risk functions to varied populations. Validation of the Framingham CHD prediction scores was achieved with data from a large number of observational data sources, representing multiple ethnic groups (4). This workshop was restricted to American studies and most of the data were derived from observational trials which were predominantly white: The Atherosclerosis Risk in Communities ([ARIC] three white cohorts, one black cohort), the Physicians Health Study, and the Cardiovascular Health Study. In addition, data were analyzed from the Honolulu Heart Program (Japanese American men), the Puerto Rican Heart Study (Puerto Rican residents), and the Strong Heart Study (Native Americans).

As part of the proceedings of the CHD workshop, D'Agostino showed that the relative effects of most CHD risk factors were similar across the different study groups (4). The first step undertaken in the workshop was identification of future CHD cases from non-cases with each study using their own data. The area under the Receiver Operating Characteristic (ROC) curve was used to assess the discriminatory capabilities of these risk predictions. By this approach, an area of 0.50 indicates no predictive capability and an area of 1.00 indicates complete identification of cases versus non-cases during follow-up. Prediction algorithms for heart disease that use traditional CHD risk variables have typically provided an ROC area of approximately 0.70. External calibration was the second step in testing the CHD risk estimation. This process tested whether equations developed from an individual site could reliably predict CHD outcomes in other locales. The equations derived in Framingham were tested in each site and showed good predictive capabilities in outcomes for the various ethnic groups and ages represented, with some exceptions. In regions where CHD risk was low, such as in the Honolulu Heart Program, the Framingham risk algorithms overestimated the CHD experience of the participants.

The third step in the validation assessment of CHD risk equations in the 1999 CHD Risk Workshop was estimation of absolute risk in different population groups. Results for the Honolulu men using the Framingham risk

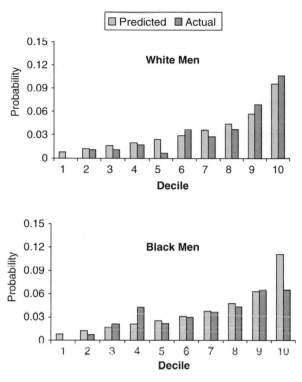

Fig. 2. Predicted versus actual estimates of hard CHD events in the arteriosclerosis risk in communities men according to decile of CHD risk. After D'Agostino (*JAMA* 2001).

equations are shown in Fig. 2. Persons were ranked according to estimated sex-specific decile of CHD risk over 5 years, each estimated decile was matched with the actual CHD experience, and goodness of fit was determined with the Hosmer–Lemeshow chi-square test *(4)*. The results were significantly different and the Framingham equations systematically overestimated CHD risk in the Hawaiian men. It was possible, however, to markedly improve the estimation if the Framingham CHD risk equations were adjusted for the overall CHD rates in Hawaii and if the estimating equations used the mean levels of the risk factor levels from the Hawaiian participants. The full details of these adjustments are provided in the D'Agostino paper. Alternatively, the Framingham Heart Study equations were able to reliably predict CHD risk in black men and white men who participated in the ARIC study (Fig. 3). No additional corrections were needed to provide accurate CHD risk estimates for the ARIC men. Good predictive capability was also shown for the ARIC white women and black women, without any need for adjustments. Overall, these results suggested that Framingham CHD equations provided reasonable estimates for CHD risk in black American population groups.

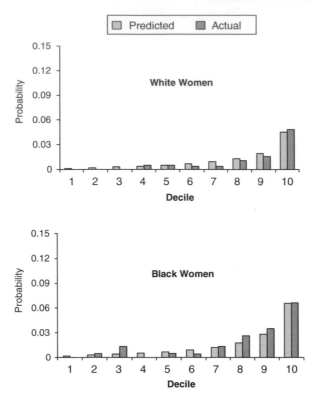

Fig. 3. Predicted versus actual estimates of hard CHD events in the arteriosclerosis risk in communities women according to decile of CHD risk. After D'Agostino (*JAMA* 2001).

The NCEP published new guidelines in 2001 that included using the Framingham risk approach to estimate the absolute risk for initial CHD events in some individuals. Persons with diabetes mellitus were considered to be at a very high risk for an initial CHD event and the committee recommended aggressive risk factor management of persons with type 2 diabetes mellitus (T2DM), treating them as if they had already developed CHD (*3*). A new CHD risk equation based on the Framingham experience was developed for the NCEP report, excluding persons with diabetes. Hard CHD risk was estimated, including interaction terms for age multiplied by cholesterol, age multiplied by smoking, and blood pressure level multiplied by blood pressure treatment.

2. EUROPEAN COMPARATIVE OUTLOOK

By the late 1990s, concern had risen among European scientists as to how well Framingham algorithms predicted CHD risk in their region. A large-scale, multinational European study was undertaken to address this issue – the Systematic Coronary Risk Estimation (SCORE) project – assembling data from 12 primarily Caucasian, European countries. The investigators analyzed data sets from several observational studies, with more than 200,000 men and women represented, totaling 2.7 million person-years of follow-up. The large number of countries, varied collection methods, and difficulty in assuring accuracy in CHD events across regions led to limitations, such as the inclusion of only fatal cardiovascular disease as estimated outcome, as there were not enough data to assess CHD morbidity.

The SCORE Project undertook validation efforts within their participating groups and they reported that risk of CVD death could be estimated with good statistical identification of cases. The area under the ROC curve ranged from 0.71 to 0.84 for the participating countries. The SCORE scientists also reported that HDL cholesterol information did not markedly improve the capability of CHD risk estimation in their data, a result that differed from the North American experience. They showed that CHD mortality risk varied considerably across Europe, and population samples from higher latitude typically experienced greater risk than those closer to the equator. Because of these differences, they provided two CVD death risk algorithms and recommended that the high-risk algorithm be used for persons from high-risk countries (Russia, Scotland, Sweden, and the United Kingdom) and a different CVD risk algorithm be used for regions where CVD risk was lower (France, Southern Germany).

Investigators from SCORE have noted limitations in vascular disease risk estimation, including the error related to use of measurements from a single clinic visit, the potential effects of a regression-dilution bias, the use of principal risk factors only, and absence of information such as family history of premature vascular CHD. The SCORE system, unfortunately, only included CVD mortality experience and little representation of minority groups, which may limit its utility outside of Europe.

Some efforts have been made more recently to develop cardiovascular risk assessment that includes evaluation of risk for first CHD events similar to what has been undertaken in Framingham, ARIC, and other North American studies. The Prospective Coronary Artery Muenster (PROCAM) Study developed a risk algorithm to predict myocardial infarction in a cohort followed in Muenster, Germany, and their prognostic variables were very similar to those included in the Framingham approach (5). Similarly, Italian researchers have undertaken analyses that tested the relative utility of Framingham and Muenster algorithms to predict the risk of heart disease in an Italian population. They compared the accuracy of their own equation to that developed by Framingham and PROCAM. They generally found that the German and American approaches overestimated heart disease risk, but identification of cases was relatively good and precision of the predictions improved considerably with calibration (6).

3. III CARDIOVASCULAR RISK ESTIMATION IN ASIANS

The experience for estimating CHD risk in Asian-Americans has been discussed above. In addition, Framingham and Chinese investigators collaborated in 2004, determining that the Framingham risk equations greatly overestimate risk of CHD in the Chinese cohort of adults. The identification of future cases for using Framingham equations in this setting was relatively good, however. Data for the male population of this study are shown in Fig. 4. With calibration, the risk of CHD was reasonably precise and the observed CHD rates were similar to what was expected *(7)*.

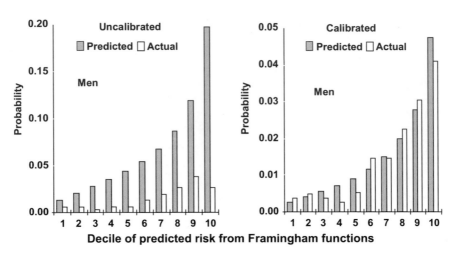

Estimation of 10 Year Hard CHD Risk in Chinese Cohort Using Framingham CHD Functions

Fig. 4. Predicted versus actual estimates of CHD events in Chinese cohort according to decile of CHD risk. After Liu (*JAMA* 2004; 299:2591).

4. CARDIOVASCULAR DISEASE RISK ESTIMATION IN THE AFRICAN-AMERICAN POPULATION

A variety of issues relating to CHD risk estimation are of particular importance to high-risk population groups such as African-Americans. Most standard CHD risk variables exhibit some differences in effects, prevalence, or treatment in blacks versus whites, and these differences can affect the accuracy of prediction.

For example, in comparisons of the relative risks for CHD in the ARIC participants, the relative risk in persons with diabetes was significantly increased in men (2.19 whites, 1.60 black) and women (2.95 whites, 1.86 blacks), as show in Figs. 5 and 6. Different results were evident for the

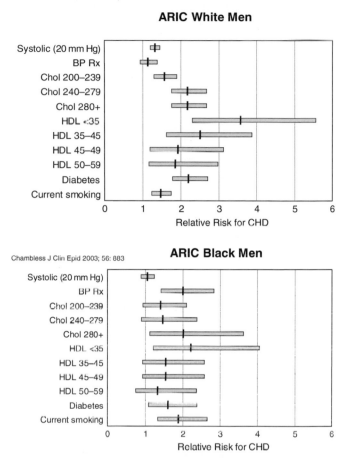

Fig. 5. Age-adjusted relative risks for CHD in the atherosclerosis risk in communities study men. After Chambless (*J Clin Epidemiol* 2003; 56:880).

effects of blood pressure on CHD risk in white versus black participants. The relative risk for CHD associated with a 20 mmHg difference for systolic pressure was 1.31 in white men, statistically greater than 1.00. Alternatively, the relative risk for a 20 mmHg difference in black men was only 1.05, not statistically significant. The lower relative risk in black men might lead a reader to conclude that systolic pressure exerts a less important effect in black men. However, the relative risk related to hypertension therapy was 2.00 in black men and only 1.13 in white men, indicating that hypertension treatment in black men was associated with much greater risk than anticipated. A reasonable interpretation of this result is that hypertensive black men were treated inadequately and may have received therapy later in the course of the hypertension. This potential for undertreatment or inadequate treatment of hypertension is discouraging, as clinical trials have

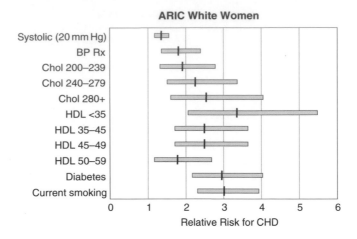

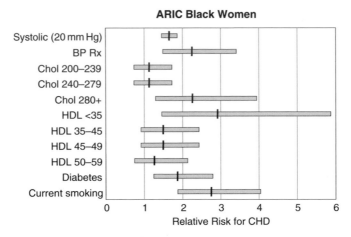

Fig. 6. Age-adjusted relative risks for CHD in the Aaherosclerosis risk in communities study women. After Chambless (*J Clin Epidemiol* 2003; 56:880).

convincingly demonstrated beneficial effects of hypertension therapy on CHD risk in white and black populations. These results also suggest that caution should be exercised when implementing CHD risk algorithms, especially when effects in observational studies are not congruent with the experience of controlled clinical trials.

Blood pressure elevation has been consistently shown to be an important CHD risk predictor and levels are typically higher in black American populations. These differences may be particularly important at higher blood pressure categories. For example, JNC 7 hypertension grades III and IV are uncommon in the Framingham Heart Study experience for whites, but are more frequently seen in black populations. A second consideration is the role of blood pressure treatment, where there may be a greater degree of no treatment, under-treatment, and late treatment of hypertension along blacks compared to whites in the United States.

A third element related to blood pressure is the myocardium itself, considering left ventricular mass and electrocardiographic left ventricular hypertrophy (ECG-LVH). In the 1991 formulation of Framingham CHD risk, ECG-LVH was included as a risk factor. Its prevalence was low, only a few percent, and the JNC 7 and NCEP have not recommended ECG determinations or echocardiographic evaluations when screening for CHD risk (2,3). This recommendation may hold for white population groups, but the greater prevalence of ECG-LVH in blacks, even at the same blood pressure levels, suggest biological differences may be operative, and more pronounced adverse effects on CHD risk are possible. Data from observational studies have consistently shown that ECG-LVH leads to a five-fold or greater risk for CHD. Overall, the data suggest that ECG-LVH is a CHD risk equivalent and should be assessed in population groups where it is reasonably common so that aggressive therapy can be instituted and maintained.

Blood cholesterol levels in whites and blacks are roughly similar but a tendency toward higher HDL cholesterol levels has typically been reported for blacks (8). However, this difference may not be obtained among blacks in a higher socioeconomic class, or if obesity or T2DM – more common in this population – is present (9). Additionally, levels of lipoprotein (a), a lipid particle that includes an apolipoprotein (a) linked to a low-density lipoprotein moiety, are typically greater in persons of African ancestry (10).

Finally, CHD risk has not been well characterized for this group. In the black ARIC participants from Jackson, Mississippi, most of the CHD risk factors appeared to operate along the lines observed for white Americans. It has been reported, however, that greater duration of diabetes and microalbuminuria can augment risk of initial CHD events in persons with diabetes (11). These issues may be particularly important to blacks with T2DM and have not been well assessed.

A variety of cardiovascular techniques are now available to assess subclinical arteriosclerosis. Examples of these methods include the ankle brachial index, carotid intima–media thickness, and assessment of arterial calcium with computed tomographic techniques (12). Investigators have suggested that subclinical assessments can improve the prediction of later clinical CHD events, but many of the investigations are limited because the population groups were self-referred (13). Caution is needed when interpreting these studies and large-scale investigations are underway to assess the utility of this new approach, especially considering the possibility of serial testing. By this strategy, individuals would undergo a screening evaluation and selected persons would undergo additional testing to refine CHD risk estimates. Caution, however, is particularly appropriate for African-American individuals, as it has been noted that they generally have less arterial calcification and higher CHD event rates. The tendency toward less arterial calcification in the black population has the potential to provide false assurances of low CHD risk for individuals who might undergo testing.

5. FUTURE DIRECTIONS FOR CHD RISK ESTIMATION

Estimation of risk for cardiovascular events is a dynamic field and it is expected the approaches will undergo modification, as better information is obtained and more contemporary data become available. There is tremendous enthusiasm for the incorporation of newer items into CHD and CVD risk estimation, but a variety of issues require examination. A primary consideration is that more clinical data may provide only small improvements in risk estimates. Novel risk factors stimulate interest in the pathophysiology of disease, but their use may be limited by lack of standardized testing, large variability in the measurements, high correlation with existing risk factors, and lack of validation across multiple studies. In addition, cost and benefit for any new test must be considered with great care. It is more likely that low-cost tests that are easy to standardize will be incorporated into CHD and CVD risk estimating approaches more rapidly than expensive tests which require technical expertise, specialized equipment, and have limited availability.

6. SUMMARY

In summary, data from black American populations suggest that Framingham risk estimations are reasonably predictive of cardiovascular outcomes in this population. As mentioned above, however, a variety of factors may be operative that could lead to a greater degree of misclassification than might have been anticipated. These include differences in blood pressure treatment, predilection toward left ventricular hypertrophy and greater left ventricular mass, different distributions of HDL cholesterol and lipoprotein (a), a greater tendency toward end-organ kidney damage, and less arterial calcification.

REFERENCES

1. Anderson KM, Wilson PW, Odell PM, Kannel WB. An updated coronary risk profile. A statement for health professionals. *Circulation* 1991; 83:356–362.
2. Lenfant C, Chobanian AV, Jones DW, Roccella EJ; Joint National Committee on the Prevention, Detection, Evaluation, and Treatment of High Blood Pressure. Seventh report of the Joint National Committee on the Prevention, Detection, Evaluation, and Treatment of High Blood Pressure (JNC 7): resetting the hypertension sails. *Hypertension* 2003; 41(6):1178–1179.
3. Executive Summary of the Third Report of The National Cholesterol Education Program (NCEP) Expert Panel on Detection, Evaluation, and Treatment of High Blood Cholesterol in Adults (Adult Treatment Panel III). *JAMA* 2001; 285(19):2486–2497.

4. D'Agostino RB, Sr, Grundy S, Sullivan LM, Wilson P. Validation of the Framingham Coronary Heart Disease Prediction Scores: results of a Multiple Ethnic Groups Investigation. *JAMA* 2001; 286(2):180–187.

5. Assmann G, Cullen P, Schulte H. Simple scoring scheme for calculating the risk of acute coronary events based on the 10-year follow-up of the prospective cardiovascular Munster (PROCAM) study. *Circulation* 2002; 105(3):310–315.

6. Ferrario M, Chiodini P, Chambless LE, Cesana G, Vanuzzo D, Panico S, Sega R, Pilotto L, Palmieri L, Giampaoli S; CUORE Project Research Group. Prediction of coronary events in a low incidence population. Assessing accuracy of the CUORE Cohort Study prediction equation. *Int J Epidemiol* 2005; 34(2):413–421.

7. Liu J, Hong Y, D'Agostino RB, Sr, Wu Z, Wang W, Sun J, Wilson PW, Kannel WB, Zhao D. Predictive value for the Chinese population of the Framingham CHD risk assessment tool compared with the Chinese Multi-Provincial Cohort Study. *JAMA* 2004; 291(21):2591–2599.

8. Watkins LO, Neaton JD, Kuller LH. Racial differences in high-density lipoprotein cholesterol and coronary heart disease incidence in the usual-care group of the Multiple Risk Factor Intervention Trial. *Am J Cardiol* 1986 Mar 1; 57(8):538–545.

9. Wilson PW, Savage DD, Castelli WP, Garrison RJ, Donahue RP, Feinleib M. HDL-cholesterol in a sample of black adults: the Framingham Minority Study. *Metabolism* 1983; 32(4):328–332.

10. Mooser V, Seabra MC, Abedin M, Landschulz KT, Marcovina S, Hobbs HH. Apolipoprotein(a) kringle 4-containing fragments in human urine. Relationship to plasma levels of lipoprotein(a). *J Clin Invest* 1996; 97(3):858–864.

11. Stevens RJ, Coleman RL, Adler AI, Stratton IM, Matthews DR, Holman RR. Risk factors for myocardial infarction case fatality and stroke case fatality in type 2 diabetes: UKPDS 66. *Diabet Care* 2004; 27(1):201–207.

12. Wilson PW, Smith SC, Jr, Blumenthal RS, Burke GL, Wong ND. 34th Bethesda Conference: Task force #4–How do we select patients for atherosclerosis imaging? *J Am Coll Cardiol* 2003; 41(11):1898–1906.

13. Raggi P, Cooil B, Callister TQ. Use of electron beam tomography data to develop models for prediction of hard coronary events. *Am Heart J* 2001; 141(3):375–382.

12

Cardiovascular Imaging in Racial/Ethnic Populations: Implications for the Adequate Application of Cardiovascular Imaging Techniques Guided by Racial/Ethnic Risk Factor Variations

A.N. Makaryus, MD, J.H. Mieres, MD, and L.J. Shaw, PhD

CONTENTS

Abstract

Over the last decade, the increased research focus on cardiovascular imaging for the identification of patients at risk for and with significant coronary artery disease (CAD) has augmented clinician awareness and ability to properly risk

From: *Contemporary Cardiology: Cardiovascular Disease in Racial and Ethnic Minorities*
Edited by: K.C. Ferdinand and A. Armani, DOI 10.1007/978-1-59745-410-0_12
© Humana Press, a part of Springer Science+Business Media, LLC 2009

stratify and categorize patients. Cardiac imaging has now become a technique not only for assessing patients with established CAD but also for the identification of patients with subclinical CAD who are at risk for ischemic heart disease and cardiac events of death and myocardial infarction. The Multi-Ethnic Study of Atherosclerosis (MESA) is a 10-year longitudinal study supported by the National Heart, Lung, and Blood Institute with the goals of identifying and quantifying risk factors for subclinical atherosclerosis, and for transition in patients from subclinical disease to clinically apparent events. Cardiac imaging findings from MESA with respect to racial/ethnic differences reveal that the incidence and prevalence of CAD differ among some racial/ethnic groups in the United States. The large number of patients affected by CAD has driven the development of effective, non-invasive methods to identify and risk-stratify patients with and at risk for CAD. When patients are properly identified, the appropriate treatment strategies can be applied to individual patients to prevent future events, such as death or myocardial infarction. Historically, exercise treadmill testing (ETT) with electrocardiogram (ECG) monitoring was the initial test applied to patients suspected of having CAD. Today, non-invasive cardiovascular testing with imaging has become the gold standard for the diagnostic and prognostic assessment of patients with suspected or known cardiovascular disease.

Most of the diagnostic non-invasive imaging tests currently available are based on assessment of regional and global function (echocardiography, radionuclide angiography, magnetic resonance imaging [MRI]), myocardial perfusion (single-photon emission computed tomography (CT), contrast-enhanced MRI), or coronary anatomy (CT angiography, magnetic resonance angiography) under resting conditions, stress conditions, or both. Diagnostic techniques such as electron beam CT, multi-slice cardiac CT scanning, and measurement of carotid intimal–medial thickness have emerged in recent years for detecting asymptomatic coronary or carotid atherosclerosis. Recent data on the assessment of long-term prognosis based upon the results of imaging tests to define false results has been shown to be reliable and helpful in risk prediction of cardiac events. In daily clinical practice, the assessment of risk allows for the identification of subsets of patients.

Key Words: Cardiovascular imaging; Multi-Ethnic Study of Atherosclerosis; Single-photon emission computed tomography; Magnetic resonance imaging; Electron beam computed tomography; Carotid intima media thickness.

1. INTRODUCTION

Significant progress has been made toward increasing awareness of the risks of heart disease in the area of cardiovascular research. Yet, coronary artery disease (CAD) remains the leading cause of death in the western world in both men and women, and in all ethnic groups that have been evaluated (1). An editorial by Bonow et al. (2) summarizes and highlights the issue of disparities in cardiovascular care in the United States, and hence the need to focus on differences in atherosclerotic burden among the different racial/ethnic subpopulations. Bonow states "...individuals in specific subgroups defined by race, ethnicity, socioeconomic status, and geography have a disproportionate burden of myocardial infarction, heart failure, stroke, and other cardiovascular events. These individuals also have a worse outcome after these events, including higher mortality rates, and a higher prevalence of unrecognized and untreated risk factors which places them at greater likelihood of experiencing these events." He further points out that "...differences such as these arise not only from disparities in access to care and quality of care but also from disparities in awareness and access to knowledge." (2)

Over the last decade, the increased research focus on cardiovascular imaging for the identification of patients at risk for and with significant CAD has augmented clinician awareness and ability to properly risk stratify and categorize patients. This research and application of the ever-increasing imaging modalities have allowed for the identification of differences among patients with respect to disease progression, presentation, location, and assessment. These differences have been noted in large prospective epidemiologic studies (most prominently the Multi-Ethnic Study of Atherosclerosis [MESA] trial (3)) that have employed imaging techniques to examine racial/ethnic differences in the presentation of CAD.

Cardiac imaging has now become a technique not only for assessing patients with established CAD but also for the identification of patients with subclinical CAD who are at risk for ischemic heart disease and cardiac events of death and MI. Cardiac imaging can do this by providing accurate, quantifiable measures of early CAD; characterizing CAD before it has become clinically manifest, and optimizing study of the progression of subclinical disease. With this background, the literature is reviewed regarding the diagnostic and prognostic evaluation of CAD in racial/ethnic subpopulations with respect to imaging assessment of heart disease.

2. PROSPECTIVE EPIDEMIOLOGIC ANALYSIS

2.1. THE MESA TRIAL: Study Design with Respect to Cardiovascular Imaging

The Multi-Ethnic Study of Atherosclerosis (MESA) (3) is a 10-year longitudinal study supported by the National Heart, Lung, and Blood Institute with the goals of identifying and quantifying risk factors for subclinical atherosclerosis and for transition in patients from subclinical disease to clinically apparent events. The MESA study cohort includes 6,814 men and women between the ages of 45 and 84 years at baseline. The patient population was recruited from six US cities: Baltimore, MD; Chicago, IL; Forsyth

County, NC; Los Angeles, CA; New York, NY; and St Paul, MN. The MESA trial has a wide variety of racial/ethnic groups and makes it ideal for the evaluation of differences between these groups. Self defined racial/ethnic categories in this study include approximately 40% whites, 30% blacks, 20% Hispanics, and 10% Chinese. Only persons free of clinical cardiovascular disease at baseline were recruited. The study sample includes 27% of subjects who were 45–54 years of age, 28% who were 55–64 years of age, 30% who were 65–74 years of age, and 16% who were ≥75 years of age at enrollment. In this study, assessment of patients with respect to disease development and progression was assessed. The center of this assessment in MESA was accomplished using imaging techniques including coronary calcium scoring *(4,5)*, MRI left ventricular function and strain assessment *(6–9)*, MRI thoracic aorta thickness, and carotid artery intima–media thickness *(8)*.

Cardiac imaging findings from MESA with respect to racial/ethnic differences reveal that the incidence and prevalence of CAD differ among some racial/ethnic groups in the United States. African-Americans tend to have higher CAD rates than do whites, particularly among women. Hispanic populations in the United States tend to have lower rates of CAD and general mortality than the general population does, despite high-risk factor levels. Pacific Asians (particularly Chinese Americans, Japanese Americans, and immigrants from Southeast Asia) have lower morbidity and mortality rates than do whites, but there are few data available on this group, particularly Pacific-Asian women in the United States *(1)*.

2.2. The Third National Health and Nutrition Examination Survey (NHANES III): Racial/ethnic Risk Factor Variations as the Reason for Cardiovascular Imaging Differences

Cardiovascular disease risk factors are present in varying percentages in different racial/ethnic populations. NHANES III data show increased rates of obesity, hypertension, smoking, and diabetes among blacks and Hispanics *(10)*. These risk factors have differing effects in different ethnic groups, with hypertension exerting a particularly deleterious effect among blacks, while diabetes disproportionately affects Hispanics. The impact of these risk factors is varied with increased cardiovascular mortality demonstrated in some ethnic minorities in the presence of less obstructive coronary disease. It is these differences that our advanced cardiac imaging modalities are able to assess and differentiate. Strategies focusing on these issues of differential disease can be very clearly assessed by the choice of proper imaging modalities to adequately risk stratify and give adequate prognostic management information *(10–12)*.

3. IDENTIFICATION OF THE PRESENCE OF CAD

The large number of patients affected by CAD has driven the development of effective, non-invasive methods to identify and risk-stratify patients with and at risk for CAD. When patients are properly identified, the appropriate treatment strategies can be applied to individual patients to prevent future events, such as death or myocardial infarction. Historically, exercise treadmill testing (ETT) with electrocardiogram (ECG) monitoring was the initial test applied to patients suspected of having CAD. Today, non-invasive cardiovascular testing with imaging has become the gold standard for the diagnostic and prognostic assessment of patients with suspected or known cardiovascular disease. The emerging technologies supporting these techniques vary widely, are in constant evolution, and require significant training of physicians who supervise and interpret test results *(13)*.

The clinical indications for these imaging modalities are guided by practice guidelines from the major scientific bodies such as the American College of Cardiology and the American Heart Association. Although one test modality have higher specificity for the detection of disease than a competing test aimed at identifying the same pathophysiology, the skill of performance and interpretation of different centers also needs to be considered *(14–19)*.

Most of the diagnostic non-invasive imaging tests currently available are based on assessment of regional and global function (echocardiography, radionuclide angiography, and magnetic resonance imaging [MRI]), myocardial perfusion (single-photon emission computed tomography [SPECT] and contrast-enhanced MRI), or coronary anatomy (computed tomography [CT] angiography and magnetic resonance angiography) under resting conditions, stress conditions, or both. The cardiovascular system is stressed by either exercise or pharmacological means, such as the infusion of a vasodilator or an inotropic agent *(20)*.

Diagnostic techniques such as electron beam CT (EBCT), multi-slice cardiac CT scanning, and measurement of carotid intimal–medial thickness have emerged in recent years for detecting asymptomatic coronary or carotid atherosclerosis. These technologies are aimed at detecting occult vascular disease in the coronary or peripheral circulation. This is especially important in high-risk racial/ethnic populations *(20)*.

4. IMAGING TECHNIQUES

4.1. Nuclear Stress Imaging – Pharmacologic and Exercise

SPECT myocardial perfusion imaging (MPI) has been demonstrated to be a powerful indicator of future cardiac events with a high diagnostic accuracy for CAD. Specifically, MPI is valuable in assessing risk for MI and cardiac

death, and evaluating the severity of disease and myocardial viability, as
a guide to future therapy, and for pre-operative risk assessment *(21–24)*.
SPECT MPI adds incremental value beyond clinical information and stress
ECG data *(21–24)*. Differences in risk factors and obstructive coronary disease prevalence between ethnic groups suggest that there be a discrepancy
in the expression of cardiovascular disease in these groups, and it is this
discrepancy which can be delineated through imaging.

Few studies have been performed assessing SPECT MPI in racial/cultural
minorities. Alkeylani et al. *(25)* analyzed a multi-center registry for cardiovascular death and myocardial infarction among 864 Caucasian and 222
African-American patients referred for nuclear stress testing. In patients
with normal perfusion imaging, they found a two-fold higher cardiac
death and MI rate in African-Americans. Patients with abnormal perfusion
imaging had similar cardiac event rates. All-cause mortality for African-
Americans with normal SPECT MPI was significantly greater than that in
Caucasians (Fig. 1). Both ethnic groups demonstrated a strong relationship
of multi-vessel perfusion defects and cardiac events. Akinboboye et al. *(26)*
studied an urban population of African-Americans with normal stress thallium SPECT MPI and they found a 2% cardiac event rate at 1 year. Among
the 35% of patients undergoing pharmacologic MPI, the cardiac event rate
was 5% at 1 year. The authors concluded that normal exercise MPI in this
population was associated with low cardiac event rates, similar to that found
in other populations, however, a 2% per year event rate is the same as 20%
over a 10-year period which is the number given to the CAD risk equivalent
group by the National Cholesterol Education Program. Patients undergoing

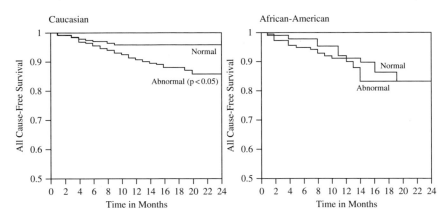

Source: Alkeylani A, Miller DD, Shaw LJ, Travin MI, Stratmann HG, Jenkins R, Heller GV. Influence of race on the prediction of
cardiac events with stress technetium-99m sestamibi tomographic imaging in patients with stable angina pectoris. Am J
Cardiol. 1998 Feb 1;81(3):293–7.

Fig. 1. Variations in Racial all-cause event-free survival in Caucasian and African-
American patients by Tc-99m sestamibi SPECT imaging results.

pharmacologic rather than exercise stress had higher cardiac event rates as has been noted in other large studies *(26)*.

Shaw et al. *(27)* studied a total of 1,993 African-American, 464 Hispanic, and 5,258 Caucasian non-Hispanic patients who underwent stress technetium-99m tetrofosmin gated single-photon emission computed tomography myocardial perfusion imaging. These investigators found that African-American and Hispanic patients more often had a history of stroke, peripheral arterial disease, angina, heart failure, diabetes, hypertension, and smoking at a younger age. Moderate or severely abnormal SPECT scans were noted in 21, 17, and 13% of African-American, Hispanic, and Caucasian non-Hispanic patients, respectively. Cardiovascular death rates were highest for ethnic minority patients ($p < 0.0001$). Annual rates of ischemic heart disease death ranged from 0.2 to 3.0% for Caucasian non-Hispanic and 0.8 to 6.5% for African-American patients with low risk to severely abnormal SPECT scans ($p < 0.0001$). For post-stress ejection fraction <45%, annualized risk-adjusted death rates were 2.7% for Caucasian non-Hispanic patients vs 8.0 and 14.0% for African-American and Hispanic patients ($p < 0.0001$). They conclude that their results provide further evidence that certain ethnic minority patient populations have a worsening outcome related to cardiovascular disease and can be accurately evaluated by SPECT MPI *(27)*.

4.2. Echocardiography – Transthoracic, Transesophageal, Stress Echocardiography, and Carotid Intima/Media Thickness Assessment

Of all the non-invasive techniques, echocardiography is the most versatile and provides the most ancillary information at the lowest cost. 2D echocardiography provides excellent images of the heart and great vessels as well as the assessment of regional and global left and right ventricular function. Stress echocardiography with exercise or dobutamine stress can assess for the presence of left ventricular systolic or diastolic dysfunction, valvular heart disease, and the extent of infarction and stress-induced ischemia *(15)*. Sonography can also be used to assess for atherosclerosis in the carotid artery as a marker for disease elsewhere. Recently, epidemiologic studies have used carotid ultrasonography to measure carotid intima/media thickness (IMT). Several prospective studies have shown that carotid IMT accurately predicts prevalent disease, incident disease, cardiac events, and cerebrovascular events. In addition, changes in carotid IMT be used as a measure of efficacy of pharmacologic intervention *(28)*.

Chapman et al. *(29)* used echocardiography to assess for left ventricular hypertrophy (LVH) in African-American and white hypertensives. They found that LVH is more prevalent in black than white hypertensives, but that this difference is greater when identified by ECG than by echocardiography. In a retrospective cross-sectional study, 408 subjects (271 white and 137 black) referred to a hypertension clinic for assessment of hypertension underwent measurement of blood pressure, ECG voltages, and echocardiographic left ventricular mass index (LVMI). Black subjects had greater ECG voltages than whites, even when closely matched for LVMI. In black subjects, current ECG criteria were twice as sensitive as in whites, but were less specific in blacks when compared to echocardiography. Willens et al. *(30)* reviewed echocardiograms and clinical data of 337 Hispanics and 279 non-Hispanic whites, aged 45–75 years to assess the difference in mitral annular calcification (MAC) and its relationship to CAD in these groups. In Hispanics, MAC was significantly associated with CAD, age, female sex, smoking, and having multiple (>2) risk factors. In non-Hispanic whites, MAC was associated with CAD, age, and having multiple risk factors. They conclude that among Hispanics referred for echocardiography, MAC is associated with CAD and multiple risk factors, but that in contrast to non-Hispanic whites, it was also associated with more factors, namely female sex and a smoking history.

McDermot et al. *(6)* reported data from the MESA trial regarding carotid IMT. They found that in patients with peripheral arterial disease (PAD), there was a strong association with significantly higher carotid IMT, but not necessarily increased high-grade lesions. In the Atherosclerosis Risk in Communities Study, in patients with PAD, there was higher carotid IMT among African-American women and white men after adjustment for age, low-density lipoprotein cholesterol, hypertension, and diabetes *(31)*.

4.3. *Computed Tomography Cardiac-Gated Electron-Beam Computed Tomography or Multi-detector ECG-Triggered Acquisition CT Scanning for Coronary Calcium Scoring and Coronary Angiography*

Cardiac-computed tomography detects and quantifies the amount of coronary artery calcium (CAC), a marker of atherosclerotic disease burden, using either electron beam tomography (EBT) or multi-detector CT. Coronary calcium scores approximate the total atherosclerotic plaque burden. In patients with moderate (CAC ≥ 100) or higher (CAC ≥ 400) calcium scores, there is a greater prevalence of obstructive coronary disease. CAC grades correlate well with the total atherosclerotic burden and strongly predict future cardiac events. The new generation of multi-slice CT scanners permits the non-invasive acquisition of coronary CT angiograms of very high quality *(32)*.

Bild et al. *(4)* presented CAC data from the MESA trial (Fig. 2). Using computed tomography, they measured coronary calcification in 6,814 white,

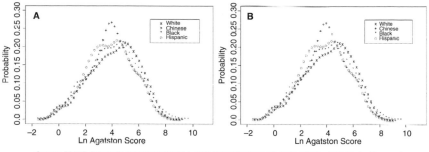

Source: Bild DE, Detrano R, Peterson D, Guerci A, Liu K, Shahar E, Ouyang P, Jackson S, Saad MF. Ethnic differences in coronary calcification: the Multi-Ethnic Study of Atherosclerosis (MESA). Circulation. 2005;111(10):1313–1320.

Fig. 2. Distribution of coronary calcification among those with detectable calcification by ethnicity in men (**A**) and women (**B**).

black, Hispanic, and Chinese men and women aged 45–84 years with no clinical cardiovascular disease. The prevalence of coronary calcification (Agatston score >0) in these four ethnic groups was 70.4, 52.1, 56.5, and 59.2%, respectively. After adjustment for age, education, lipids, body mass index, smoking, diabetes, hypertension, treatment for hypercholesterolemia, gender, and scanning center, compared with whites, the relative risks for having coronary calcification were 0.78 in blacks, 0.85 in Hispanics, and 0.92 in Chinese. After similar adjustments, the amount of coronary calcification among those with an Agatston score >0 was greatest among whites, followed by Chinese, Hispanics, and blacks. They conclude that the observed ethnic differences in the presence and quantity of coronary calcification were not explained by coronary risk factors and that identification of the mechanism underlying these differences would further the understanding of the pathophysiology of coronary calcification and its clinical significance *(4)*.

Budoff et al. *(33)* studied 782 symptomatic subjects who underwent both EBCT and angiography. They observed substantial ethnic differences in prevalence of both CAC and angiographic stenosis. In whites ($n = 453$), prevalence of CAC (score >0) was 84%, and significant obstruction on angiogram was 71%. Compared with whites, blacks ($n = 108$) had a significantly lower prevalence of CAC (62%, $p < 0.001$) and angiographic disease (49%, $p < 0.01$). Hispanics ($n = 177$) also had a lower prevalence of CAC (71%, $p < 0.001$) and angiographic obstruction (58%, $p < 0.01$). Asians ($n = 44$) were not significantly different in regard to CAC (73%, $p = 0.06$) or angiographic stenosis (64%, $p = 0.30$). These ethnic differences remained after controlling for age, gender, and cardiac risk factors. They conclude that compared with whites, blacks and Hispanics had significantly lower prevalence of CAC and obstructive coronary disease. Similar to other studies, ethnic differences in risk-factor profiles do not explain these differences *(33)*.

A recent analysis by Nasir et al. *(34)* assessed mortality rates in a large, ethnically diverse cohort of 14,812 patients. They examined calcium score as a predictor of mortality in this population of 637 African-Americans; 1,334 Hispanics; 1,065 Asians; and 11,776 non-Hispanic whites. They found that ethnic minority patients were generally younger (0.3–4 years), more often had diabetes ($p < 0.0001$), hypertensive ($p < 0.0001$), and female ($p < 0.0001$). The prevalence of CAC scores ≥ 100 was highest in non-Hispanic whites (31%) and lowest for Hispanics (18%) ($p < 0.0001$). Overall survival was 96, 93, and 92% for Asians, non-Hispanic whites, and Hispanics, respectively, as compared with 83% for African-Americans ($p < 0.0001$). When comparing prognosis by CAC scores in ethnic minorities as compared with non-Hispanic whites, relative risk ratios were highest for African-Americans with CAC scores ≥ 400 ($p < 0.0001$). Hispanics with CAC scores ≥ 400 had relative risk ratios from 7.9 to 9.0, whereas Asians with CAC scores $\geq 1,000$ had relative risk ratios 6.6-fold higher than non-Hispanic whites ($p \geq 0.0001$). These data are consistent with population evidence that African-Americans with an increasing burden of subclinical coronary artery disease are the highest-risk ethnic minority population. These data further support a growing body of evidence noting substantial differences in cardiovascular risk by ethnicity *(34)*.

4.4. Cardiac Magnetic Resonance Imaging—Function and Delayed Enhancement as well as Stress Perfusion

Cardiac MRI (CMR) is an excellent non-invasive technique for evaluating right and left ventricular function, cardiac masses, and congenital heart disease. CMR has the ability to evaluate the presence of coronary artery disease by multiple techniques including evaluation of myocardial perfusion by first-pass imaging, assessment of abnormal wall motion during stress, and identification of infarcted myocardium using delayed hyperenhancement imaging. Current studies are also underway using high-resolution, non-invasive MR imaging to provide exhaustive 3D anatomical information about the coronary lumen and vessel wall. MR imaging has the ability to characterize plaque composition and microanatomy and therefore to identify lesions vulnerable to rupture or erosion *(35,36)*.

Natori et al. *(37)* report on CMR data from the MESA trial of 800 participants (400 men and 400 women) in four age strata (45–54, 55–64, 65–74, and 75–84 years) that were chosen at random. Participants with known cardiovascular risk factors were excluded. Cardiac MR images were analyzed and they found significant differences in LV volumes and mass between men and women. LV mass was the largest in the African-American group and was smallest in the Asian-American group. They conclude that the normal LV differs in volume and mass between sexes and among certain ethnic groups. Further they recommend that studies that assess cardiovascular risk factors in relationship to cardiac function and structure need to account for these normal variations in the population (37).

Li et al. (8) report on data from the MESA trial using CMR to assess aortic wall thickness. In this study, 196 participants (99 black, 97 white; 98 men, 98 women) underwent fast spin-echo double inversion recovery MRI to measure thoracic aortic wall thickness. Blacks had greater mean maximal wall thickness than whites (3.74 vs 3.42 mm, $p = 0.023$). They conclude that aortic wall thickness increases with age and also varies by race (8).

Edvardsen et al. (7) reported on CMR data assessing left ventricular strain and strain rate by tagged MRI in the corresponding vascular territories of calcified coronary vessels in 509 participants (136 white, 85 African-American, 222 Hispanic, and 66 Chinese subjects) in the MESA trial. Greater coronary calcification in the LAD, LCX, and right coronary arteries were related to worse function in their respective perfusion. Participants with 1- and 2-vessel coronary artery calcium had better myocardial function in the remote area compared with the territory supplied by the diseased artery. The conclusions were that high-local calcium score is related to regional dysfunction in the corresponding coronary territory among individuals without a history of previous heart disease. These results indicate a link between atherosclerosis and subclinical regional left ventricular dysfunction (7).

5. IMPLICATIONS FOR CARDIAC IMAGING IN RACIAL/ETHNIC POPULATIONS

5.1. Technique Selection

In today's medical environment, a wide array of imaging tests can be used to evaluate the cardiovascular system. The proper cardiac evaluation starts with detailed history taking and physical examination. Evaluation of the patient's history will reveal the presence of cardiac risk factors, which include hypertension, diabetes, smoking, and the presence of a family history in any first-degree relative at an age of 55 years or less. The presence of chest pain or angina, the character and location of discomfort, discomfort radiation, associated symptoms, and precipitating, exacerbating, or alleviating factors should be assessed. Other important features of the history are the patient's estimate of functional capacity and the presence of additional coronary artery disease risk factors (16).

Through this evaluation and the knowledge of ethnic cultural differences in CAD, patients can be initially risk stratified using the Framingham risk score (FRS), a global risk score that includes traditional risk factors for CAD including age, smoking, blood pressure, and cholesterol values. From the FRS, patients with low, intermediate, and high-risk scores have expected annual rates of CAD death or myocardial infarction (MI) of <0.6% (low risk), 0.6–2.0% (intermediate risk), and >2.0% (high risk), respectively (20).

5.2. Diagnostic Bias and Prognostication

The aim of the diagnostic evaluation is to diagnose CAD with optimal accuracy and reproducibility. However, this accuracy is hampered by a bias in which patients with abnormal imaging test results are the ones referred to cardiac catheterization (which is currently felt to be the gold standard for documenting the presence of CAD), thus resulting in enhanced diagnostic sensitivity and diminished specificity (38). Recent data on the assessment of long-term prognosis based upon the results of imaging tests to define false results have been shown to be reliable and helpful in risk prediction of cardiac events. The availability of prognostic information promotes a change from a simply anatomy-based treatment strategy to a risk factor-based strategy as defined by interpretation of the results of the non-invasive test (38). In daily clinical practice, the assessment of risk allows for the identification of subsets of patients based on cultural and ethnic differences who are at increased risk for a cardiac event and should therefore be referred for testing and more intensive treatment. It at the same time identifies patients at low

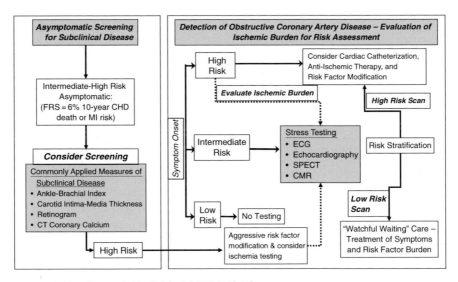

Adapted from Shaw et al. *J Am Coll Cardiol.* 2006;47:4S-20S.

Fig. 3. Cardiac-testing algorithm for symptomatic and asymptomatic patients for the detection of subclinical and obstructive coronary artery disease (38).

risk for cardiac events who can be managed with medical therapy, risk factor modification, and no further testing.

5.3. Clinical Application of Cardiac Imaging Techniques in High-Risk Ethnic Groups

Knowledge of the diverse and increased risk factors associated with the different ethnic groups allows the clinician to guide the proper management of the cardiac patient. This management is applied in the case of both the patient at risk for cardiac disease who needs primary prevention and the patient with established cardiac disease who needs follow-up and proper secondary prevention. Figure 3 provides an algorithm for the step-wise management of symptomatic and asymptomatic patients for the detection of subclinical and obstructive coronary artery disease (39).

6. CONCLUSIONS

Cardiovascular disease remains the leading cause of death and disability in the United States, with blacks having a higher mortality rate compared to white Americans. In the past, clinicians and researchers have been comfortable extracting data from large epidemiological surveys which mostly focused on Caucasians and people of the male gender. Clinically naive assumptions have been made that the data found would be applicable to all persons, irrespective of gender, race, or ethnicity. However, current literature now strongly suggests that certain dissimilarities between cardiovascular disease in white populations and the other racial/ethnic populations in the United States do exist and that these differences are indeed clinically relevant (Table 1). Today, it is prudent to be more cognizant of the differences among cultural and ethnic groups and large studies such as the MESA trial are underway to assess the differences among these groups applying the latest in imaging technology. Further research is needed in this area to assess

Table 1.
Chapter Highlights

Coronary artery disease (CAD) remains the leading cause of death in the western world in both men and women, and in all ethnic groups that have been evaluated

Research and application of the ever-increasing imaging modalities have allowed for the identification of differences among patients of varying racial/ethnic backgrounds with respect to disease progression, presentation, location, and assessment

Table 1.
(Continued)

The Multi-Ethnic Study of Atherosclerosis (MESA), a 10-year longitudinal
  study supported by the National Heart, Lung, and Blood Institute with the
  goals of identifying and quantifying risk factors for subclinical
  atherosclerosis, and for transition in patients from subclinical disease to
  clinically apparent events, has and continues to shed light on the utility of the
  various imaging modalities (coronary calcium scoring, MRI left ventricular
  function and strain assessment, MRI thoracic aorta thickness, and carotid
  artery intima-media thickness) in the diverse patient population studied
  (6,814 men and women between the ages of 45 and 84 years at baseline;
  self-defined racial/ethnic categories in this study include approximately 40%
  whites, 30% black, 20% Hispanic, and 10% Chinese

Another report, the Third National Health and Nutrition Examination Survey
  (NHANES III) examined racial/ethnic risk factor variations as the reason for
  cardiovascular imaging differences. This data shows increased rates of
  obesity, hypertension, smoking, and diabetes among blacks and Hispanics. It
  is these differences that our advanced cardiac imaging modalities are able to
  assess and differentiate. Strategies focusing on these issues of differential
  disease can be very clearly assessed by the choice of proper imaging
  modalities to adequately risk stratify and give adequate prognostic
  management information

Knowledge of the diverse and increased risk factors associated with the
  different ethnic groups allows the clinician to guide the proper management
  of the cardiac patient. This management is applied in the case of both the
  patient at risk for cardiac disease who needs primary prevention and the
  patient with established cardiac disease who needs follow-up and proper
  secondary prevention. An integrated step-wise management approach (Fig. 3)
  of symptomatic and asymptomatic patients for the detection of subclinical
  and obstructive coronary artery disease is essential

disparities in referral patterns for non-invasive testing and to better delineate the ideal imaging modality for patients of different ethnic and racial backgrounds.

REFERENCES

1. Heart Disease and Stroke Statistics—2008 Update: A Report From the American Heart Association Statistics Committee and Stroke Statistics Subcommittee. *Circulation* 2008; 117: e25–e146.
2. Bonow RO, Grant AO, Jacobs AK. The cardiovascular state of the union: confronting healthcare disparities. *Circulation* 2005; 111(10):1205–1207.
3. Bild D, Bluemke D, Burke G, et al. The Multi-Ethnic Study of Atherosclerosis (MESA): objectives and design. *Am J Epidemiol* 2002; 156:871–881.

4. Bild DE, Detrano R, Peterson D, et al. Ethnic differences in coronary calcification: the Multi-Ethnic Study of Atherosclerosis (MESA). *Circulation* 2005; 111(10):1313–1320.

5. McClelland RL, Chung H, Detrano R, Post W, Kronmal RA. Distribution of coronary artery calcium by race, gender, and age: results from the Multi-Ethnic Study of Atherosclerosis (MESA). *Circulation* 2006; 113(1):30–37.

6. McDermott MM, Liu K, Criqui MH, et al. Ankle-brachial index and subclinical cardiac and carotid disease: the multi-ethnic study of atherosclerosis. *Am J Epidemiol* 2005; 162(1):33–41.

7. Edvardsen T, Rosen BD, Pan L, et al. Regional diastolic dysfunction in individuals with left ventricular hypertrophy measured by tagged magnetic resonance imaging— The Multi-Ethnic Study of Atherosclerosis (MESA). *Am Heart J* 2006; 151(1): 109–114.

8. Li AE, Kamel I, Rando F, Anderson M, Kumbasar B, Lima JA, Bluemke DA. Using MRI to assess aortic wall thickness in the multiethnic study of atherosclerosis: distribution by race, sex, and age. *Am J Roentgenol* 2004; 182(3):593–597.

9. Wang L, Jerosch-Herold M, Jacobs DR Jr, Shahar E, Detrano R, Folsom AR. Coronary artery calcification and myocardial perfusion in asymptomatic adults. The MESA (Multi-Ethnic Study of Atherosclerosis). *J Am Coll Cardiol* 2006; 48(5): 1018–1026.

10. Centers for Disease Control and Prevention. The Third National health and Nutrition Survey, (NHANES III, 1988-94); www.cdc.gov/nchs/nhanes.htm.

11. Cooper R, Cutler J, Desvigne-Nickens P, et al. Trends and disparities in coronary heart disease, stroke, and other cardiovascular diseases in the United States: findings of the national conference on cardiovascular disease prevention. *Circulation* 2000; 102(25):3137–3147.

12. Jones DW, Chambless LE, Folsom AR, et al. Risk factors for coronary heart disease in African Americans: the atherosclerosis risk in communities study, 1987-1997. *Arch Intern Med* 2002; 162(22):2565–2571.

13. Beller GA. A proposal for an advanced cardiovascular imaging training track. *J Am Coll Cardiol* 2006; 48(7):1299–1303.

14. Klocke FJ, Baird MG, Bateman TM, et al. ACC/AHA/ASNC guidelines for the clinical use of cardiac radionuclide imaging– executive summary: a report of the American College of Cardiology/American Heart Association Task Force on Practice Guidelines (ACC/AHA/ASNC Committee to Revise the 1995 Guidelines for the Clinical Use of Cardiac Radionuclide Imaging). *Circulation* 2003; 108(11):1404–1418.

15. Cheitlin MD, Armstrong WF, Aurigemma GP, et al. ACC/AHA/ASE 2003 guideline update for the clinical application of echocardiography: summary article: a report of the American College of Cardiology/American Heart Association Task Force on Practice Guidelines (ACC/AHA/ASE Committee to Update the 1997 Guidelines for the Clinical Application of Echocardiography). *Circulation* 2003; 108(9):1146–1162.

16. Greenland P, Bonow RO, Brundage BH, et al. ACCF/AHA 2007 clinical expert consensus document on coronary artery calcium scoring by computed tomography in global cardiovascular risk assessment and in evaluation of patients with chest pain: a report of the American College of Cardiology Foundation Clinical Expert Consensus Task Force (ACCF/AHA Writing Committee to Update the 2000 Expert Consensus Document on Electron Beam Computed Tomography) developed in collaboration with the Society of Atherosclerosis Imaging and Prevention and the Society of Cardiovascular Computed Tomography. *J Am Coll Cardiol* 2007; 49(3):378–402.

17. Gibbons RJ, Balady GJ, Bricker JT, et al. ACC/AHA 2002 guideline update for exercise testing: summary article: a report of the American College of Cardiology/American Heart Association Task Force on Practice Guidelines (Committee to Update the 1997 Exercise Testing Guidelines). *Circulation* 2002; 106(14):1883–1892.

18. Gibbons RJ, Abrams J, Chatterjee K, et al.; American College of Cardiology; American Heart Association Task Force on practice guidelines (Committee on the Management of Patients With Chronic Stable Angina). ACC/AHA 2002 guideline update for the management of patients with chronic stable angina–summary article: a report of the American College of Cardiology/American Heart Association Task Force on practice guidelines (Committee on the Management of Patients with Chronic Stable Angina). *J Am Coll Cardiol* 2003; 41(1):159–168.
19. Mieres JH, Shaw LJ, Arai A, et al. Role of noninvasive testing in the clinical evaluation of women with suspected coronary artery disease: consensus statement from the Cardiac Imaging Committee, Council on Clinical Cardiology, and the Cardiovascular Imaging and Intervention Committee, Council on Cardiovascular Radiology and Intervention, American Heart Association. *Circulation* 2005; 111(5):682–696.
20. Mieres JH, Makaryus AN, Redberg RF, Shaw LJ. Noninvasive cardiac imaging. *Am Fam Physician* 2007; 75(8):1219–1228.
21. Hachamovitch R, Berman DS, Kiat H, Cohen I, Friedman JD, Shaw LJ. Value of stress myocardial perfusion single photon emission computed tomography in patients with normal resting electrocardiograms: an evaluation of incremental prognostic value and cost-effectiveness. *Circulation* 2002; 105(7):823–829.
22. Eagle KA, Berger PB, Calkins H, et al. ACC/AHA guideline update for perioperative cardiovascular evaluation for noncardiac surgery–executive summary. A report of the American College of Cardiology/American Heart Association Task Force on Practice Guidelines (Committee to Update the 1996 Guidelines on Perioperative Cardiovascular Evaluation for Noncardiac Surgery). *Anesth Analg* 2002; 94(5):1052–1064.
23. Allman KC, Shaw LJ, Hachamovitch R, Udelson JE. Myocardial viability testing and impact of revascularization on prognosis in patients with coronary artery disease and left ventricular dysfunction: a meta-analysis. *J Am Coll Cardiol* 2002; 39(7):1151–1158.
24. Hachamovitch R, Berman DS, Kiat H, et al. Exercise myocardial perfusion SPECT in patients without known coronary artery disease: incremental prognostic value and use in risk stratification. *Circulation* 1996; 93(5):905–914.
25. Alkeylani A, Miller DD, Shaw LJ, et al. Influence of race on the prediction of cardiac events with stress technetium-99m sestamibi tomographic imaging in patients with stable angina pectoris. *Am J Cardiol* 1998; 81(3):293–297.
26. Akinboboye OO, Idris O, Onwuanyi A, Berekashvili K, Bergmann SR. Incidence of major cardiovascular events in black patients with normal myocardial stress perfusion study results. *J Nucl Cardiol* 2001; 8(5):541–547.
27. Shaw LJ, Hendel RC, Cerquiera M, et al. Ethnic differences in the prognostic value of stress technetium-99m tetrofosmin gated single-photon emission computed tomography myocardial perfusion imaging. *J Am Coll Cardiol* 2005; 45(9):1494–1504.
28. O'Leary DH, Polak JF, Kronmal RA, Manolio TA, Burke GL, Wolfson SK Jr. Carotid-artery intima and media thickness as a risk factor for myocardial infarction and stroke in older adults. Cardiovascular Health Study Collaborative Research Group. *N Engl J Med* 1999; 340(1):14–22.
29. Chapman JN, Mayet J, Chang CL, Foale RA, Thom SA, Poulter NR. Ethnic differences in the identification of left ventricular hypertrophy in the hypertensive patient. *Am J Hypetens* 1999; 12(5):437–442.
30. Willens HJ, Chirinos JA, Hennekens CH. Prevalence and clinical correlates of mitral annulus calcification in Hispanics and non-Hispanic whites. *J Am Soc Echocardiogr* 2007; 20(2):191–196.
31. Zheng ZJ, Sharrett AR, Chambless LE, et al. Associations of ankle-brachial index with clinical coronary heart disease, stroke, and preclinical carotid and popliteal atherosclerosis: The Atherosclerosis Risk In Communities (ARIC) Study. *Atherosclerosis* 1997; 131:115–125.

32. Greenland P, LaBree L, Azen SP, Doherty TM, Detrano RC. Coronary artery calcium score combined with Framingham score for risk prediction in asymptomatic individuals. *JAMA* 2004; 291(2):210–215.
33. Budoff MJ, Yang TP, Shavelle RM, Lamont DH, Brundage BH. Ethnic differences in coronary atherosclerosis. *J Am Coll Cardiol* 2002; 39(3):408–412.
34. Nasir K, Shaw LJ, Liu ST, et al. Ethnic differences in the prognostic value of coronary artery calcification for all-cause mortality. *J Am Coll Cardiol* 2007; 50(10):953–960.
35. Budoff MJ, Achenbach S, Duerinckx A. Clinical utility of computed tomography and magnetic resonance techniques for noninvasive coronary angiography. *J Am Coll Cardiol* 2003; 42:1867–1878.
36. Nagel E, Klein C, Paetsch I, et al. Magnetic resonance perfusion measurements for the noninvasive detection of coronary artery disease. *Circulation* 2003; 108:432–437.
37. Natori S, Lai S, Finn JP, et al. Cardiovascular function in multi-ethnic study of atherosclerosis: normal values by age, sex, and ethnicity. *AJR Am J Roentgenol* 2006; 186(6 Suppl. 2):S357–S365.
38. Douglas PS. Is noninvasive testing for coronary artery disease accurate? *Circulation* 1997; 95:299–302.
39. Shaw LJ, Bairey Merz CN, Pepine CJ, et al. Insights from the NHLBI-Sponsored Women's Ischemia Syndrome Evaluation (WISE) Study: Part I: gender differences in traditional and el risk factors, symptom evaluation, and gender-optimized diagnostic strategies. *J Am Coll Cardiol* 2006; 47(3 Suppl.):S4–S20.

13 Unique Aspects of Vascular and Cardiac Ultrasound in Racial/Ethnic Groups

Robert L. Gillespie, MD
and Icilma V. Fergus, MD

CONTENTS

Abstract

Cardiac ultrasound is a portable, relatively inexpensive primary tool which assists the clinician with evaluation of several conditions found disproportionately in minority populations. Left ventricular hypertrophy (LVH) is more prevalent in African-Americans and this is a precursor to increased cardiovascular morbidity and mortality in this population. Left ventricular systolic and diastolic dysfunction are also power predictors of morbidity and mortality, often presenting with clinical features and etiologies that are different than non

From: *Contemporary Cardiology: Cardiovascular Disease in Racial and Ethnic Minorities*
Edited by: K.C. Ferdinand and A. Armani, DOI 10.1007/978-1-59745-410-0_13
© Humana Press, a part of Springer Science+Business Media, LLC 2009

African-American populations. Abnormalities of diastolic function also develop from infiltrative processes found in specific minority populations, including amyloidosis and sarcoidosis.

Other cardiomyopathies including hypertrophic cardiomyopathy in athletes and left ventricular noncompaction are important areas of clinical research in the application of cardiac ultrasound. Obesity, a well-described potent risk factor for cardiovascular disease, is increased in certain racial/ethnic populations and has certain echocardiographic features that can be identified. Kawasaki disease is seen predominantly in children, with a high incidence in Asians, and along with certain constitutional symptoms, demonstrates unique echocardiographic findings.

Key Words: Left ventricular hypertrophy; Systolic and diastolic dysfunction; Left ventricular noncompaction; Hypertrophic cardiomyopathy in athletes; Diastolic heart failure; Systolic heart failure; Kawasaki disease.

1. INTRODUCTION

The intent of this chapter is to describe some of the major diseases that confront minority patients and clinicians, as well as to highlight a few novel conditions that have specific implications in minority patients. Echocardiography is a portable and relatively inexpensive modality that allows rapid and accurate assessment of multiple cardiac features, including systolic and diastolic function, wall thickness, valvular function, chamber size, and pericardial disease. It has also been used as a primary tool to assess a number of cardiac diseases, many of which disproportionately affect minority populations. Left ventricular hypertrophy (LVH), in addition to hypertrophic cardiomyopathy, and sarcoid are major contributors to poor outcomes in the African-American population, leading to diastolic and systolic dysfunctions. In certain Asian populations, Kawasaki disease is much more prevalent. The cardiac implications of diet and obesity are well known and cardiac ultrasound can be used to assess increased cardiovascular disease (CVD) risk markers that may disproportionately effect minority populations particularly Hispanic and African-American patients. Furthermore, serial assessment of children may also prove to be very informative in high-risk minority patients with hypertension, diabetes, and obesity.

2. LEFT VENTRICULAR HYPERTROPHY

Left ventricular hypertrophy has been associated with increased morbidity and mortality (Figs. 1 and 2) and its detection also has therapeutic implications. The Seventh Report of the Joint National Committee on Prevention, Detection, Evaluation, and Treatment of High Blood Pressure (JNC 7) correctly categorizes patients with LVH as higher risk and strongly endorses aggressively treating hypertension in these patients (1). Clinicians, however,

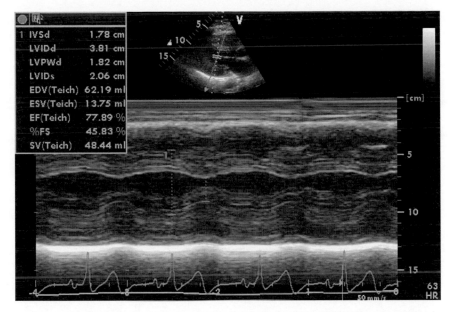

Fig. 1. An M-mode recording from a patient with concentric left ventricular hypertrophy.

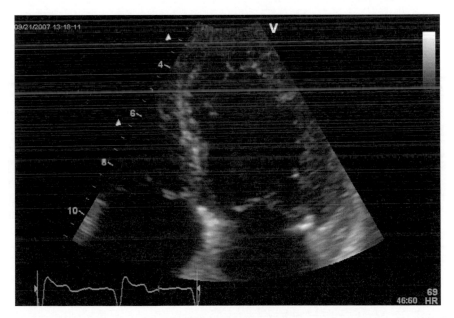

Fig. 2. A two-dimensional long-axis echocardiogram of a patient with concentric left ventricular hypertrophy.

should differentiate between the healthy, eccentric LVH seen in athletes and the unhealthy concentric LVH associated with hypertension. In the Massa Ventricolare sinistra nell'Ipertensione study, over 1033 Italian hypertensive patients were studied (2). After adjusting for multiple factors including renal function, diabetes and tobacco use, LVH was associated with a two-fold increased risk of major cardiovascular events. Each 39 g/m increase in left ventricular (LV) mass resulted in a 40% increase in cardiovascular events. Framingham data for the 3220 predominantly white patients who underwent cardiac ultrasound showed that the 4-year age-adjusted incidence of cardiovascular events increased as LV mass increased (3). Moreover, LVH has been shown to result in larger infarctions and increased incidence of sudden death in the setting of coronary occlusion (4). The prevalence of LVH has long been suspected to be much greater in the African-American population (5) in addition to a higher incidence of renal disease relative to the degree of hypertension when compared to whites (6).

It was unclear whether the increased prevalence of LVH in African-Americans remained after adjustment for body habitus. This question appears to have been definitively answered in the Dallas Heart Study (7) of 1335 African-American participants. Compared to the 858 white patients, the prevalence of LVH using the accurate modality of magnetic resonance imaging (MRI) showed a two- to three-fold increased incidence in both black men and black women. This study used multiple variables, including fat free mass, height, and body surface area. The study investigators concluded that these same factors were associated with markedly increased prevalence of LVH in the black population. Therefore, LVH may also reflect increased risk in African-Americans beyond that due to BMI per se.

It has been commonplace to use electrocardiography (ECG) to assess for the presence of LVH due to its minimal expense and widespread availability. Although simple and readily available, ECG has been shown to be a suboptimal modality for the assessment of LVH. Until recently, its accuracy has been primarily assessed in white populations, and studies using ECG in nonwhite populations have shown to have even less specificity. A study performed by Jaggy et al. (8) showed that in a population of 334 East African patients, the accuracy of classic criteria for LVH using ECG when compared to echocardiography was diminished in this population relative to previous studies in white populations. Thus, the authors caution the use of these criteria particularly in nonwhite patients. Okin et al. (9) in a subset of white and African-American hypertensive patients in the Losartan Intervention For Endpoint (LIFE) trial, also showed that using standard non-ethnicity-specific criteria led to disparate findings when comparing ECG and cardiac ultrasound. They furthermore suggested this difference was eliminated with ethnicity specific ECG criteria.

While the use of ECG has been a helpful modality, in the usual clinical setting, echocardiography has become the gold standard. The American

Society of Echocardiography *(10)* defines LVH as an end diastolic thickness of the septum or posterior wall greater than 10 mm in females and greater than 11 mm in males. Increased LV mass is defined as greater than 150 g in females and greater than 200 g in males. LV mass index, less commonly used clinically, has been validated and often cited as a standard in the literature. In clinical practice, the typical cardiac ultrasound laboratory will define LVH as a septum or posterior wall 11 mm or greater, regardless of gender. Therefore, even with a modality utilized in daily clinical practices, there remains a significant variability in defining LVH. Likewise, there are variable definitions applied to studies in the literature and it is important to recognize these differences in criteria when evaluating data. Also, it is not fully known if there are echocardiographic criteria that should be applied differently depending on race, since there are potentially profound differences in outcomes between whites and African-Americans with current thresholds for LVH. This conundrum, perhaps, warrants a lower threshold in diagnosing LVH in African-Americans, particularly those with risk factors such as hypertension. Other imaging techniques such as MRI and computed tomography (CT) are also very accurate but are impractical for the routine clinical assessment of LVH.

The detection of LVH by cardiac ultrasound in young African-Americans with hypertension is disproportionately high. For example, in one study of 309 male residents of Baltimore, Maryland, aged 18–54 years, the prevalence of LVH was 30%. There was, furthermore, a 9% incidence of systolic dysfunction in African-American men with poorly controlled hypertension *(11)*. These data are consistent with the large clinical trials on systolic dysfunction in heart failure which demonstrate predominance of hypertension as a primary etiology of heart failure in African-American patients *(12,13)*. Even higher is the prevalence of LVH in patients with mild to moderate renal insufficiency. While this in itself is not surprising, the extent of echocardiographic LVH is remarkable. In a substudy of 599 patients from the African American Study of Kidney Disease (AASK), 67% of men and 74% of women had echocardiographic criteria consistent with LVH *(14)*. This high incidence is undoubtedly associated with the high prevalence of stroke and heart failure in this population, as evidenced in the Atherosclerosis Risk in Communities (ARIC) study. In ARIC, of the 1792 black patients, those with an increased LV mass index had a significant increase in the incidence of stroke *(15)*. A study of 77 African-American patients with normal LV ejection fractions compared echocardiography in patients with hypertensive heart disease without heart failure versus those with clinical heart failure (i.e., diastolic heart failure). Findings demonstrated similar features in these populations, including abnormalities of systolic, diastolic, and vascular functions. However, the distinguishing factor in the heart failure group was the degree of LVH and the extent of left atrial enlargement. Moreover, the product of LV mass index

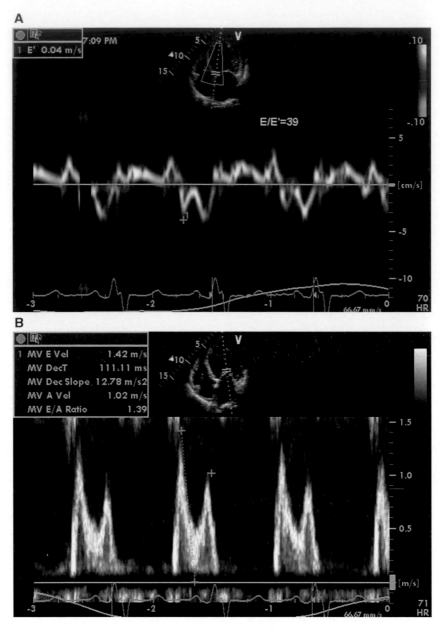

Fig. 3. Tissue Doppler imaging of the medial mitral valve anulus (**A**) and pulsed Doppler imaging of mitral valve inflow (**B**). Pulmonary vein flow with diastolic predominance is also shown (**C**). This patient has severe diastolic dysfunction as noted by a short deceleration time of mitral valve inflow and markedly elevated E/E′ with tissue Doppler imaging. Severe left atrial enlargement (**D**) is also noted.

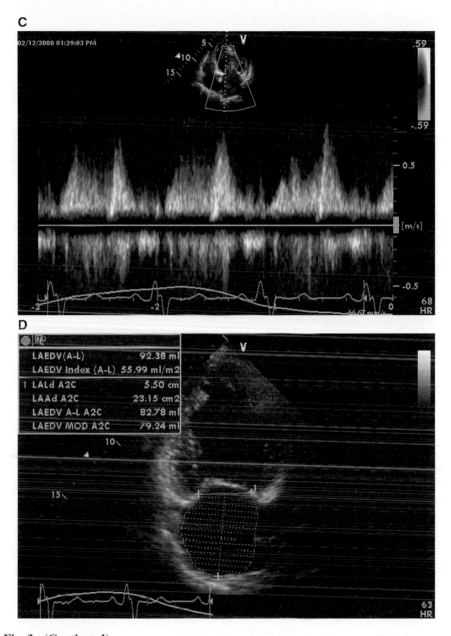

Fig. 3. (Continued)

and maximum left atrial volume best distinguished the patients with heart failure from the hypertensive non-failing hearts *(16)*.

These data support the use of quantitative measures of diastolic dysfunction and LV morphology. This is, in part, done by combining the information obtained from measuring left atrial volume, assessing the left ventricle itself (including LVH and systolic function), and using diastolic parameters such as tissue Doppler, mitral valve inflow patterns, and pulmonary vein flow patterns (Fig. 3). The use of quantitative assessment of diastolic and systolic parameters in the daily assessment of patients in the cardiac ultrasound laboratory is now the standard of care and can no longer be considered too difficult and time consuming. Updated software packages and advances in harmonic imaging, as well as other technical advances in the ever growing field of echocardiography, have made it much easier to obtain this valuable information. The American Society of Echocardiography has put forth specific guidelines which address the importance of quantitative echocardiographic parameters including measurement of left atrial volume instead of the commonly accepted method of using measurements in a single dimension.

3. SYSTOLIC AND DIASTOLIC LEFT VENTRICULAR HEART FAILURE

When patients present with symptoms and signs of heart failure, it is always important to distinguish between systolic and diastolic heart failure. The presence of systolic heart failure is typically defined as a reduced LV ejection fraction (Fig. 4), while diastolic heart failure is typically defined as heart failure in the setting of preserved LV ejection fraction. The commonly accepted belief is that patients with systolic heart failure have a worse prognosis than those with diastolic heart failure. However, long-term follow-up shows a very similar poor prognosis in these patients *(17)*. There is a great deal of overlap between the two types of heart failure, and diastolic dysfunction is present to some degree in all patients with systolic heart failure. It is important to note that diastolic dysfunction and diastolic heart failure are not the same. Diastolic dysfunction is an abnormality of diastology, but does not necessarily denote clinical heart failure. While these abnormalities of diastolic function such as E/A reversal are present, the patient may not have the clinical features of heart failure. The use of LV ejection fraction clearly is an oversimplification of the disease, but it has been useful in guiding therapy.

The overwhelming majority of major heart failure clinical trials thus far have been directed at treating patients with systolic dysfunction and there have been significant advances in treatment of systolic heart failure over the last 15–20 years. Large clinical trials such as the African-American Heart Failure Trial *(12)*, Vasodilator Heart Failure Trials 1 and 2 *(18,19)*, the Study of Left Ventricular Dysfunction *(20)*, Cooperative North Scandinavian Enalapril Survival Study *(21)*, U.S. Heart Failure Trials *(22)*, the Metoprolol CR/XL Randomized Intervention Trial in Chronic Heart Failure *(23)*, Randomized Aldactone Evaluation Study *(24)*, and others have shown significant benefits for the treatment of systolic

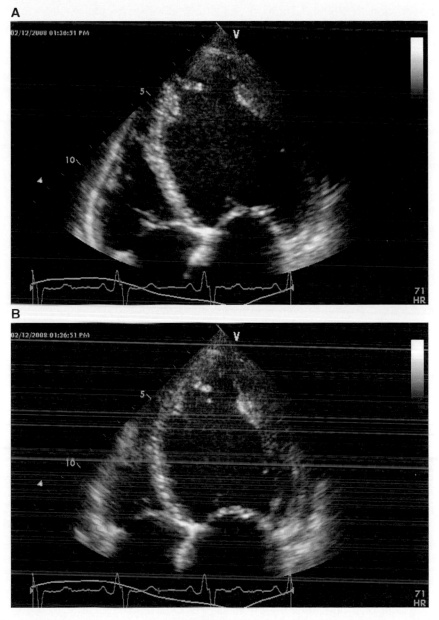

Fig. 4. Diastolic (**A**) and systolic (**B**) images of a patient with a dilated cardiomyopathy and a severely reduced left ventricular ejection fraction. Note tenting of the mitral valve leaflets which is commonly seen in patients with a dilated cardiomyopathy.

dysfunction. Through afterload reduction, renin–angiotensin–aldosterone system modulation, including angiotensin-converting enzyme inhibitors and angiotensin receptor blockers, aldosterone antagonists and beta blockers, significant benefits in morbidity and mortality have been achieved. None of these studies have examined therapy for diastolic heart failure. Additional studies are ongoing but to date, there are no proven therapies demonstrating reduction in total or cardiovascular mortality for diastolic heart failure except treating the underlying cause such as hypertension and coronary artery disease. The use of diuretics provides symptomatic relief without proven prognostic benefit. Nevertheless, in the Candesartan in Heart Failure-Assessment of Mortality and Morbidity (CHARM) trial, patients with preserved LV function treated with candesartan appeared to have a decrease in hospitalization without mortality benefit (25).

Most of the aforementioned studies relied heavily on echocardiography as a means to assess LV ejection fraction. These studies also showed a significant difference in the etiology of heart failure with an increased incidence of hypertensive heart disease as a precursor to the development of systolic dysfunction in the African-American population. Presumably, the presence of diastolic dysfunction preceded systolic dysfunction in most, if not all of these patients. This has important therapeutic implications since aggressive treatment of the underlying cause for the diastolic dysfunction, usually hypertension, may have a significant influence on eventual outcomes.

It is important to appreciate that diastolic dysfunction may occur in the presence of long-standing hypertension even without LVH (26). The National Heart, Lung, and Blood Institute (NHLBI), Jackson Heart Study, and ARIC evaluated 1849 African-American subjects to evaluate the determinants and distribution of geometric patterns of LVH and how they relate to LV function (27). Diastolic dysfunction was more likely to be present in patients with concentric hypertrophy and systolic dysfunction present in patients with eccentric hypertrophy. Concentric remodeling was not associated with either systolic or diastolic dysfunction. A study conducted in 505 Afro-Caribbean subjects revealed that the underlying cardiomyopathy associated with LVH tended to be secondary to diastolic dysfunction in approximately 57% of the subjects (28). Review of clinical trials which examine diastolic function demonstrates that subjects are usually middle aged and older and disproportionately African-American and Hispanic. In a recent study of the New York Heart Failure Registry, which evaluated 400 subjects with heart failure and preserved ejection fraction, the subject profile was similar, but mainly female (29).

Diastolic abnormalities may also develop from several other processes including infiltrative processes. Furthermore, intramyocardial fibrin, protein, and collagen deposition may result in increased myocardial stiffness along with reduced compliance. The prototypical disease process is amyloidosis of the heart, which will be subsequently discussed. In addition, patients can present with acute diastolic abnormalities in the presence of acute ischemia. Though hypertension is a major factor in CVD in African-Americans, coronary artery disease is also very prevalent. In ischemia, the mismatch in myocardial oxygen supply and demand leads to increased myocardial noncompliance, hence the diastolic abnormality. An increase in LV end diastolic pressure because of impaired compliance results in exertional dyspnea and orthopnea and may ultimately lead to pulmonary edema; thus volume overload, per se, may not be the only precursor for heart failure in patients with diastolic dysfunction *(28)*.

The ability to directly treat diastolic dysfunction, regardless of etiology, would also provide a significant benefit to patients, particularly African-Americans who have higher degrees of heart failure and possibly decreased outcomes. Recent advances in echocardiography have made it much easier to assess diastolic indices. As briefly mentioned previously, there are a number of parameters used to assess diastolic function. A highly recommended report from the Mayo Clinic refers to three key recommended measurements for the clinical assessment of diastolic function: a quantitative assessment of left atrial volume, assessment of the mitral valve inflow profile, and lastly the assessment of LV function *(30)*.

4. ULTRASOUND IMAGING IN INFILTRATIVE DISEASE

There are certain diseases, such as sarcoidosis, which are known to cause infiltrative cardiomyopathies and have a predilection for African-Americans and darker-skinned Europeans. The incidence of sarcoidosis is higher in African-Americans and although it is typically manifested by a worsening chronic lung disease, there is involvement of the heart at autopsy in 20–30% of cases. Sarcoidosis usually manifests in the heart as nodules composed of fibrin and other protein which affect the conduction system and may result in various dysrhythmia, mainly heart block. Echocardiographic imaging may reveal that the ejection fraction is normal or near normal, and abnormal diastolic relaxation may be found. However, it rarely causes a restrictive physiology. The left ventricle may appear dilated with regional wall motion abnormalities at the mid and basal levels and there may be evidence of right-sided failure and pulmonary hypertension. The nodular deposition in the heart and the mediastinal lymphadenopathy cannot be seen by echocardiography; therefore, MRI may be a useful imaging modality for this entity.

Amyloid disease may be primary or secondary. Primary amyloid is a rapidly fatal disease especially if it involves the heart, with time of diagnosis of disease to demise of ~10 months. There is also an autosomal dominant type of amyloidosis, formerly described as pre-albumin amyloidosis and now referred to as Trans Thyretin protein or TTR amyloid, which may be potentially treatable even if it involves the heart, affecting

African-Americans 3.5–4% more frequently and predominantly seen in older males *(31)*. The effects, outcomes, and treatability are still being researched. On the echocardiogram, the typical speckled pattern with a significantly thickened left ventricle in the correct clinical setting is highly suggestive of amyloid. Using harmonic imaging, which is standard on modern echocardiography equipment, will often give a speckled appearance on many studies and switching to fundamental imaging when amyloid is suspected will often be helpful to minimize over diagnosing amyloid. Additionally, the presence of significant "hypertrophy" on echocardiography without increased voltage on ECG is highly suspicious for amyloid heart disease. In many African-Americans with hypertension and renal disease, secondary amyloid of the heart can develop but may remain undiagnosed as there will be evidence of LVH and LV dysfunction, independent of whether or not amyloid is involved. A small pericardial effusion can be common to both chronic renal disease and cardiac amyloid. This pericardial effusion may be an innocent bystander and the patient may not necessarily have manifestation of pericarditis. The other possibility is that this is an effusive low-grade chronic pericarditis or an effusion secondary to heparin used during dialysis.

5. OTHER CARDIOMYOPATHIES

5.1. Hypertrophic Cardiomyopathy in Athletes

Sudden death in young athletes is devastating. The attention to this highly reported condition was initiated after the anguish and disbelief that accompanied the unexpected death of Hank Gathers in 1989 while playing basketball for Loyola Marymount, California. His autopsy subsequently showed that he died from hypertrophic cardiomyopathy which is thought to be the most common cause of nontraumatic death in young athletes (Fig. 5). The disease has extensive diastolic abnormalities and has a particular interest for many physicians particularly caring for African-American athletes. It must be noted that these patients also have significant systolic abnormalities despite often having normal LV ejection fractions. Sudden death in young athletes disproportionately affects African-Americans as compared to whites *(32)*. The use of tissue Doppler imaging and diastolic filling patterns are specifically beneficial in distinguishing the pathology in these patients and are very useful in identifying the normal changes accompanying the athletic heart versus the pathologic heart of hypertrophic cardiomyopathy.

5.2. Left Ventricular Noncompaction

Left ventricular noncompaction is a disorder of the myocardium that is characterized by very prominent trabeculations (Fig. 6), typically only

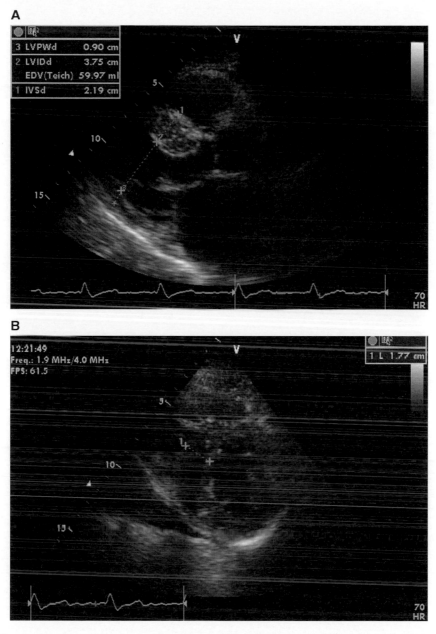

Fig. 5. Parasternal long axis (**A**) and a parasternal short-axis (**B**) images of a patient with hypertrophic cardiomyopathy. An outflow tract gradient (**C**) with a the character-istic *dagger* shape and systolic anterior motion of the mitral valve (**D**) are also noted.

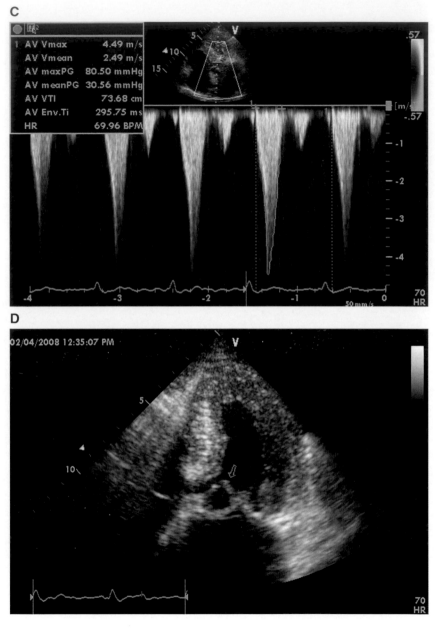

Fig. 5. (Continued)

seen in utero. This condition has been associated with progressive decline
in LV function and a higher incidence of thromboembolism and ventricu-

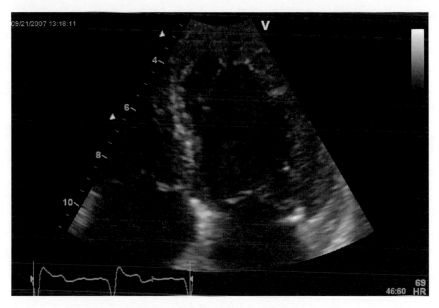

Fig. 6. Four chamber echocardiogram of a patient with left ventricular noncompaction. Note the sinusoidal trabeculations present most prominently at the left ventricular apex.

lar arrhythmia *(33)*. More recent studies suggest a more benign outcome than previously suspected *(34)*, although it is thought to be familial with an autosomal-dominant inheritance, which makes the diagnosis important for the purpose of screening first-degree relatives. As knowledge of this condition increases and image quality improves with current cardiac ultrasound equipment, frequency of diagnosis has also become more common. Increased awareness with wider utilization of cardiac ultrasound may lead to more widespread recognition of this condition. Current diagnostic criteria are controversial *(35–37)* although the echocardiographic features often are not subtle. Also, there has been data that suggest an increased incidence of cardiomyopathy secondary to noncompaction in black children *(38, 39)*. Alternatively, Kohli et al. recently suggested that current diagnostic criteria are too sensitive, particularly in black patients *(40)*. They found that the incidence based on current criteria in a control group of healthy black patients was higher than expected. Furthermore, the diagnosis in blacks using current criteria was more than twice that of whites. This again highlights the importance of studying both white and nonwhite populations to recognize important differences between these groups.

Systemic lupus erythematosus (SLE) occurs in about 2% of the African-American population, is more likely to involve young women between the ages of 19 and 25 years old, and may also result in a cardiomyopathy or pericardial process. The cardiomyopathy is often manifested as congestive heart failure with systolic dysfunction, and diastolic dysfunction may coexist. There may also be evidence of a myopericarditis with elevated troponins and other cardiac markers, secondary to an inflammatory process, although cardiac catherization may demonstrate normal coronaries. There may be a wall motion abnormality on echo which may be global or segmental. Additionally, an effusive pericardial effusion may be present also manifested by chest discomfort and dyspnea. Valvular disease may be separate or concomitant; this is manifested by cardiac ultrasound as wart-shaped verucous vegetations on the underside of the mitral valve or non-infectious endocarditis.

Hemosiderosis is another type of infiltrative disease. This condition is more prominent in Asians and mainland Europeans. It may also be secondary, in the case of hemophiliacs and patients with sickle cell disease who have received multiple transfusions. The incidence in sickle cell anemia is directly related to the amount of blood transfusion received and the diagnosis may be made with echocardiography or MRI and confirmed with cardiac biopsy.

6. OBESITY

The prevalence of obesity has doubled over the last 25 years in the United States (41). Obesity, defined as a body mass index (BMI) greater than 30 in adults, has emerged as the most concerning problem as it relates to combating CVD in the United States, particularly in Hispanic and African-American patients. According to the National Health and Nutrition Examination Survey, 40% of Mexican American women and 50% of African-American women are obese (42). Patients who are obese have increased risk of developing sleep apnea, hypertension, cardiometabolic syndrome, and diabetes. They have higher incidence of diastolic dysfunction and LVH and are at greater risk for developing overt heart failure (43). The Bogalusa Heart Study evaluated 467 young adults aged 20–38 and showed that the elevated BMI as a child correlated with increased LV mass as an adult, thereby linking childhood obesity to subsequent increased cardiac morbidity and mortality in adults (44). Furthermore, compared with whites, blacks had greater LV mass (indexed to height). In addition, this same cohort of young patients has demonstrated that as clinical risk factors for cardiac disease increase, so does carotid intima medial thickness by ultrasound, particularly in the carotid bifurcation (45).

Black women tend to have extreme obesity (BMI >40 kg/m^2), three- to four-fold more than white or Hispanic women (46). In general, first-generation Asians do not have the problem of obesity. However, it is increasing in second-generation Asians in the United States. In one study, the Framingham Cohort was followed over 32 years and the investigators determined that incidence of obesity was 57% if a friend was obese, 40% if a sibling was obese, and 37% if a spouse was obese. Of course the

Framingham study is not a multiethnic study but we may draw inferences that the spread of obesity may be linked to social relations or contacts *(47)*.

Echocardiographic features seen in cardiomyopathy of obesity are often related to eccentric hypertrophy and markers of abnormal relaxation or early diastolic dysfunction. In addition, a prominent pericardial fat pad, usually apical or anterior to heart, may be seen. This may be misconstrued as pericardial effusion or pericarditis.

Arrythmogenic right ventricular dysplasia (ARVD) is a potentially lethal arrythmogenic disease with areas of right ventricular fatty infiltration and outpouchings or pseudoaneurysmal formation with a different appearance than normal pericardial fat. ARVD has a predilection for Asian patients but is not associated with obesity. The gold standard for examination of ARVD is cardiac MRI but it can also be diagnosed by a two-dimensional or three-dimensional echocardiography.

7. KAWASAKI DISEASE

Kawasaki disease, also known as mucocutaneous lymph node disease, was initially described by Tomisaku Kawasaki in 1967. The vast majority of Kawasaki disease patients are children younger than 5 years of age and it is usually self-limiting. However, the cardiac complications related to this inflammatory condition can be life threatening. There is a high incidence in children of Asian ancestry, with Japan reporting annual incidence of 500 cases per million children under the age of 5 *(48)*. The incidence is much lower in the United States, but the disease persists in some Asian American populations, such as in California where there are approximately 35 cases per 100,000 Asian children under the age of 5, over twice as high as the general population of the country *(49)*. Kawasaki disease has been described in many other groups throughout the world though none as high as in Japan. Echocardiography has assumed a primary role in the diagnosis of cardiac involvement with this illness. Establishing a diagnosis early is crucial to minimize the long term complications associated with those not treated with acetylsalicylic acid and intravenously administered immunoglobulin. The detection of aneurysms typically in the proximal segment of the major coronary arteries is often diagnostic (Fig. 7). While visualizing the coronary arteries in adults can be challenging, this is typically not difficult in the young population that this condition typically affects. Since many patients present atypically and do not fit the diagnostic criteria for Kawasaki disease, it is important to have a high incidence of suspicion particularly in children less than 5 years of age with unexplained fever.

Typical clinical features – including oral changes, arthralgia, thombocytocis, conjunctivitis, rash, or adenopathy – are often lacking. Patients under the age of 6 months are particularly prone to presenting atypically *(50,51)*. On occasion, these patients are treated for other conditions such as meningitis

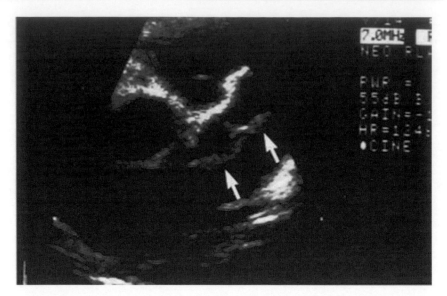

Fig. 7. Echocardiogram showing a large coronary aneurysm in a patient with Kawasaki disease.
Figure courtesy of Jane Burns-Department of Pediatrics, University of California, San Diego.

and the correct diagnosis is not established until autopsy demonstrates coronary aneurysms with thrombosis *(52)*. In those patients in which the diagnosis is suspected, echocardiography should be performed early. The incidence of coronary anomalies, which includes uniform dilatation and aneurysm, is greater than 50% in one series *(53)* and typically 18–25% in most reviews in the pediatric population. The incidence of coronary aneurysm formation is possibly related to the recognition of disease at earlier stages, thus prompt treatment is likely to decrease the incidence of aneurysm formation. It has been demonstrated that coronary aneurysms typically develop in the second week of illness and increase to the maximal diameter by the third to eighth week *(54)*. Additionally, normalizing coronary artery size to body surface area may increase the recognition of coronary anomalies in Kawasaki disease *(55)*.

Rarely recognized in adults, a Kawasaki disease diagnosis is determined almost exclusively on the constellation of clinical features described earlier. The incidence of coronary abnormalities in adults is low and recognized in only 5% of documented cases *(56)*. Using transesophageal echocardiography may increase the diagnostic yield, particularly in the adult population when there is a high clinical suspicion of Kawasaki disease with a negative transthoracic echocardiogram *(57)*. Stress echocardiography has also been used to diagnose ischemia in patients with a diagnosis of Kawasaki disease *(58)* and a recent study has shown that three-dimensional echocardiography may be superior to two-dimensional echocardiography for the evaluation of these patients *(59)*. Though less commonly reported, valvular pathology has been seen in patients with Kawasaki disease. One study showed the presence of valvular regurgitation that resolved in several patients after the acute phase of the disease *(60)*. Additionally the incidence of valvular involvement was higher in patients with coronary aneurysms.

8. FUTURE CONSIDERATIONS

The utility of cardiac ultrasound for assessing cardiac disease will continue to expand as the imaging quality increases and technical advances proceed. The use of strain imaging and other techniques will allow for better characterization of LV function both systolic and diastolic. Many trials including some discussed in this chapter have highlighted significant differences between racial and ethnic groups. Presently, and going forward, studying and recognizing these differences can only be accomplished by emphasizing the importance of including large numbers of minorities in trials using cardiac ultrasound to assess cardiac anatomy and function.

REFERENCES

1. Chobanian AV, Bakris GL, Black HR, Cushman WC, Green LA, Izzo JL, Jr, et al. The Seventh Report of the Joint National Committee on Prevention, Detection, Evaluation, and Treatment of High Blood Pressure: the JNC 7 Report. *JAMA* 2003; 289:2560–2572.
2. Verdecchia P, Carini G, Circo A, et al.; MAVI (MAssa Ventricolare sinistra nell'Ipertensione) Study Group. Left ventricular mass and cardiovascular morbidity in essential hypertension: the MAVI study. *J Am Coll Cardiol* 2001; 38:1829–1835.
3. Levy D, Garrison RJ, Savage DD, Kannel WB, Castelli WP. Prognostic implications of echocardiographically determined levt ventricular mass in the Framingham Heart Study. *N Engl J Med* 1990; 322:1561–1566.
4. Burke AP, Farb A, Liang YH, Smialek J, Virmani R. Effect of hypertension and cardiac hypertrophy on coronary artery morphology in sudden cardiac death. *Circulation* 1996; 94:3138–3145.
5. Savage DD. Hypertensive heart disease in African Americans. *Circulation* 1991; 83:1472–1474.
6. Martins D, Tareen N, Norris KC. The epidemiology of end stage renal disease among African Americans. *Am J Med Sci* 2002; 323:65–71.
7. Drazner MH, Dries DL, Peshock RM, et al. Left ventricular hypertrophy is more prevalent in blacks than whites in the general population. *Hypertension* 2005; 46:124–128.
8. Jaggy C, Perret F, Bovet P, et al. Performance of classic electrocardiographic criteria for left ventricular hypertrophy in an African population. *Hypertension* 2000; 36:54–61.
9. Okin PM, Wright JT, Nieminen MS, et al. Ethnic differences in electrocardiographic criteria for left ventricular hypertrophy: the LIFE study. Losartan intervention For End-point. *Am J Hypertens* 2002; 15:663–671.
10. Schiller NB, Shah PM, Crawford M, et al. Recommendations for quantification of the left ventricle by two-dimentional echocardiography. American Society of Echocardiography Committee on Standards, Subcommittee on Quantification of Two Dimensional Echocardiograms. *J Am Soc Echo* 1989; 2:358–367.

11. Post WS, Hill MN, Dennison CR, Weiss JL, Gerstenblith G, Blumenthal RS. High prevalence of target organ damage in young, African American inner-city men with hypertension. *J Clin Hypertens* 2003; 5:24–30.
12. Taylor AL, Ziesche S, Yancy C, et al.; African-American Heart Failure Trial Investigators. Combination of isosorbide dinitrate and hydralazine in blacks with heart failure. *N Engl J Med* 2004; 351:2049–2057.
13. The SOLVD Investigators. Effects of enalapril on survival in patients with reduced left ventricular ejection fractions and congestive heart failure. *N Engl J Med* 1991; 325: 293–302.
14. Peterson GE, de Backer T, Gabriel A, et al.; African American Study of Kidney Disease Investigators. Prevalence and correlates of left ventricular hypertrophy in the African American study of kidney disease cohort study. *Hypertension* 2007; 50:1033–1039.
15. Fox ER, Alnabhan N, Penman AD, et al. Echocardiographic left ventricular mass index predicts incident stroke in African Americans. *Stroke* 2007; 38:2686–2691.
16. Melenovsky V, Borlaug BA, Rosen B, et al. Cardiovascular features of heart failure with preserved ejection fraction versus nonfailing hypertensive left ventricular hypertrophy in The Urban Baltimore Community. *J Am Coll Cardiol* 2007; 49:198–207.
17. Bhatia RS, Tu JV, Lee DS, et al. Outcomes of heart failure with preserved ejection fraction in a population based study. *N Engl J Med* 2006; 355:260–269.
18. Cohn JN, Archibald DG, Ziesche S, et al. Effect of vasodilator therapy on mortality in chronic congestive heart failure. Results of a Veterans Administration Cooperative Study. *N Engl J Med* 1986; 325:303–310.
19. Cohn JN, Johnson G, Ziesche S, et al. A comparison of enalapril with hydralazine-isisorbide dinitrate in the treatment of congestive heart failure. *N Engl J Med* 1991; 325:303–310.
20. The SOLVD Investigators. Effect of enalapril on mortality and the development of heart failure in asymptomatic patients with reduced left ventricular ejection fractions. *N Engl J Med* 1992; 327:685–691.
21. The CONSENSUS Trial Study Group. Effects of enalapril on mortality in severe congestive heart failure. Results of Cooperative North Scandinavian enalapril survival study. *N Engl J Med* 1987; 316:1429–1435.
22. Cohn JN, Fowler MB, Bristow MR, et al. Safety and efficacy of carvedilol in severe heart failure. The US Carvedilol Heart Failure Study Group. *J Card Fail* 1997; 173–179.
23. Effect of metoprolol CR/XL in chronic heart failure: Metoprolol CR/XL Randomised Intervention Trial in Congestive Heart Failure (MERIT-HF). *Lancet* 1999; 353: 2001–2007.
24. Pitt B, Zannad F, Remme WJ, et al. The effect of spironolactone on morbidity and mortality in patients with severe heart failure. Randomized Aldactone Evaluation Study Investigators. *N Engl J Med* 1999; 341:709–717.
25. Yusuf S, Pfeffer MA, Swedberg K, et al.; CHARM Investigators and Committees. Effects of candesartan in patients with chronic heart failure and preserved left-ventricular ejection fraction: the CHARM-Preserved Trial. *Lancet* 2003; 362:772–776.
26. Devereux, R. Management of hypertensive patients with left ventricular hypertrophy and diastolic dysfunction. Hypertension Primer 2008, 4th ed. 501–504.
27. Fox ER, Taylo, J, Taylor H et al. Left ventricular geometric patterns in the Jackson Cohort of the Atherosclerotic Risk in communities (ARIC) study: clinical correlates and influences on systolic and diastolic dysfunction. *Am Heart J* 2007; 153(2):238–244.
28. Martin TC. Comparison of Afro-Caribbean patients presenting in heart failure with normal versus poor left ventricular systolic function. *Am J Cardiol* 2007; 100(8): 1271–1273.
29. Klapholz M, Maurer M, Lowe AM, et al.; New York Heart Failure Consortium. Hospitalization for heart failure in the presence of a normal left ventricular ejection frac-

tion: results of the New York Heart Failure Registry. *J Am Coll Cardiol* 2004; 43(8): 1432–1438.

30. Lester SJ, Tajik AJ, Nishimura RA, Oh JK, Khandheria BK, Seward JB. Unlocking the mysteries of diastolic function: deciphering the Rosetta Stone 10 years later. *J Am Coll Cardiol* 2008; 51:679–689.

31. Jacobson DR, Pastore RD, Yaghoubian R, et al. Variant-sequence transthyretin (isoleucine 122) in late-onset cardiac amyloidosis in black Americans. *N Engl J Med* 1997 Feb 13; 336(7):466–473.

32. Maron BJ, Shirani J, Poliac LC, Mathenge R, Roberts WC, Mueller FO. Sudden death in young competitive athletes. Clinical, demographic, and pathological profiles. *JAMA* 1996; 276:199–204.

33. Oechslin EN, Attenhofer Jost CH, Rojas JR, Kaufmann PA, Jenni R. Long-term follow-up of 34 adults with isolated left ventricular noncompaction: a distinct cardiomyopathy with poor prognosis. *J Am Coll Cardiol* 2000 Aug; 36(2):493–500.

34. Murphy RT, Thaman R, Blanes JG, et al. Natural history and familial characteristics of isolated left ventricular noncompaction. *Eur Heart J* 2005; 26:187–192.

35. Stöllberger C, Finsterer J, Blazek G. Left ventricular hypertrabeculation/noncompaction and association with additional cardiac abnormalities and neuromuscular disorders. *Am J Cardiol* 2002 Oct 15; 90(8):899–902.

36. Chin TK, Perloff JK, Williams RG, Jue K, Mohrmann R. Isolated noncompaction of the left ventricular myocardium. A study of eight cases. *Circulation* 1990; 82:507–513.

37. Jenni R, Oechslin E, Schneider J, Attenhofer Jost C, Kaufmann PA. Echocardiographic and pathoanatomical characteristics of isolated left ventricular noncompaction: insights from cardiovascular magnetc resonance imaging. *J Am Coll Cardiol* 2005; 46:101–105.

38. Nugent AW, Daubeney PE, Chondros P, et al. National Australian Childhood Cardiomyopathy Study. National Australian Childhood Cardiomyopathy Study. The epidemiology of childhood cardiomyopathy in Australia. *N Engl J Med* 2003; 348:1639–1646.

39. Lipshultz SE, Sleeper LA, Towbin JA, et al. The incidence of pediatric cardiomyopathy in two regions of the United States. *N Engl J Med* 2003; 348:1647–1655.

40. Kohli SK, Pantazis AA, Shah JS, et al. Diagnosis of left ventricular non compaction in patients with left ventricular systolic dysfunction: time for reappraisal of diagnostic criteria? *Eur Heart J* 2008; 29:89–95.

41. Ogden CL, Carroll MD, Curtin LR, McDowell MA, Tabak CJ, Flegal KM. Prevalence of overweight and obesity in the United States, 1999-2004. *JAMA* 2006; 13:1549–1555.

42. www.cdc.gov/nchs/data/databriefs. accessed 3/23/2008.

43. Grossman E, Oren S, Messerli FH. Left ventricular filling in the systolic hypertension of obesity. *Am J Cardiol* 1991; 68:57–60.

44. Li X, Li S, Ulusoy E, Chen W, Srinivasan SR, Berenson GS. Childhood adiposity as a predictor of cardiac mass in adulthood: the Bogalusa Heart Study. *Circulation* 2004; 110:3488–3492.

45. Berenson GS. Childhood risk factors predict adult risk associated with subclinical cardiovascular disease. The Bogalusa Heart Study. *Am J Cardiol* 2002; 90(10C):3L–7L.

46. Colin Bell A, Adair LS, Popkin BM. Ethnic differences in the association between body mass index and hypertension. *Am J Epidemiol* 2002; 155:346–353.

47. Christakis NA, Fowler JH. The spread of obesity in a large social network over 32 years. *N Engl J Med* 2007; 357(4):370–379.

48. Watts RA, Scott DG. Epidemiology of the vasculitides. *Semin Respir Crit Care Med* 2004; 25(5):455–464.

49. Chang RK. Epidemiologic characteristics of children hospitalized for Kawasaki disease in California. *Pediatr Infect Dis J* 2002; 21(12):1150–1155.

50. Burns JC, Wiggins JW, Jr, Toews WH, et al. Clinical spectrum of Kawasaki disease in infants younger than 6 months of age. *J Pediatr* 1986; 109(5):759–763.

51. Joffe A, Kabani A, Jadavji T. Atypical and complicated Kawasaki disease in infants. Do we need criteria? *West J Med* 1995; 162:322–327.
52. Huang YC, Huang FY, Lee HC. Atypical Kawasaki disease: report of two cases. *Zhonghua Min Guo Xiao Er Ke Yi Xue Hui Za Zhi* 1992; 33:206–211.
53. Marques C, Macedo A, Lima M. Changes in the coronary arteries in Kawasaki disease: echocardiographic aspects. *Rev Port Cardiol* 1990; 9:435–440.
54. Yanagisawa M, Yano S, Shiraishi H, et al. Coronary aneurysms in Kawasaki disease: follow-up observation by two-dimensional echocardiography. *Pediatr Cardiol* 1985; 6:11–16.
55. de Zorzi A, Colan SD, Gauvreau K, Baker AL, Sundel RP, Newburger JW. Coronary artery dimensions may be misclassified as normal in Kawasaki disease. *J Pediatr* 1996; 133:254–258.
56. Wolff AE, Hansen KE, Zakowski L. Acute Kawasaki disease: not just for kids. *J Gen Intern Med* 2007; 22:681–684.
57. Habon T, Toth K, Keltai M, Lengyel M, Palik I. An adult case of Kawasaki disease with multiplex coronary aneurysms and myocardial infarction: the role of transesophageal echocardiography. *Clin Cardiol* 1998; 21:529–532.
58. Noto N, Ayusawa M, Karasawa K, et al. Dobutamine stress echocardiography for detection of coronary artery stenosis in children with Kawasaki disease. *J Am Coll Cardiol* 1996; 27:1251–1256.
59. Miyashita M, Karasawa K, Taniguchi K, et al. Usefulness of real-time 3-dimensional echocardiography for the evaluation of coronary artery morphology in patients with Kawasaki disease. *J Am Soc Echocardiogr* 2007; 20(8):930–933.
60. Akagi T, Inoue O, Ohara N, et al. Valvular regurgitation in patients with Kawasaki disease and in healthy children: a pulsed Doppler echocardiographic study. *J Cardiol* 1989; 19:787–796.

14 Heart Failure in Racial/Ethnic Groups

M.R. Echols, MD
and C.W. Yancy, MD

CONTENTS

Abstract

Heart failure management continues to excel through evidence-based efforts. In relation to race/ethnicity, heart failure continues to disproportionately affect minorities, often with a significantly different phenotypical profile. As the evidence strengthens for heart failure management, there are rising concerns of differential effects of medical therapies for various minority groups. Even so, there are no data to suggest that any of the current medical therapies available have deleterious effects on any group of minority patients with heart failure.

From: *Contemporary Cardiology: Cardiovascular Disease in Racial and Ethnic Minorities*
Edited by: K.C. Ferdinand and A. Armani, DOI 10.1007/978-1-59745-410-0_14
© Humana Press, a part of Springer Science+Business Media, LLC 2009

This chapter will evaluate the evidence for the accepted chronic therapies of heart failure management as they relate to minority patients and outcome. We will also address the selective benefits of more current race-specific evidence-based therapies.

Key Words: Heart failure; Genetic polymorphisms; Beta-blockers; Angiotensin-converting enzyme inhibitors; Angiotensin receptor blockers; Aldosterone antagonists; Isosorbide dinitrate/hydralazine.

1. OVERVIEW

The United States population continues to diversify at an accelerated rate. Although the Caucasian race remains the majority, the minority population is quickly expanding so much so that there is not likely to be a majority group in the United States by 2050. The African-American and Hispanic populations are at the forefront of growth in the United States, with reported Hispanic community increases of almost 20 times that of the African-Americans since 2000 (1). Although these changes in the population continue to diversify cultural and societal background of the United States, all three of the top racial/ethnic populations share a commonality in the burden of cardiovascular disease (CVD). CVD is the most prevalent disease state for Caucasians, African-Americans, and the Hispanic population, with increased death rates in specific entities, such as heart failure, for the African-American cohort and increased prevalence of important risk factors, such as obesity and diabetes, for the Hispanic cohort with an increase in overt CVD likely to follow (2).

Although significant advances in the treatment of heart failure have occurred, certain racial/ethnic groups appear to have inexplicable differences in disease prevalence and outcomes. Some of these differences are clearly due to nuances in risk factors/physiology and to individual patient preferences but an important component of the differences among groups is due to disparate health care which reflects inherent bias in medical decision making, certain cultural insensitivities within the health-care delivery model and inadequate access to care. Whether the issues relate to risk factor prevalence, differing physiology or disparate health care, research efforts continue to lag regarding interventions within the minority community to reduce the significant differences/disparities of care and management. To further complicate this matter, the data on the Hispanic population with heart failure are scant at best, as this population has just recently become a focus of investigation relating to health-care disparities and record keeping based on surnames only is unfortunately incomplete and inaccurate. Clinical trial participation has also been problematic for the minority community, which lessens the confidence of extrapolation of positive results to these groups (3). Even so, there are no data at present that suggest the ineffectiveness of treating any minority group based on the well-recognized clinical guidelines for heart failure management *(4)*.

This chapter will review many of the societal, genetic, and clinical varia tions in the African-American and Hispanic communities, primarily pertaining to heart failure. Through critical appraisal of the available evidence, we hope to provide a much needed sense of appreciation for population-specific research in heart failure, as the opportunities for reduction of CVD dispari ties continue to persist.

2. EPIDEMIOLOGY AND VARIANCE OF HEART FAILURE IN MINORITY GROUPS

The prevalence of heart failure in African-Americans, approximately 3%, is higher than any other race/ethnic group, although data from the American Heart Association suggest that the prevalence of heart failure in Hispanic males follows closely (~2.7%) *(2)*. This increased prevalence is compounded by worrisome prognosis, as the death rates for both African-American males and females suffering with heart failure especially between the ages of 45 and 64 years, exceeds any other race/ethnic group. These findings raise several important inquiries as to why there are differences in the prevalence of heart failure between racial and ethnic groups. In order to provide reasons for these differences, the prevalence and prognosis of other CVD must be considered as these disease states often foreshadow events leading to heart failure through a variety of pathophysiologic conditions. In the African-American and Hispanic communities, diseases such as hyper tension, diabetes, and obesity occur in significantly higher proportions than in Caucasians *(5–7)*. One or a combination of these conditions are usually responsible for myocardial damage either as a result of myocyte loss due to a myocardial infarction or due to left ventricular remodeling from hyperten sive heart disease or other non-ischemic disease states. African-Americans are particularly affected by hypertension significantly more than any other racial/ethnic group in the world, which is thought to be the pre-emptive condition associated with the progression to heart failure in this group *(8)*. Remarkably, the precise pathophysiologic pathways that explain the devel opment of left ventricular systolic dysfunction from hypertensive heart dis ease have not yet been elucidated. Thus, the association of hypertension with heart failure is a certainty but the etiology of left ventricular dysfunc tion leading to heart failure when hypertension is the sole antecedent illness remains an uncertainty. Even so, the etiology of the common non-ischemic cardiomyopathy in African-Americans is most probably multi-factorial in origin, with emerging evidence pertaining to endothelial dysfunction as a significant cause of injury *(8–10)*.

The reasons for the increased prevalence of heart failure in Hispanic males are not as clear, although the prevalence of diabetes, obesity, and hypercholesterolemia certainly establishes a very high-risk environment *(2)*. With this increased prevalence of a number of cardiovascular conditions, it is not unreasonable to consider these conditions collectively representing a strong predilection for myocardial infarctions. However, the prevalence of MI in 2004 was the highest in Caucasian males (5.9%), while all other racial–ethnic gender groups had a prevalence of approximately 3–4%, with a slightly decreased prevalence of MI in Caucasian females and Hispanic females (~2%). This apparent "paradox" of risk factors vs overt episodes of myocardial infarction remains the focus of intense epidemiological investigation. Although few research efforts have evaluated possible biochemical implications in the Hispanic community, there are most likely some commonalities within their physiological/phenotypic profile that contribute to the multi-factorial reasons of significant heart failure prevalence.

The phenotypic profile of African-Americans (and likely Hispanics) with heart failure differs substantially from Caucasians. African-Americans with chronic heart failure tend to be younger, with a higher prevalence of hypertension and lower atherosclerotic burden *(8,11–15)*. Few studies have evaluated the profile and racial differences in acute decompensated *or hospitalized* heart failure. Echols and colleagues compared the African-American phenotype presentation of an acute heart failure exacerbation with their Caucasian counterparts in the OPTIME-CHF trial *(13)*. African-Americans were again younger, with higher blood pressure at the time of presentation. With respect to prognosis, the African-American patients tended to fare better in terms of intermediate survival prior to statistical adjustment. After adjustment for confounding factors, there was no difference in short-term survival between African-Americans and Caucasians. These data are promising, as an emphasis on appropriate medical therapy and access to care afforded by participation in a clinical trial seem to lessen the disparities in outcome for African-American patients with heart failure. These data also provocatively suggest that the source of true disparate care is likely not within the hospital setting but in the outpatient setting when access to care is not as readily provided. Because of the inherent bias of retrospective analyses, these data only provide hypothesis stimulating concepts without definitive evidence and prompt more research.

3. THEORIES OF DISPARATE CARDIOVASCULAR CARE

The exact reasons for the disparate prevalence and care of heart failure in various racial–ethnic groups are unknown. Several generalizable key factors have been identified as potential contributors to the disparities seen in cardiovascular disease. Bias, whether it is racial, ethnic, gender, or age-related, is a well-recognized entity in American medicine. However, many of the studies assessing potential bias in cardiovascular care have demonstrated that racial bias is only one of several potential explanations for disparate health care and is not the sole reason for disparate care. Kressin and colleagues *(16)* prospectively evaluated the possibility of patient belief as explanation of the disparities seen in cardiac catheterization in the Veteran's Administration system. In this study, Caucasian patients were significantly more likely to undergo cardiac catheterization after a positive test of myocardial ischemia on nuclear imaging when compared with the African-American patients in the study (OR 1.43, 95% CI 1.02–2.02, $p = 0.04$). All of the patients were surveyed to assess the possible reason for this occurrence. On average, the African-American patients were more likely to admit to having physician trust issues, and more often reported stronger religious connections. However, there were no significant differences seen between the African-Americans and the Caucasians pertaining to patient's belief or attitude toward health care. In this study, socio-demographic or clinical characteristics were not related to the disparity in cardiac catheterization between races. Interestingly, physician assessment of the probability of disease did differ between groups, as the physicians were less likely to feel that African-Americans had clinically significant coronary artery disease. These findings suggested that the source of bias may involve the physician's perception of the clinical situation. A more recent study evaluated the possibility of unconscious or implicit bias regarding decision making of 287 internal medicine and emergency medicine residents *(17)*. The study consisted of web-based evaluation of several clinical vignettes pertaining to decision making of thrombolysis during an acute MI compared with invasive testing. After the residents viewed the clinical vignettes, the Implication Association Test (IAT) was given. Despite the conscious denial of explicit bias toward African-American patients, the results of the IAT suggested not only favorable preference toward the Caucasian patients of the clinical vignettes but also strongly correlated an implicit bias against the African-American patients due to stereotypical beliefs of less cooperation for invasive testing. These findings were the first of its kind suggesting implicit bias of physicians against African-Americans in cardiovascular medicine. This is an important factor to recognize, as approaching each case objectively with proper application of clinical guidelines is a crucial step in the elimination of health-care disparities.

Other factors have been implicated as possible explanations for cardiovascular disease disparities. Language barriers for patients unable to communicate in English may definitely contribute to a portion of the racial disparities seen in the Hispanic population as well as in other non-English speaking populations. DuBard and colleagues *(18)* reported that primarily Spanish-speaking Hispanics were far less likely to recognize myocardial infarction or stroke symptoms, when compared with English-speaking Hispanics, African-American, and Caucasian patients. These findings persisted after adjustment for socio-demographic characteristics, health-care access, and cardiovascular risk factors. From the medical perspective, this is quite alarming as delayed diagnosis of both myocardial infarction and stroke could have untoward effects which impact prognosis.

Still other factors have also been implicated in the persistent racial disparities seen in cardiovascular care and heart failure management, such as socioeconomic status and access to health care. Socioeconomic status is the term used most commonly to describe several important factors that possibly contribute to health-care disparities, including education level of the patient, financial income, insurance status, as well as access to care *(19)*. Undoubtedly, these factors are related to the health-care disparities, but again, no single factor fully explains disparate health care. In many cases, socioeconomic status tends to become less important after adjustment for other confounders *(20)*, but this is incipient research and both limited research methods and inadequate quantifiable measures of socioeconomics may explain the underwhelming findings when socioeconomic status is evaluated as a contributor to disparate health care. Thus, socioeconomic variances may still represent possible causes of CVD disparities and further research is warranted *(21,22)*.

4. GENETIC VARIATION IN MINORITY GROUPS

4.1. Beta (β1Arg389) and Alpha (α2cDel322-325) Receptor Polymorphism

The terms "race" and "ethnicity" encompass numerous phenotypical profiles that are often categorized or described when referring to health-care disparity. However, it is clear that these terms alone do not offer either a scientific or a physiological grouping. Thus, great care must be exercised when genetic data are being evaluated along racial or ethnic lines. It should be clearly stated that race is not an appropriate proxy for genetics and that race or ethnicity is only important to the extent that it provides a grouping of individuals, admittedly heterogeneous, with certain shared environmental factors and a certain degree of shared genetic substrate due to intermarriage. Within the last decade, research efforts have accommodated the possibility of genetic variation between racial and ethnic groups as a more plausible explanation for the differences seen in therapy between racial and ethnic groups *(14)*. The β-1 adrenergic receptor (β1Arg389) and alpha$_{2c}$-adrengergic receptor (α2cDel322-325) have been targets of evaluation for several investigators pertaining to heart failure risk. Small and colleagues recognized an association of these receptor variants with an increase risk for heart failure *(23)*. The β1-adrenergic receptor variant (β1Arg389) of the cardiomyocyte has been associated with increased coupling to the stimulatory G protein, increasing intracellular cyclic AMP. This stimulation of the cardiac myocytes produce increased chronotropy and inotropy

(23). The alpha$_{2c}$-adrengergic receptor is associated with feedback regulation of norepinephrine release in the sympathetic nerves. The presence of the α2cDel322-325 allele is associated with decreased regulatory function and increased presynaptic release of norepinephrine from the sympathetic ganglion *(24)*. When the beta-1 receptor is stimulated by increased cyclic AMP and there is more release of norepinephrine, there may be apparent increase seen in the risk of left ventricular dysfunction. Small and colleagues confirmed these findings in a small cohort of African-American and Caucasian patients with and without heart failure. The African-American patients were more commonly homozygous for the α2cDel322-325 allele, which increased the risk of heart failure development in this study. The presence of both α2cDel322-325 and β1Arg389 alleles in homozygous form were also seen more commonly in African-American patients, which also significantly increased their risk for heart failure when compared with the Caucasian patients of the cohort (odds ratio 10.11, 95% CI 2.11–48.53, $p = 0.004$).

However, recent data from the Dallas Heart Study (DHS) suggest that there are no associations of these alleles with decreased systolic function in African-Americans without a known history of heart disease *(25)*. The DHS is a large population-based probability sample in Dallas County, Texas, which overestimated the African-American cohort by design, in order to increase participation and data collection of this group. Although the investigators of DHS confirmed the increased frequency of these genetic variants in African-Americans compared with Caucasian patients within the study, these findings suggest that the variants may not fully explain the associations of worse prognosis and increased risk of heart failure reported in other studies. Moreover, these contrasting findings point out that even when reasonable genetic markers of disease/risk have been identified, there may remain certain environmental factors which are necessary before the disease phenotype is expressed.

4.2. Nitric Oxide and NOS3

Nitric oxide (NO) is an endogenous compound generated by NO synthases (NOS) that convert L-arginine to L-citrulline in the presence of molecular oxygen, nicotinamide–adeninine dinucleotide phosphate (NADPH), calmodulin and other cofactors *(26,27)*. This compound is produced in the presence of NO synthase (NOS), utilizing molecular oxygen and several other cofactors in the catalytic process. Three isoforms of NOS have been identified in human and animal models, all of which are found in the human heart. Neuronal NOS (nNOS) and endothelial NOS (eNOS) are both dependent on calcium/calmodulin complex for activation. Inducible NOS (iNOS) is calcium independent and is associated with continuous production of NO, unlike the pulsatile production of NO by nNOS and eNOS. Nitric oxide produced by nNOS appears to facilitate neuronal transmission and nitric oxide produced by iNOS is important in the response to infection and in the function of leukocytes. Endothelial NO production affords relaxation of smooth muscle and prevention of proliferation, inhibition of platelet aggregation, and reduction of shear stress via decreased vascular resistance. NO has also demonstrated antihypertrophic effects on myocardium, primarily through cGMP-dependent protein kinases (28).

Dysfunctional endothelium hinders the production and bioavailability of NO which increases the production of reactive oxygen species and oxidative stress. Reduced concentrations of NO cosubstrates, such as L-arginine, promote inactivation of eNOS and 1 electron reduction of $O2$ to $O2^-$, also known as superoxide. Increased production of $O2^-$ further increases oxidative stress by reacting with available NO to form peroxynitrite ($ONOO^-$). $ONOO^-$ is responsible for several deleterious effects within the cardiovascular system, such as lipid peroxidation, increased apoptosis of myocytes, and inactivation of enzymes necessary for contractile function (29).

Investigations from the genetics substudy of the African American Heart Failure Trial (A-HeFT) regarding a NOS3 variant allele (Asp298 variant) suggest altered production and regulation of NO specific to African-Americans patients with heart failure (30). This NOS variant is also associated with worse outcome in Caucasian patients with systolic dysfunction as well (31). The Asp298 variant of the NOS3 gene has a shorter-half-life in vitro, which is thought to be responsible for reduce nitric oxide production (32). Limited data from the Genetic Risk Assessment in Heart Failure (GRAHF), subset A-HeFT study, suggest significantly higher frequency of the Asp298 variant in approximately 80% of the patients from A-HeFT (33). This frequency was significantly higher than the 56% frequency detected in a previous Caucasian cohort (31). These studies and others provide new insight into the genetic variants and outcome of the African-American population with systolic heart failure. Further evaluation of "gene-tailored" therapies is now required to assess whether this mode of treatment will alter the overall outcome and prognosis in this group.

4.3. Aldosterone Synthase (CYP11B2-C344-T)

Aldosterone has been associated with a number of deleterious effects in heart failure, including progression of cardiac remodeling and inflammation (34–37). Although limited, the data evaluating therapies emphasizing aldosterone reduction or receptor blockade have proven to be of significant benefit in the management of chronic systolic heart failure, as well as heart failure associated with acute coronary syndrome (38,39). Aldosterone is primarily produced from transcription of the gene aldosterone synthase (CYP11B2). A genetic variant of this gene, involving C to T transition at position −344 (−344C) has been implicated in the prognosis of heart failure specific to

African-Americans, as it is associated with increased aldosterone production *(40,41)*. This association was demonstrated in the aforementioned GRAHF study. McNamara and colleagues evaluated the outcome of patients with the −344C polymorphism in comparison with other *CYP11B2* genotypes. A total of 354 patients were evaluated in this study, with 22 patients having the homozygous −344C polymorphism. The patients with this genetic pattern had significantly worse heart failure hospitalization-free survival, as well as a higher rate of death. This study presented intriguing evidence that control of aldosterone activity in African-American patients with heart failure may be another importance genetic variation and target for intervention.

Although a compelling association, other data seem to curtail the significance of these results. Biolo and colleagues *(41)* evaluated the prognostic effect of the C allele frequency in 74 patients with chronic systolic heart failure. Approximately 65% of the patients were African-American; however, the C allele frequency for *CY11B2* was found much less common in the African-American cohort. There was also no significant difference in the serum level of aldosterone between allele frequencies, a finding that was not reported from the GRAHF study. In this study, the 344-C allele was actually associated with improved cardiac function in the African-American patients, while no benefit was seen with the polymorphism in the non-African-American patients. Other studies have shown similar findings, with greater improvement in cardiac function shown after implementation of angiotensin-converting enzyme inhibitors *(42)*. These findings suggest a complex interaction of the aldosterone and angiotensin system, with further delineation of the effects required. It is reasonable to consider that the conflicting findings for this polymorphism de-emphasizes the importance of the evaluation of a single polymorphism in heart failure management for certain populations and once again highlight the importance of the context in which these genetic variants occur.

Although limited studies have evaluated genetic polymorphisms for heart failure in the Hispanic community, much of the data are not associated with significant prognostic findings in this population. Several polymorphisms of the rennin–angiotensin–aldosterone system were evaluated in an African-American and Latino cohort relating to hypertension. The aldosterone synthase gene, *CYP11B2*, was also evaluated in this study and was found to have no association with pathologic disease in the Hispanic patients evaluated, unlike the African-American patients of the study *(43)*. Although this study did not show an association with hypertension in the Hispanic patients, it is conceivable that other genetic variants may have an association with cardiovascular disease in this population. Therefore, continued characterization of other polymorphisms may offer a promise for more race-based pharmacologic interventions. Much like the African-American population where considerable heterogeneity exists, the Hispanic population likewise has significant intra-group variations as the origin of certain Hispanic persons might be from Mexico, South America, Puerto Rico, etc.

5. EVIDENCE-BASED MEDICAL THERAPY FOR MINORITIES WITH HEART FAILURE

The therapeutic management evidence for heart failure in minority groups is primarily derived from large clinical trials, most of which has been incorporated into clinical guidelines for heart failure management. Much of the data characterizing medical therapy in the African-American and Hispanic populations are from retrospective analyses, which were never statistically powered for evaluation of possible differential effects of therapy between race/ethnic groups. However, the subset analyses from many of the large studies do confirm benefit in specific populations, and importantly, *no evidence-based therapy has been disqualified as being totally ineffective in non-white patients (12,44).* Much of the research evaluating differential response to therapy in minorities primarily emphasizes treatment effect in African-Americans. Clinical trial participation by minority patients has been challenging. This is especially so for African-Americans who have consistently been underrepresented in major heart failure trials. Hispanic patients have been nearly absent in most clinical trials and thus virtually no data exists regarding the magnitude of benefit of certain evidence-based therapies for this group.

5.1. Beta-Blockers

Beta-blocker therapy in the management of heart failure is regarded as one of the better medical interventions in recent decades. This drug class has been associated with improved survival and quality of life for patients living with heart failure, as well as substantial reductions in sudden cardiac death *(14,45)*. Although the larger trials of beta blocker therapy in heart failure included only a small number of African-Americans, the subset findings from most of these studies are compelling for therapy in this population. However, Shekelle and colleagues performed a meta-analysis to evaluate the effects of beta-blocker and angiotensin-converting enzyme inhibitor therapy on heart failure by gender and race and reported some very interesting findings *(46)*. According to their analysis, beta-blockers were only associated with a small benefit in African-Americans, which contrasted with the significantly larger benefits seen in the Caucasian patients in this meta-analysis. This study again highlights the difficulty of result interpretation when underpowered subset populations are used to constitute a meta-analysis. Only a few studies pertaining to heart failure have successfully enrolled a representative number of minorities. The Beta-Blocker Evaluation of Survival Trial (BEST) was the only trial to primarily evaluate a beta-blocker in heart failure that stratified randomization according to race *(44)*. For this reason, the BEST trial enrolled a significant number of African-American patients

(~23%), more than any other single beta-blocker trial for heart failure. Unfortunately, the beta-blocker used (bucindolol) did not improve the outcome of heart failure for African-Americans and was actually associated with a non-significant 17% risk of death in African-Americans. The meta-analysis performed by Shekelle included this study, which represents yet another reason why the results of the meta-analysis are so difficult to interpret. As research efforts have continued with bucindolol, this drug has been associated with intrinsic sympathomimetic activity in the myocardium and is not felt to be an appropriate drug for heart failure management (46).

Other major beta-blocker trials in heart failure have had fewer African-American participants, although no adverse effects of beta-blocker therapy have been reported specific to minorities (47–49). Although only a small number of African-Americans participants were enrolled, The US Carvedilol Heart Failure Trials and the Carvedilol Prospective Cumulative Survival trial (COPERNICUS) reported very compelling findings evaluating the drug carvedilol. In both studies, optimal medical management including an ACE-I and carvedilol was associated with increased survival and reduced hospitalizations in the African-American cohorts, findings which were comparable to the results of the non-African-American participants in the studies. The Metoprolol CR/XL Randomization Intervention Trial (MERIT-HF) did not include an acceptable number of minorities but no concerns of a lack of responsiveness were noted (49).

5.2. Angiotensin-Converting Enzyme Inhibitors (ACE-I)

The ACE-I drug class is one of the most investigated drug classes in heart failure pertaining to differential effects of therapy as a function of race. The Studies of Left Ventricular Dysfunction (SOLVD) evaluated the differential effects of enalapril on heart failure outcome for patients with both asymptomatic and symptomatic left ventricular dysfunction (12,50). These studies reported a significant increased relative risk of all-cause death and rehospitalizations for African-Americans with left ventricular dysfunction when compared with the Caucasian patients of the study. These differences persisted after several adjustments, including extensive crude adjustments for socioeconomic status. These findings fueled controversy of ACE-I efficacy in the African-American population with heart failure. A re-analysis of these data using a 1:4 case-matched design was performed, with persistent increases in rehospitalizations seen for the African-American patients, although no differences in mortality were seen between races (50). In review of these findings, it does appear that African-American patients have a reduced response to ACE-I therapy when compared with Caucasians. However, these findings as all others are still subject to the flaws of retrospective analysis and serve as only thought-provoking concepts for further research. Treating African-Americans with ACE-inhibitors for heart failure is an accepted and *strongly indicated* intervention for this group and should be initiated according to clinical guidelines of chronic heart failure management *(4)*.

The Heart Outcomes Prevention Evaluation (HOPE) Study had significantly less minority participation than the SOLVD trials, and therefore no racial subset analyses have been pursued from this database *(51)*.

5.3. Angiotensin Receptor Blockers (ARBs)

Although ARBs have non-inferiority data for heart failure when compared to ACE-Is, there is little data available regarding the effects of this drug class in minority patients with heart failure. Most of the data regarding differential effects of this class comes from antihypertensive trials, although subset analyses of such trials are consistent with evidence of lesser responsiveness of therapeutics targeted toward the rennin–angiotensin system in African-Americans patients *(52,53)*. Although most of the retrospective data regarding racial responses to medical therapies for heart failure confirm benefit for minority patients, the importance of exercising care in retrospective analyses of trials with limited minority participation cannot be over-emphasized as certain observations may detract from the use of evidence-based therapies and result in less good outcomes in a high-risk patient population.

5.4. Aldosterone Antagonists or Blockers

Neither of the two major trials evaluating an aldosterone antagonist or blocker included adequate minority participation for any meaningful analysis *(37,38)*, therefore the specific effects on the African-American or Hispanic population have not been described. At present, there are no reasons to suspect that minority patients would be harmed by appropriately initiating this drug class, excluding any contraindications for therapy *(54)*.

5.5. Isosorbide Dinitrate/Hydralazine Therapy (ISDN/HYD)

The Veterans Administration Cooperation Study (V-HeFT I) was the first double blind randomized controlled trial to examine the effects of a vasodilator regimen on heart failure management *(55)*. The initial hypothesis suggested that hemodynamic compromise in heart failure was related to elevations in systemic vascular resistance which further exacerbated heart failure symptoms. Isosorbide dinitrate and hydralazine were chosen as intended therapy based on the ability of this combination to reduce preload (venodilation) and afterload (arterial dilation), similar to the effects seen with nitroprusside *(56)*. The V-HeFT I study enrolled 642 men, of which 28% were African-American. All participants received either ISDN-HYD combination (n = 186), prazosin (n = 183), or placebo (n = 273). Approximately 55% of the ISDN-HYD group achieved the maximum dose, which consisted of 160 mg of ISDN and 300 mg of HYD. At 1 year, there was a 38% reduction in mortality for the patients receiving ISDN-HYD, compared to placebo (mortality rates: 12.1% vs 19.5%, respectively). At the end of the pre-specified time point of 2 years, there was a 25% reduction in mortality (25.6% for the ISDN-HYD group compared to 34.3% for the placebo group, $p < 0.028$). Although there was significant blood pressure reduction in the prazosin group, the mortality rate was similar to the placebo group. At the end of the trial, the overall cumulative mortality reduction for the ISDN-HYD group was of borderline statistical significance ($p \sim 0.05$). Despite the marginal statistical signal, this trial was the first trial to demonstrate improved survival with drug therapy for any heart failure population.

The effects of the ISDN-HYD combination therapy were further evaluated against enalapril in V-HeFT II *(57)*. Enalapril had previously demonstrated reduction in mortality when compared to placebo in the Cooperative North Scandinavian Enalapril Survival Study (The CONSENSUS Trial Study Group 1987) in class IV heart failure *(58)*. The V-HeFT II trial enrolled 804 patients and compared the use of ISDNHYD (maximum dose 160 and 300 mg, respectively, divided into four daily doses) to enalapril (maximum dose 20 mg daily). At the pre-specified end point of 2 years, enalapril reduced mortality 28% more than the ISDN-HYD therapy. Although death from worsening heart failure did not differ between the groups, there was a significant reduction in sudden cardiac death with enalapril compared to the ISDN-HYD group. The results from this study suggested that patients benefited from enalapril therapy more than ISDN-HYD for improved survival in the setting of mild to moderate heart failure.

Further inspection of specific drug therapies began to suggest differential effects between African-Americans and Caucasian heart failure patients, primarily after the results of the SOLVD analysis for racial outcomes. A retrospective analysis of V-HeFT I and II revealed a interesting racial differences in outcomes for the African-Americans who were administered ISDN-HYD therapy *(10)*. In V-HeFT I, there was a 47% reduction in mortality for African-Americans receiving ISDN-HYD combination when compared with the African-American patients in the placebo group (9.7% vs 17.3%, respectively, $p = 0.04$). When the use of ISDN-HYD was compared to enalapril in African-American patients from V-HeFT II, there was no significant difference in mortality (12.9% vs 12.8%, $p = NS$). However, the Caucasian patients had a 26% reduction in mortality with the use of enalapril when compared with the Caucasian patients receiving ISDN-HYD therapy (11% vs 14.9%, respectively, $p = 0.02$). Results of this analysis suggested that African-Americans patients with heart failure had a heightened response to ISDN-HYD therapy, similar to that seen with the use of ACE-inhibitors. The reasons for these findings of differential response in V-HeFT I and II were not well understood at the time. There were several baseline differences in the African-American patients when compared with their Caucasian counterparts. As seen through a number of race-specific analyses for heart failure, African-American patients were younger, had less CAD, and had a significantly higher incidence of hypertension. Although there were no differences in plasma rennin activity, the Caucasian patients had higher plasma norepinephrine when compared with the African-American patients. The exclusion criteria deemed patients with uncontrolled hypertension or hypertension requiring more than diuretic therapy ineligible for both V-HeFT I and II. This exclusion undoubtedly eliminated a population in which persistent hypertension may have been the nidus for left ventricular systolic impairment.

The focus of differential effects for African-American patients with heart failure soon consisted of evaluating the effects of nitric oxide (NO) and its relationship to endothelial function in African-Americans. Previous studies evaluating the response of innate vasodilatory stimuli on forearm arterial resistance suggested differential effects between African-Americans and Caucasians (8,9). Cardillo and colleagues evaluated the differences in NO mediated vasodilation on forearm arterial resistance in relation to mental stress between African-American and Caucasian patients. Mental stress, in the form of serial seven subtractions, was used as a standard measure to increase forearm blood flow (8). The increase in forearm blood flow was easily demonstrated in the Caucasian subjects but not in the African-American subjects. Use of a NO synthesis (NOS) inhibitor NG-monomethyl-L-arginine (L-NMMA) infusion significantly reduced forearm blood flow in Caucasian patients, where the forearm blood flow in African-American patients was unaffected. These results suggested a preexisting state of nitric oxide deficiency, most probably secondary to impaired endothelial cell function in African-Americans. Use of methacholine, a parasympathetic agonist, in hypertensive patients also demonstrated less vasodilatory response of forearm blood flow in African-American patients compared with Caucasians (9). These results confirmed previous findings suggesting impaired endothelial vasomotor function in African-American patients.

There are strong suggestions of reduced endothelium-derived NO bioavailability in normotensive African-Americans as well (59). These data are also accompanied with findings of increased oxidative stress, i.e., increased production of superoxide and peroxynitrite, further increasing the likelihood of endothelial impairment in African-Americans. Ironically, total eNOS protein also appears to be increased in African-Americans, but there is lack of biologically active NO production (25). It is reasonable to presume that reduced NO bioavailability may alter myocyte function and increase cardiac hypertrophy. However, these concepts are controversial, as higher or "supernormal" levels of NO (perhaps related to iNOS activation), appear to induce caspase activation, DNA fragmentation, and cell death (27). This is a thought-provoking hypothesis, as the majority of evidence suggests that a relative NO deficiency is present in African-Americans.

HYD has been emphasized among research efforts suggesting that use of the drug therapy with nitrates reduce oxidative stress and nitrate tolerance, which are likely associated with the clinical benefit seen in patients with heart failure (28,60,61). HYD acts as a free radical scavenger in vitro, primarily from dose-dependent reduction of superoxide and peroxynitrite signaling (28). In a dose-dependent fashion, HYD suppresses the production of the free radicals, suggesting that HYD attenuated oxidative stress in a nitrate rich environment.

The effects of HYD on nitrate tolerance in the setting of heart failure have been reported in previous studies (28,29,55,57,61,62). Gogia and colleagues described the hemodynamic effects of intravenous nitroglycerin with HYD in a small number of patients with heart failure. A total of 28 patients (two groups of 14) received a 24-hour infusion of nitroglycerin either with or without oral HYD administration. Although the group-receiving nitroglycerin only did not have sustained effects, the use of HYD was associated with sustained reductions in blood pressure, pulmonary artery pressure, and mean

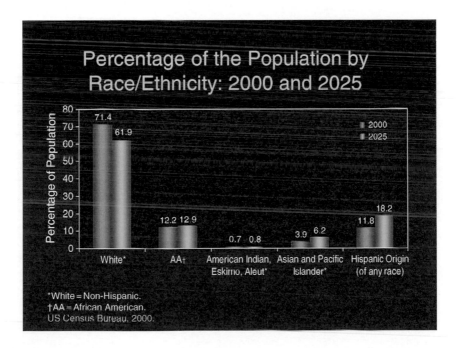

Fig. 1.

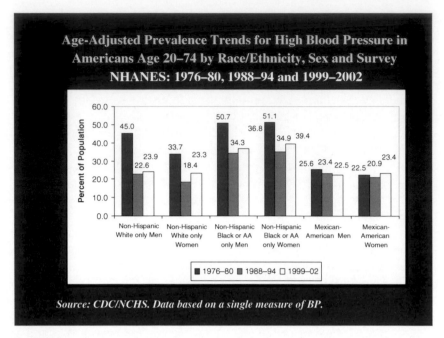

Fig. 2.

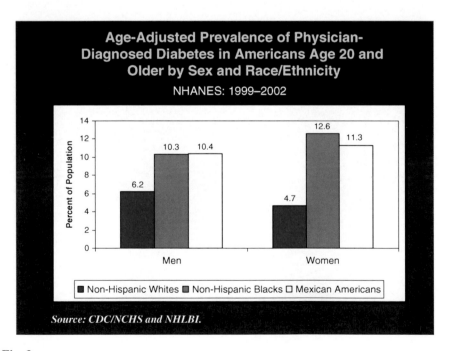

Fig. 3.

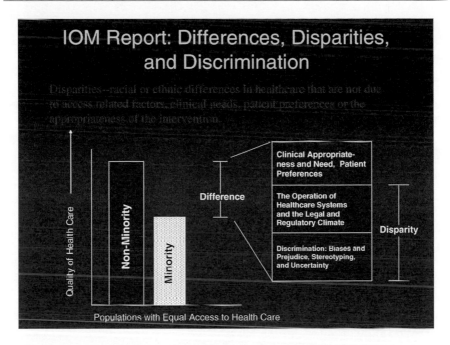

Fig. 4.

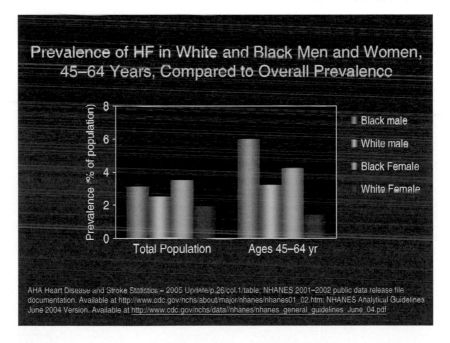

Fig. 5.

pulmonary artery wedge pressure, whereas these effects quickly weaned in the group receiving only nitroglycerin *(61)*. Based on the background of basic science from a number of previous studies and provocative mechanistic data and clinical observation, the African American Heart Failure Trial (A-HeFT) was initiated to evaluate the use of ISDN-HYD in African-American patients with advanced systolic heart failure already treated with evidence-based neurohormonal blockade.

6. THE A-HeFT EXPERIENCE

The African American Heart Failure Trial (A-HeFT) evaluated the effects of ISDN-HYD in African-American patients with moderate to severe heart failure *(29,63,64)*. A fixed-dose tablet of HYD 37.5 mg and ISDN 20 mg was administered three times daily (total daily dose HYD 112.5 mg and ISDN 60 mg). The dose was titrated to two tablets three times daily, for a total dose of HYD 225 mg and ISDN 120 mg. The maximum doses and frequency of ISDN-HYD were lower in the A-HeFT trial when compared with V-HeFT I and II (HYD 300 mg, ISDN 160 mg). The majority of all patients within the trial were taking diuretics, ACE-I/angiotensin receptor blockers, beta-blockers, and digoxin. Approximately 38–40% of the patients were receiving aldosterone antagonists at the time of enrollment. The average ejection fraction for both groups was 24%. At the end of the trial, approximately

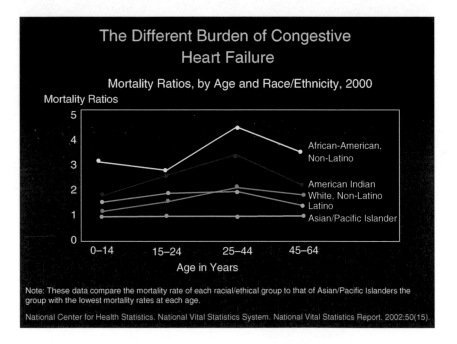

Fig. 6.

68% of the patients achieved maximal therapy in the ISDN-HYD group. The primary end point was a composite score composed of weighted values for death from any cause, first hospitalization for heart failure, and quality of life at 6 months. The Minnesota Living with Heart Failure questionnaire was used to assess quality of life. This was the first heart failure trial that utilized this composite endpoint. The composite system was designed to consider all mortality/morbidity events that contribute to heart failure outcomes (63). Secondary outcome included the separate components of the composite system, death from cardiovascular causes, the total number of hospitalizations for any reason, the total number of days of hospitalization, the overall quality of life throughout the trial, the number of unscheduled emergency room and clinic visits, the change in B-type natriuretic peptide level at 6 months, new need for cardiac transplantation, and change in myocardial remodeling at 6 months (29). The study was terminated early as there was a significantly lower mortality in the ISDN-HYD group (6.2% vs 10.2% in the placebo group, $p = 0.02$). The mean duration of follow-up was 10 months. Overall, there was a 43% reduction in mortality with the use of ISDN-HYD therapy (10.2% in the placebo group vs 6.2% in the ISDN-HYD group; Hazard Ratio 0.57, $p = 0.01$). The primary end point composite score was also significantly improved in the ISDN-HYD group. Based on the prespecified end points, quality of life was improved as well. There was a 33% reduction

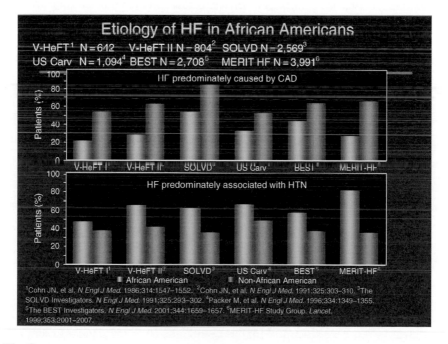

Fig. 7.

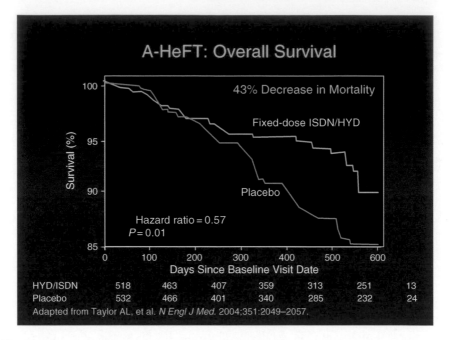

A-HeFT: Overall Survival

43% Decrease in Mortality

Fixed-dose ISDN/HYD

Placebo

Hazard ratio = 0.57
P = 0.01

HYD/ISDN	518	463	407	359	313	251	13
Placebo	532	466	401	340	285	232	24

Adapted from Taylor AL, et al. *N Engl J Med.* 2004;351:2049–2057.

Fig. 8.

in the rate of first hospitalization in the ISDN-HYD group compared with the placebo group, as well as a reduced rate of severe heart failure exacerbations in the treatment group. These findings of the A-HeFT study firmly establish the use of ISDN-HYD combination in addition to evidence-based neurohormonal blockade in African-Americans with moderately severe to severe heart failure. The data are less clear for the use of this combination vasodilator therapy in patients with mild heart failure (NYHA I or II), as there was virtually no enrollment of these populations in the A-HeFT study. Unfortunately, there is no data available for the treatment effect of this drug combination in other racial/ethnic groups.

More recent analyses from A-HeFT studies show that the ISDN-HYD combination was associated with sustained benefit in a number of subgroups. Use of the therapy was also associated with significantly relative risk reduction of approximately 75% for death related to pump failure *(65)*.

7. DEVICE AND SURGICAL THERAPY FOR HEART FAILURE

Sudden cardiac death (SCD) is a condition with a well-described association to heart failure, occurring in approximately 450,000 patients per year. The death rates for African-Americans men and women due to sudden cardiac death (?) are significantly higher than Caucasian men and women, and the sudden death rates for Hispanic patients with cardiovascular disease are slightly higher than for Caucasian women *(2)*. Gillum estimated the rates of SCD in Hispanic and African-American patients in 1997 and found significantly higher rates of SCD in African-American patients, although Hispanic patients with coronary artery disease had the lowest death rate for SCD of all racial/ethnic groups evaluated *(66)*. Other studies have shown similar findings *(67)*. It is reasonable to assume that SCD remains a significant health burden and is associated with a worrisome incidence in the minority population. However, the majority of the information pertaining to defibrillator device therapy in African-Americans is subject to critique once again due to the use of retrospective analyses. Racial differences have been evaluated from two major trials of implantable cardiac defibrillator (ICD) therapy. The Multicenter Unsustained Tachycardia Trial (MUSTT) evaluated use of ICD therapy in patients with coronary artery disease, left ventricular ejection fraction of ≤40%, and induced ventricular arrhythmia during an electrophysiology study *(68)*. The patients with inducible arrhythmias received ICD therapy, as the patients not selected for EP-guided approach received medical therapy, which included a beta-blocker and an ACE-I. African-American patients represented approximately 11% of the participants within the study, with Hispanic patients only comprising 3% of the participants. Due to the fairly low number, an analysis for the Hispanic patients of the trial was not performed. The African-American patients within the trial did

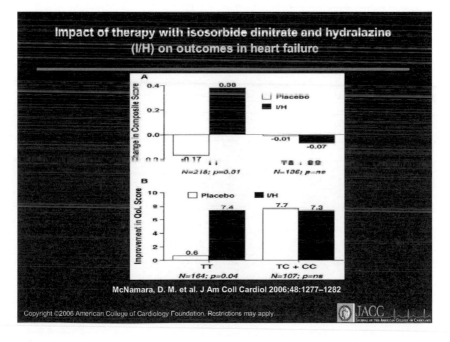

Fig. 9.

not receive benefit from the EP-guided testing and ICD placement. The Caucasian patients who received EP-guided ICD therapy had a lower mortality at
5 years when compared to the African-American patients in the study (60%
vs 37%, respectively, $p = 0.051$). These results may have been skewed significantly as a much lower percentage of African-American patients actually
received ICD therapy when compared with the Caucasian patients in the
trial (50% vs 28%, respectively) and importantly, the number of African-
Americans in the trial was too low to provide truly meaningful data.

Racial differences were also described from the Multicenter Automated
Defibrillator Trial II (MADIT-II), which highlighted similar findings (69).
African-Americans represented only 8% of the patients participating in this
trial. The African-American cohort that received ICDs in this trial did not
receive any mortality benefit, as opposed to a significantly lower mortality rate in the Caucasian patients who received ICDs (Hazard Ratio 0.29,
95% CI 0.17–0.49). Once again, due to the significantly lower numbers
of minorities in this trial, it is difficult to surmise any definite conclusions from this study. There is very little data regarding racial differences
in patients after receiving heart transplantation. However, the data do suggest that racial disparities in care may lessen or resolve after receiving such
high-intensity intervention for end-stage heart failure (70,71). Pamboukian
and colleagues (70) demonstrated this in a retrospective review of the Rush

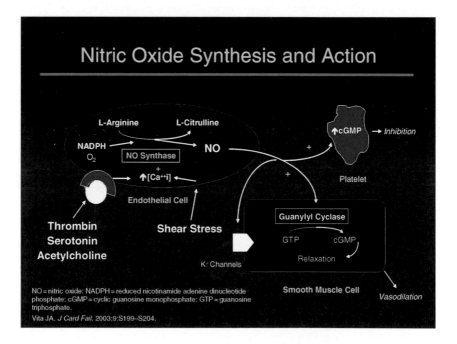

Fig. 10.

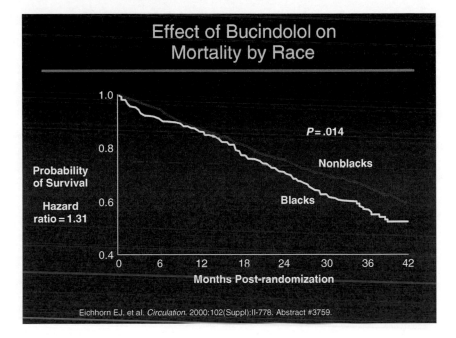

Fig. 11.

Heart Failure and Cardiac Transplant Database. Twenty-eight percent of the patients in this registry were African-American. Although there were no significant differences in mortality between the African-American and Caucasian patients after transplantation, the African-American patients did have significantly higher rehospitalizations and outpatient resource utilization during the period of follow-up. These results are promising, although issues with access to care and financial limitations are emphasized as heart transplantation is a very resource-intense service. As heart transplantation patients receive great scrutiny and close follow-up, selection bias may actually underestimate any differential in outcomes for minority patients. Further evaluation of the financial burdens of transplantation care and the psychosocial factors pertaining to management may be required to identify the reason for higher resource utilization for minority patients receiving heart transplant.

8. CONCLUSION

Heart failure therapy continues to benefit from evidence-based discoveries. It is imperative that such discoveries represent the entire cohort of patients affected by heart failure and incorporate certain unique sensitivities to racial and ethnic populations. Regardless of race or ethnicity, the most important take home message is that adherence to recognized guidelines of

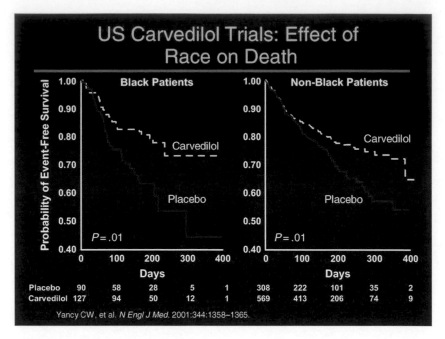

Fig. 12.

the American Heart Association/American College of Cardiology is crucial for all patients and there should be no differential application of these measures for any reason. This is likely the most important effort that may ultimately reduce and possibly even eliminate racial disparities in heart failure care.

REFERENCES

1. US Census Bureau. Available at: http://factfinder.census.gov/servlet/ACSSAFFPeople? _submenuId=people_10&_sse=on Accessed April 2007.
2. American Heart Association. 2007 Heart and Stroke Statistical Update. Dallas, TX. American Heart Association, 2007.
3. Shaya FT, Gbarayor CM, Yang HK, et al. A perspective on African American participation in clinical trials. *Con Clin Trials* 2007; 28:213–217.
4. Hunt SA, Abraham WT, Chin MH, et al. ACC/AHA 2005 Guideline Update for the Diagnosis and Management of Chronic Heart Failure in the Adult: a report of the American College of Cardiology/American Heart Association Task Force on Practice Guidelines (Writing Committee to Update the 2001 Guidelines for the Evaluation and Management of Heart Failure): developed in collaboration with the American College of Chest Physicians and the International Society for Heart and Lung Transplantation: endorsed by the Heart Rhythm Society. *Circulation* 2005; 112:e154–e235.
5. Centers for Disease Control Diabetes fact sheet. Available at http://www.cdc.gov/ diabetes/pubs/estimates05.htm. Accessed July 2007.

6. Centers For Disease Control Hypertension fact sheet. Available at http://www.cdc.gov/nchs/data/hus/tables/2003/03hus066.pdf. Accessed July 2007.
7. American Obesity Association. Available at http://obesity1.tempdomainname.com/subs/fastfacts/Obesity_Minority_Pop.shtml. Accessed July 2007.
8. Ferdinand KC. African American Heart Failure Trial: role of endothelial dysfunction and heart failure in African Americans. *Am J Cardiol* 2007; 99:3D–6D.
9. Cardillo C, Kilcoyne CM, Cannon RO, et al. Racial difference in nitric oxide-mediated vasodilator response to mental stress in the forearm circulation. *Hypertension* 1998; 31:1235–1239.
10. Kahn DF, Duffy SJ. Effects of black race on forearm resistance vessel function. *Hypertension* 2002; 40:195–201.
11. Carson P, Ziesche S, Johnson G, et al. Racial differences in response to therapy for heart failure: Analysis of the Vasodilator-Heart Failure Trials. *J Card Fail* 1999; 5: 178–187.
12. Dries DL, Exner DV, Gersh BJ, et al. Racial differences in the outcome of left ventricular dysfunction. *N Engl J Med* 1999; 340:609–616.
13. Echols, MR, Felker GM, Thomas KL, et al. Racial differences in the characteristic of patients admitted for acute decompensated heart failure and their relation to outcomes: results from the OPTIME-CHF trial. *J Card Fail* 2006; 12:684–688.
14. Yancy CW. Heart failure in African Americans. *Am J Cardiol* 2005; 96:3i–12i.
15. Yancy CW. The prevention of heart failure in minority communities and discrepancies in health care delivery systems. *Med Clin North Am* 2004; 94:595–601.
16. Kressin NR, Chang BH, Whittle J, et al. Racial differences in cardiac catheterization as a function of patients' beliefs. *Am J Public Health* 2004; 94:2091–2097.
17. Green AR, Carney DR, Pallin DJ, et al. Implicit bias among physicians and its prediction of thrombolysis decisions for black and white patients. *J Gen Inter Med* 2007; 9: 1231–1238.
18. DuBard CA, Garrett J, Gizlice Z. Effect of language on heart attack and stroke awareness among U.S. Hispanics.*Am J Prev Med* 2006; 30:189–196 .
19. Mensah GA, Mokdad AH, Ford ES, Greenlund KJ, Croft JB. State of disparities in cardiovascular health in the United States.*Circulation* 2005; 111:133–141.
20. Rathore SS, Masoudi FA, Wang YF. Socioeconomic status, treatment, and outcomes among elderly patients hospitalized with heart failure: findings from the National Heart Failure Project. *Am Heart J* 2006; 152:371–378.
21. Conard MW, Heidenreich P, Rumsfeld JS, Weintraub WS, Spertus J Patient-reported economic burden and the health status of heart failure patients. *J Card Fail* 2006; 12:369–374.
22. Hamner JB, Ellison KJ. Predictors of hospital readmission after discharge in patients with congestive heart failure. *Heart Lung* 2005; 34(4):231–239.
23. Small KM, Wagoner LE, Levin AM, et al. Synergistic polymorphisms of b1- and a2c-adrenergic receptors and the risk of congestive heart failure. *N Engl J Med* 2002; 347:1135–1142.
24. Hein L, Altman JD, Kobilka BK. Two functionally distinct a2-adrenergic receptors regulate sympathetic neurotransmission. *Nature* 1999; 402:181–184.
25. Canham RM, Das SR, Leonard D, et al. Alpha2cDel322-325 and beta1Arg389 adrenergic polymorphisms are not associated with reduced left ventricular ejection fraction or increased left ventricular volume. *J Am Coll Cardiol* 2007; 49:274–276.
26. Malinski T. Understanding nitric oxide physiology in the heart: a nanomedical approach. *Am J Cardiol* 2005; 96(Suppl):13–24.
27. Prabhu SD. Nitric oxide protects against pathological ventricular remodeling: reconsideration of the role of NO in the failing heart.*Circ Res* 2004; 94:115–157.

28. Wollert KC, Drexler H. Regulation of cardiac remodeling by nitric oxide: focus on cardiac myocyte hypertrophy and apoptosis. *Heart Fail Rev* 2002; 7:317–325.
29. Diaber A, Oleze M, Coldeway M, et al. Hydralazine is a powerful inhibitor of peroxynitrite formation as a possible explanation for its beneficial effects on prognosis in patients with congestive heart failure. *Biochem Biophys Res Commun* 2005; 338(4): 1865–1874.
30. Taylor AL, Ziesche S, et al. Combination of isosorbide dinitrate and hydralazine in blacks with heart failure. *N Engl J Med* 2004; 351:2049–2057.
31. McNamara DM, Holubkov R, Postava L, et al. Effect of Asp298 variant of endothelial nitric oxide synthase on survival for patients with congestive heart failure. *Circulation* 2003; 107:1598–1602.
32. Tesauro M, Thompson WC, Rogliani P, et al. Intracellular processing of the endothelial nitric oxide synthase isoforms associated with differences in severity of cardiopulmonary diseases: cleavage of proteins with aspartate vs. glutamate at position 298. *Proc Natl Acad Sci U S A* 2000; 97:2832–2835.
33. McNamara DM, Tam SW, Sabolinski ML, et al. The genetic risk sub-study of the African American heart failure trial (A-HeFT): impact of genetic variations of NOS3. Abstract presented at the 2005 Heart Failure Society of America national conference. Retrieved June 22, 2006 from http://www.abstracts2view.com/hfsa05/view.php?nu=HFSA5L1_232
34. Weber KT. Aldosterone in congestive heart failure. *N Engl J Med* 2001; 345:1689–1697.
35. Struthers AD. Aldosterone escape during angiotensin-converting enzyme inhibitor therapy in chronic heart failure. *J Cardiol Fail* 1996; 2:47–54.
36. Sun Y, Zhang J, Lu L, et al. Aldosterone-induced inflammation in the rat heart: role of oxidative stress. *Am J Pathol* 2002; 161:1773–1781.
37. Kotlyar E, Vita JA, Winter MR, et al. The relationship between aldosterone, oxidative stress, and inflammation in chronic, stable human heart failure. *J Card Fail* 2006; 12:122–127.
38. Pitt B, Zannad F, Remme WJ, et al. The effect of spironolactone on morbidity and mortality in patients with severe heart failure. Randomized Aldactone Evaluation Study Investigators. *N Engl J Med* 1999; 341:709–717.
39. Pitt B, Remme W, Zannad F, et al. Eplerenone, a selective aldosterone blocker, in patients with left ventricular dysfunction after myocardial infarction. *N Engl J Med* 2003; 348:1309–1321.
40. McNamara DM, Tam W, Sabolinski ML, et al. Aldosterone synthase promoter polymorphism predicts outcome in African Americans with heart failure. *J Am Coll Cardiol* 2006; 48:1277–1282.
41. Biolo A, Chao T, Duhaney TS, et al. Usefulness of the aldosterone synthase gene polymorphism to predict cardiac remodeling in African-American and non-African-Americans with chronic systolic heart failure. *Am J Cardiol* 2007; 100:285–290.
42. Tiago AD, Badenhorst D, Skudicky D, Woodiwiss AJ, et al. An aldosterone synthase gene variant is associated with improvement in left ventricular ejection fraction in dilated cardiomyopathy. *Cardiovasc Res* 2002; 54:584–589.
43. Henderson SO, Haiman CA, Mack W. Multiple polymorphisms in the renin-angiotensin-aldosterone system (ACE, CYP11B2, AGTR1) and their contribution to hypertension in African Americans and Latinos in the multiethnic cohort. *Am J Med Sci* 2004; 328: 266–273.
44. The Beta-Blocker Evaluation of Survival Trial Investigators. A trial of the beta-blocker bucindolol in patients with advanced chronic heart failure. *N Engl J Med* 2001; 344:1659–1667.
45. Shekelle PG, Rich MW, Morton SC, et al. Efficacy of angiotensin-converting enzyme inhibitors and beta-blockers in the management of left ventricular systolic dysfunction

according to race, gender, and diabetic status: a meta-analysis of major clinical trials. *J Am Coll Cardiol* 2003; 41:1529–1538.

46. Andreka P, Aiyar N, Olson LC, et al. Bucindolol displays intrinsic sympathomimetic activity in human myocardium. *Circulation* 2002; 105:2429–2434.

47. Yancy CW, Fowler MB, Colucci WS, et al. Race and the response to adrenergic blockade with carvedilol in patients with chronic heart failure. *N Engl J Med* 2001; 344: 1358–1365.

48. Packer M, Coats AJS, Fowler MB, et al for the Carvedilol Prospective Randomized Cumulative Survival Study Group. Effect of carvedilol on survival in severe chronic heart failure. *N Engl J Med* 2001; 344:1651–1658.

49. MERIT-HF Study Group. Effect of metoprolol CR/XL in chronic heart failure: Metoprolol CR/XL Randomised Intervention Trial in Congestive Heart Failure (MERIT-HF). *Lancet* 1999; 353:2001–2007.

50. Exner DV, Dries DL, Domanski MJ, Cohn JN. Lesser response to angiotensin-converting-enzyme inhibitor therapy in black as compared with white patients with left ventricular dysfunction. *N Engl J Med* 2001; 344:1351–1357.

51. The Heart Outcomes Prevention Evaluation Study Investigators. Effects of an angiotensin-converting-enzyme inhibitor, ramipril, on cardiovascular events in high-risk patients. *N Engl J Med* 2000; 342:145–153.

52. Julius S, Alderman MH, Beevers G, et al. Cardiovascular risk reduction in hypertensive black patients with left ventricular hypertrophy: the LIFE study. *J Am Coll Cardiol* 2004; 43:1047–1055.

53. Julius S, Kjeldsen SE, Weber M, Brunner HR, et al for the VALUE Trial Group. Outcomes in hypertensive patients at high cardiovascular risk treated with regimens based on valsartan or amlodipine: the VALUE randomized trial. *Lancet* 2004; 363: 2022–2031.

54. Cavallari LH, Fashingbauer LA, Beitelshees AL, et al. Racial differences in patients' potassium concentration during spironolactone therapy for heart failure. *Pharmacotherapy* 2004; 24:750–756.

55. Cohn JN, Archibald MP, Ziesche S, et al. Effect of vasodilator therapy on mortality in chronic congestive heart failure. *N Engl J Med* 1986; 314:1547–1552.

56. Pierpont GL, Cohn JN, Franciosa JA, et al. Combined oral Hydralazine-nitrate therapy in left ventricular failure: hemodynamic equivalency to sodium nitroprusside. *Chest* 1978; 73:8–13.

57. Cohn JN, Johnson G, Ziesche S., et al. A comparison of enalapril with hydralazine-isosorbide dinitrate in the treatment of chronic congestive heart failure. *N Engl J Med* 1991; 325:303–310.

58. The CONSENSUS Trial Study Group. Effects of enalapril on mortality in severe congestive heart failure: results of the Cooperative North Scandinavian Enalapril Survival Study (CONSENSUS). *N Engl J Med* 1987; 316:1429–1435.

59. Kalinowski L, Dobrucki IT, Tomasian D, et al. Race-specific differences in endothelial function: Predisposition of African Americans to vascular disease. *Circulation* 2004; 109:2511–2517.

60. Unger P, Berkenboom G, Fontaine J interaction between hydralazine and nitrovasodilators in vascular smooth muscle. *J Cardiovasc Pharmacol* 1993; 21:478–483.

61. Gogia H, Mehra A, Parikh S, et al. Prevention of tolerance to hemodynamic effects of nitrates with concomitant use of hydralazine in patients with chronic heart failure. *J Am Coll Cardiol* 1995; 26:1575–1580.

62. Elkayam U, Bitar F. Effects of nitrates and hydralazine in heart failure. Clinical evidence before the African American heart failure trial. *Am J Cardiol* 2005; 96:37i–43i.

63. Taylor AL. The African American heart failure trial (A-HeFT): rationale and methodology. *J Card Fail* 2003; 9:S216–S219.

64. Taylor AL. The African American heart failure trial. A clinical trial update. *Am J Cardiol* 2005; 96:44i–48i.
65. Taylor AL, Ziesche S, Yancy CW, et al. Early and sustained benefit on event-free survival and heart failure hospitalization from fixed-dose combination of isosorbide dinitrate/hydralazine: consistency across subgroups in the African-American Heart Failure Trial. *Circulation* 2007; 115:1747–1753.
66. Gillum RF. Sudden cardiac death in Hispanic Americans and African American. *Am J Public Health* 1997; 87:1461–1466.
67. Zheng ZJ, Croft JB, Giles WH, Mensah GA. Sudden cardiac death in the United States, 1989 to 1998. *Circulation* 2001; 104:2158–2163.
68. Russo AM, Hafley GE, Lee KL, et al. Racial differences in outcome in the multicenter unsustained tachycardia trial (MUSTT): a comparison of whites versus blacks. *Circulation* 2003; 108:67–72.
69. Vorobiof G, Goldenberg I, Moss AJ, Zareba W, McNitt S. Effectiveness of the implantable cardioverter defibrillator in blacks versus whites (from MADIT-II). *Am J Cardiol* 2006; 98:1383–1386.
70. Pamboukian SV, Costanzo MR, Meyer P, et al. Influence of race in heart failure and cardiac transplantation: mortality differences are eliminated by specialized, comprehensive care. *J Card Fail* 2003; 9:80–86.
71. Moore DE, Feurer ID, Rodgers S Jr, et al. Is there racial disparity in outcomes after solid organ transplantation? *Am J Surg* 2004; 188:571–574.

15 Minority Women and Cardiovascular Disease

A.L. Taylor, MD
and L. Bellumkonda, MBBS

CONTENTS

Abstract

Large epidemiological studies have helped define differences in majority and minority population health risks and outcomes. The National Health and Nutrition Examination Survey (NHANES) observed African American, Mexican American, and white non-Hispanic women from 1988 to 1994 and found a striking prevalence of abdominal obesity and metabolic syndrome in both African-Americans and Mexican Americans. The Multi-Ethnic Study of Atherosclerosis (MESA) was designed to study the prevalence and progression of sub-clinical CVD in multiple ethnicities including whites. The rate of awareness of CVD as the leading cause of death has nearly doubled among women since 1997.

From: *Contemporary Cardiology: Cardiovascular Disease in Racial and Ethnic Minorities*
Edited by: K.C. Ferdinand and A. Armani, DOI 10.1007/978-1-59745-410-0_15
© Humana Press, a part of Springer Science+Business Media, LLC 2009

Awareness of heart disease is independently correlated with increased physical activity and weight loss. The NHANES study shows that the prevalence of obesity, which can be associated with insulin resistance, is highest in non-Hispanic black women.

The Women's Health Initiative (WHI) has shown that the major correlates of HTN among postmenopausal women were black race, CVD, physical inactivity, and excess alcohol consumption. There was also evidence that blood pressure control decreased with age. The Dallas Heart Study has shown that left ventricular hypertrophy (LVH) is two- to three-fold more common in African-American women compared to Caucasian women. About 30% of women in America do not perform any leisure-time physical activity (Centers for Disease Control and Prevention. http://www.cdc.gov/nchs/data/nhis/earlyrelease/200709_07.pdf;). This percentage is higher in women with less than a high school education or lower income groups. Women respond better to lifestyle physical activity recommendations vs structured exercise recommendations. For many women, a home-based format for physical activity which would accommodate their caregiver and work roles would be more advantageous over more traditional sessions in a gym or health club.

When adjustment for lipids, diabetes, and HTN were made, elevated levels of CRP still remained a predictor of increase risk of CAD with a RR Of 1.68 (Pai et al. *N Engl J Med* 351:2599–2610, 2004). Anemia, which is much more prevalent in women, is associated with adverse CV consequences by increasing preload and reducing afterload and in the long term, resulting in LVH. The WHS found no benefit of adding 600 IU of vitamin E supplementation every other day on reduction of major CV events or cancer, as well as overall survival benefits. The Primary Prevention Project enrolled 4495 patients (2583 women with a mean age of 64.4 years) with one or more risk factors for CVD. This trial found that 100 mg of aspirin/day lowered CV death by 44% and total CV events by 23%. By contrast, the WHS found that in healthy women 45 years and above, 100 mg of aspirin every other day did not affect the risk of myocardial infarction or death from CV causes but lowered the risk of stroke. Compared to the WHS, the Primary Prevention Project was an open label study which enrolled older patients (mean age 64.4 years compared to 54.6 in WHS), with at least one CV risk. These factors may explain the variable effect of aspirin found in these two studies.

Multiple observational studies suggested that estrogen replacement in postmenopausal women decreased heart disease risk by 50%. However, new randomized studies have addressed the issue of hormone replacement in menopausal women. Exercise electrocardiographic evaluation has lower sensitivity and specificity in detecting obstructive CAD in women: 61 and 70% as compared to 70 and 77% in men. Despite this, prognostic information can be derived from exercise testing. Exercise duration is the strongest predictor of long-term outcomes. Because of the limitations of exercise stress electrocardiography in women, concomitant imaging has been tested. The positive predictive value is lower in women compared to men (66% vs 84%) which may be a reflection of the lower prevalence of obstructive CAD in women who were tested. Pharmacologic stress testing such as dobutamine stress echocardiography (DSE) can be done in patients that cannot exercise. Women who cannot exercise should undergo pharmacologic stress testing or dobutamine echocardiography, which has the highest combination of sensitivity and specificity. Cardiovascular disease in women is very unique in that there is greater symptom burden, despite a lower prevalence of obstructive CAD by coronary angiography as compared to men. The pathophysiology of chest pain with non-obstructive epicardial CAD is very variable. Some patients have non-cardiac chest pain, while others have endothelial dysfunction, variant angina, or an overlap of these conditions. Even though women bear about 50% of the burden of heart failure in the United States, their representation in the randomized controlled heart failure trials has been about 20% and it has not changed over the past two decades.

Key Words: Minority women; Risk factors; Hypertension; Left ventricular hypertrophy; Diabetes; C-reactive protein; Anemia; Vitamin E; Aspirin; Hormone replacement; Stress testing; Endothelial dysfunction.

1. INTRODUCTION

In the United States, cardiovascular disease (CVD) remains the number one cause of mortality for men and women; however, mortality, particularly for coronary artery disease (CAD), has declined significantly in men with little decrease in women. In addition, cardiovascular (CV) morbidity and mortality varies by ethnicity with minorities having a greater disease burden *(1)*.

2. EPIDEMIOLOGY OF CARDIOVASCULAR DISEASE IN MINORITY WOMEN

Large epidemiological studies have helped define differences in majority and minority population health risks and outcomes. The National Health and Nutrition Examination Survey (NHANES) observed African-American, Mexican American, and white non-Hispanic women from 1988 to 1994 and found a striking prevalence of abdominal obesity and metabolic syndrome in both African-Americans and Mexican Americans *(2)*. The Strong Heart Study included more than 4500 Native American participants and demonstrated that diabetes is a particularly prevalent risk factor in the Native American population, and the outcomes of CVD in these patients are poor *(3)*. The Multi-Ethnic Study of Atherosclerosis (MESA) was designed to study the prevalence and progression of sub-clinical CVD in multiple ethnicities including whites, African-Americans, Hispanics, and Chinese *(4)* and found that whites had the highest prevalence of coronary calcification measured by computed tomography. The prevalence was 70.4% in whites followed by 59.2% in Chinese, 56.5% in Hispanics, and 52.1% in African-Americans *(4)*.

According to recent American Heart Association (AHA) statistics in 2003, overall preliminary death rate from CVD was 256.2 per 100,000 for white women and 354.8 per 100,000 for African-American women. In 2002, the age-adjusted death rates for heart disease in American Indian or Alaska Native women was 123.6 per 100,000, Asian or Pacific Islander women was 108.1 per 100,000, and for Hispanic or Latino women the rate was 149.7 per 100,000 *(5)*. The trends in mortality from CVD have been encouraging in general, but over the past two decades the decrease in mortality has been slowest in African-American women *(5)*.

The decreasing trend in mortality in general may be a reflection of both improvements in therapeutic interventions and increasing awareness of heart disease. The rate of awareness of CVD as the leading cause of death has nearly doubled among women since 1997, but this was significantly greater among whites vs African-Americans vs. Hispanics (62% vs. 38% vs. 34%) *(6)*. Lack of English language proficiency is associated with less awareness of heart attack and stroke warning symptoms among Hispanics *(7)*. Other issues such as educational status, socioeconomic status, and health-care access all play a role in patient awareness *(7)*. Awareness of heart disease is independently correlated with increased physical activity and weight loss *(8)*. Most women took steps to lower risk not only for themselves but also in their family members. This suggests that increased educational interventions, especially in racial and ethnic minority women, will lead to preventative actions in the individuals and potentially the whole family *(8)*.

Physician awareness of CVD in women also has limitations. Mosca et al. found that physicians from different specialties including primary-care physicians, obstetrics/gynecology, and even cardiologists underestimated the CV risk in women *(9)*. They also found that assignment of risk level significantly predicted recommendations for lifestyle and preventative pharmacotherapy. Thus, underestimation of women's risk of CVD may result in prescription of less stringent preventive measures in women compared to men. This suggests increasing educational interventions not only for patients but also for physicians are needed *(9)*.

3. RISK FACTORS

3.1. Traditional Risk Factors

3.1.1. OBESITY AND METABOLIC SYNDROME

The prevalence of traditional risk factors and their impact on CV outcomes varies by racial/ethnic groups. The NHANES study shows that the prevalence of obesity, which can be associated with insulin resistance, is highest in non-Hispanic black women (49%) compared to Mexican

American women (38.4%) and non-Hispanic white women (30.7%) *(10)*. Traditionally, obesity has been characterized by measurement of body mass index (BMI). Waist–hip ratio (WHR) is an indicator of regional adipose tissue distribution and predicts insulin resistance and coronary heart disease (CHD) in women better *(11)*. We now have data that suggests that visceral adipocytes differ from peripheral adipocytes. Visceral fat contributes significantly to the circulating free fatty acids and cytokines or adipokines *(11)*. Their response to lipolytic activity, response to insulin, sex hormones, adrenergic, and angiotensin stimulation is different than non-visceral adipocytes *(11)*. Lipid accumulation patterns are also different in men and women. Premenopausal women usually have peripheral obesity with subcutaneous accumulation of fat while men and postmenopausal women have central or visceral obesity *(12)*. Adipocytes produce proinflammatory adipokines such as tumor necrosis factor (TNF)-alpha, leptin, plasminogen activator inhibitor (PAI)-1, angiotensinogen, interleukin (IL)-6, C-reactive protein (CRP) and resistin, and anti-inflammatory cytokines such as adiponectin. These proinflammatory adipokines exert their influence on insulin resistance and atherosclerosis and endothelial function *(13)*.

Certain ethnicities such as South Asians have insulin resistance at lower BMI levels probably due to the "thin-fat phenotype" (muscle thin but body fat). Hence in these populations BMI cutoff for obesity has been lowered to <25 kg/m^2. This amplifies the need for population specific correlates of CV risk factors and outcomes *(14)*.

Among African-Americans, women had a 57% higher prevalence of metabolic syndrome compared to men, and among Mexican Americans, women had a 26% higher prevalence than men. African-American women had the highest prevalence of high blood pressure and Mexican American women had the highest prevalence of hypertriglyceridemia, low HDL, and hyperglycemia *(2,4)*.

3.1.2. HYPERTENSION

The prevalence of hypertension (HTN) is much greater in African-Americans than other groups in the United States. It also has a very aggressive course with earlier age of onset, higher rates of CV mortality, cerebral vascular accident, hypertensive heart disease, congestive heart failure, and end-stage renal disease compared to Caucasians *(15)*. The progression from initial diagnosis of HTN to end organ damage is also more rapid. African-Americans and American Indians with HTN have four- to five-fold greater incidence of end-stage renal disease compared to Caucasians *(15)*.

The Women's Health Initiative (WHI) has shown that the major correlates of HTN among postmenopausal women were black race, CVD, physical inactivity, and excess alcohol consumption. There was also evidence that blood pressure control decreased with age *(16)*.

The Antihypertensive and Lipid-Lowering Treatment to Prevent Heart Attack Trial (ALLHAT) has shown that angiotensin-converting enzyme inhibitors (ACEI) have lesser antihypertensive effect in African-Americans and that thiazide diuretic and calcium channel blockers may be better agents *(17)*. In light of the poor prognosis with HTN, these patients should be treated aggressively and early initiation of combination therapy should be considered *(18)*.

3.1.3. LEFT VENTRICULAR HYPERTROPHY

The Dallas Heart Study has shown that left ventricular hypertrophy (LVH) is two- to three-fold more common in African-American women compared to Caucasian women *(19)* and is an independent predictor of all-cause mortality and CV mortality. Left ventricular mass assessed by echocardiogram was associated with relative risk (RR) of 2.12 for death from CVD and 2.01 for all-cause mortality in women and LVH has also been associated with decreasing ejection fraction on follow-up *(20,21)*.

3.1.4. DIABETES

Diabetes has particularly severe CV consequences in women. Lee et al. *(22)* found that women with diabetes had a RR of coronary death of 2.58 compared to 1.85 in diabetic men. Franco et al. built life-time tables using the Framingham data and found that the risk of CVD is increased due to diabetes (hazard ratio 2.5 for women and 2.4 for men). The risk of dying when CVD was present was also higher in women compared to men (2.2 for women and 1.7 for men) *(23)*. Diabetes decreases the vascular protection afforded to premenopausal women, presumably by endogenous estrogen. Steinberg demonstrated that premenopausal women with diabetes exhibit impaired endothelium-dependent vasodilation compared to non-diabetic women. This was similar to the endothelial dysfunction in diabetic men *(24)*. Estrogen administration to postmenopausal diabetic women was shown to lower low-density lipoprotein (LDL) levels and increase high-density lipoprotein (HDL) but did not have any effect on improving nitric oxide bioavailability as measured by brachial artery flow-mediated vasodilation *(25)*.

In addition, some of the differences in CV outcomes in diabetic women may be due to less aggressive treatment of risk factors. In a cross sectional analysis of diabetic patients in five academic centers, Wexler et al. *(26)* found that compared to men, women were less likely to have HbA1c < 7% and less likely to be on lipid-lowering medication or aspirin.

3.1.5. TOBACCO

The risk of CHD among women increases linearly with the number of cigarettes smoked in a day, total number of years of smoking, the degree of inhalation, and age at initiation of smoking *(27)*. The Nurses Health Study suggests smoking even as few as one to four cigarettes a day was associated with a two-fold increase in risk of fatal CHD or nonfatal infarction compared to women who never smoked *(28)*. The age-adjusted RR for CHD mortality among current smokers compared to those who never smoked was 2.3 for black women, 2.2 for Asian women, and 1.6 for white women *(28)*. On stopping smoking, one-third of the excess risk of CHD was eliminated by 2 years, and the risk was decreased to that of women who never smoked by 10–14 years of cessation *(29)*. Those women who do not smoke, but are exposed to secondhand smoke are also at risk. There is a 15% increased risk of dying from heart disease among non-smoking women exposed to environmental tobacco smoke compared to non-smoking women not exposed to secondhand smoke *(30)*.

3.1.6. SEDENTARY LIFE STYLE

About 30% of women in America do not perform any leisure time physical activity *(31)*. This percentage is higher in women with less than a high school education or lower income groups *(32)*. A case–control study suggests that the risk of myocardial infarction among postmenopausal women is decreased by 50% with modest leisure-time energy expenditures, equivalent to 30–45 minutes of walking for exercise three times a week *(33)*. Women respond better to lifestyle physical activity recommendations vs structured exercise recommendations. For many women, a home-based format for physical activity which would accommodate their caregiver and work roles would be more advantageous than more traditional sessions in a gym or health club *(34)*.

3.2. Non-traditional Risk Factors

3.2.1. HIGH-SENSITIVITY C-REACTIVE PROTEIN

One hundred and twenty-two participants who had suffered a CV event in the Women's Health Study (WHS) were compared to 244 matched participants, and it was noted that women with highest CRP at baseline had a five-fold increase in risk of any vascular event and a seven-fold increase in myocardial infarction or stroke. This was independent of other risk factors *(35)*.

These results were later confirmed when CRP and LDL were tested in all 27,939 women in WHS. Higher quintiles of CRP correlated well with CV events and it was shown to be a stronger predictor than LDL alone *(36)*. This adds prognostic information to the Framingham risk score *(36)*. The Justification for the Use of Statins in Primary Prevention: an Intervention Trial Evaluating Rosuvastatin (JUPITER) trial is underway and will examine whether treating healthy patients with LDL <130 mg/dl but CRP > 2 mg/L with rosuvastatin will improve their CV outcomes *(37)*.

Analysis of the inflammatory markers from women participating in the Nurse's Health Study revealed that high levels of IL-6 and CRP were also significantly related to increased risk of CAD. Higher levels of soluble TNF-alpha receptors were significant among women. When adjustment for lipids, diabetes, and HTN were made, elevated levels of CRP still remained a predictor of increase risk of CAD with a RR Of 1.68 *(38)*.

3.2.2. ANEMIA

Anemia, which is much more prevalent in women, is associated with adverse CV consequences by increasing preload and reducing afterload and in the long term, resulting in LVH. This can also exacerbate ischemia by increasing the demand for oxygen and decreasing the supply. Anemia is thought to result in hypoxia induced vasodilation or altered nitric oxide activity and can result in development of cardiac failure *(39)*. In a pooled data analysis of community-based studies, anemic patients with diabetes and chronic renal insufficiency had a higher rate of CV events than patients without anemia *(39)*. The Atherosclerosis Risk in Communities (ARIC) trial shows a RR of 1.96 for CHD in patients with anemia and chronic kidney disease *(40)*. There was an independent association between the presence of anemia and the adverse CV outcomes in women presenting with symptoms of ischemia in the Women's Ischemia Syndrome Evaluation (WISE) *(41)*. This association was seen regardless of the presence or severity of CAD on angiogram. Although the exact pathophysiology of this association is not known, there seem to be higher levels of inflammatory markers like CRP and TNF-alpha in women with anemia. It is postulated that this may play a role in microvascular disease resulting in CVD *(41)*.

3.2.3. RETINAL ARTERY

The degree of retinal artery atherosclerosis on fundoscopic examination has been shown to correlate with extent and severity of atherosclerotic changes in the coronaries *(42)*. Retinal arterial narrowing with lower arteriole–venule ratio was shown to be independently associated with new incident diabetes at a 3.5-year follow-up *(43)*. A similar relationship with incident CHD and arteriole–venule ratio was found in women but not men in the ARIC trial *(44)*. These data may suggest a more important role for microvascular disease in women than men.

3.2.4. RACE-SPECIFIC RISK FACTORS

In a study comparing young healthy women college students of African-American, Asian Indian American, and Caucasian American descent, it was found that African-American women had lower triglyceride levels and higher apolipoprotein A [apo(a)]-1, HDL, lipoprotein (a) [Lp(a)], fibrinogen, and fasting insulin levels. They also consumed more fat and had higher percentage of body fat and less physical activity compared to Caucasians. Asian Indian American women also had higher Lp(a), HDL and fibrinogen levels and less physical activity compared to their Caucasian peers (45).

The exact physiologic role of Lp(a) is as yet not known, thus it is not considered an established factor. Several meta-analyses have found an association between Lp(a) and CAD, mostly seen in white populations. The association has been harder to prove in African-Americans, who generally have higher Lp(a) levels. More specifically, elevated Lp(a) levels with small apo(a) isoforms were associated with increased CAD in African-American and Caucasian men but not in African-American women. Some suggest it is only a marker for CVD and others suggest a pro-atherogenic, thrombotic role (46).

3.2.5. VITAMIN E

Supplemental vitamin E was evaluated for primary CV prevention along with aspirin in the Primary Prevention Project which was an open label 2×2 factorial trial including patients with at least one risk factor for CVD. This trial did not find any benefit from using vitamin E (47). This was later substantiated by the WHS which found no benefit of adding 600 IU of vitamin E supplementation every other day on reduction of major CV events or cancer, as well as overall survival benefits; however, there was 24% RR of CV mortality noted (48).

3.2.6. ASPIRIN FOR PRIMARY PREVENTION

The Primary Prevention Project enrolled 4495 patients (2583 women with a mean age of 64.4 years) with one or more risk factors for CVD. This trial found that 100 mg of aspirin/day lowered CV death by 44% and total CV events by 23% (47). By contrast, the WHS found that in healthy women 45 years and above, 100 mg of aspirin every other day did not affect the risk of myocardial infarction or death from CV causes but lowered the risk of stroke. There was a significant reduction of these risks in women over 65 years of age according to a subgroup analysis (49).

A meta-analysis of 51,342 women concurred with the WHS and showed 17% RR of stroke with no beneficial effect on myocardial infarction or CV mortality. There was a significant risk of bleeding with aspirin in women (OR 1.68; 95% CI 1.13–2.52; $p = 0.01$) (50) which was similar in men. These results were not confirmed in the WHS. Compared to the WHS, the

Primary Prevention Project was an open label study which enrolled older patients (mean age 64.4 years compared to 54.6 in WHS), with at least one CV risk. These factors may explain the variable effect of aspirin found in these two studies.

3.2.7. HORMONE REPLACEMENT

Multiple observational studies suggested that estrogen replacement in postmenopausal women decreased heart disease risk by 50%. The Postmenopausal Estrogen/Progestin Interventions (PEPI) showed that estrogen alone or in combination with progestin lowered CV risk factors such as fibrinogen levels improved HDL levels and reduced LDL levels in 875 healthy postmenopausal women aged 45–64 years *(51)*. However, hard end points were not analyzed. In randomized, blinded, placebo-controlled trials such as the Heart and Estrogen/Progestin Replacement Study (HERS) and the Estrogen Replacement and Atherosclerosis (ERA) study, which examined secondary prevention, and WHI, which was a primary prevention trial, there was an increased risk of cardiovascular events, especially in the first year of hormone replacement therapy, despite an improvement in the lipid profile *(52,53)*.

The discordant findings between observational and randomized trials may be explained by the fact that observational studies mostly included perimenopausal women, while randomized studies enrolled postmenopausal women, in addition to lower cohort numbers in the randomized studies compared to observational studies. However, new randomized studies are currently addressing the issue of hormone replacement in perimenopausal women *(54)*. Analysis of the WHI study showed a trend toward lower CHD risk and overall mortality when hormone replacement was started in perimenopause, with increase in risk if hormone replacement therapy was started more distant from menopause. The risk of stroke was elevated irrespective of when the hormone replacement therapy was started *(55)*.

4. ASSESSMENT IN WOMEN

4.1. Stress Testing

Exercise electrocardiographic evaluation has lower sensitivity and specificity in detecting obstructive CAD in women: 61 and 70% as compared to 70 and 77% in men. Premenopausal women have a low-to-intermediate likelihood of CAD and so using the Bayes theorem the utility of noninvasive testing decreases. There are many proposed mechanisms for this disparities including digoxin- like effect of estrogen on ST segments, inappropriate catecholamine response to exercise, also the lower functional capacity in women decreasing the sensitivity of the test *(56,57)*. Other factors that lower the specificity in women are greater prevalence of mitral valve prolapse and endothelial dysfunction and vasospasm in women *(57)*. Estrogen with its vasodilatory properties has an influence on the stress testing *(57)*. A cyclic variation in endothelial function as noted by flow-mediated dilation of brachial artery corresponding to the changing estrogen levels during the menstrual cycle *(57)*. In premenopausal women, angina, myocardial ischemia, and exercise performance were highly dependent on the time of the menstrual cycle. Ischemia was more easily induced during low estrogen periods as in early follicular phase and the women's performance was best during mid-cycle when estrogen concentrations were highest *(58)*.

Despite this, prognostic information can be derived from exercise testing. Exercise duration is the strongest predictor of long-term outcomes. This is a good indicator of functional capacity. In the WISE study, using a self-reported functional capacity the Duke Activity Status Index (DASI) women with DASI-estimated metabolic equivalents (METs) ≥ 4.7 were more likely to have indeterminate exercise testing as compared to women achieving >4.7 METs. This index can be used to risk stratify and identify functionally impaired women and advise pharmacologic stress testing instead *(59)*.

A 20-year follow-up of 2994 women who underwent treadmill testing suggests that low exercise capacity, low heart rate recovery (<22 bpm), and not achieving target heart rate were independent predictors of increased all-cause and CV mortality *(60)*.

4.2. SPECT Imaging

Because of the limitations of exercise stress electrocardiography in women, other forms of imaging have been tested. Stress myocardial perfusion imaging provides independent and additional prognostic information over exercise treadmill test alone. Pancholy et al. *(61)* showed in 212 women who underwent thallium single photon emission computed tomography (SPECT) imaging and coronary angiography, increasing age and large thallium abnormality greater than or equal to 15% of myocardium were independent predictors of events. Unfortunately, planar imaging and SPECT with thallium (Tl) 201 have some limitations in women. There is a higher rate of false-positive rates in women due to breast attenuation, higher incidence of obesity, and smaller ventricular chamber size causing greater effect on image blurring *(62)*. In one meta-analysis comparing exercise electrocardiogram, exercise thallium, and exercise echocardiogram testing in women, it was found that exercise thallium had a weighted mean sensitivity and specificity of only 0.78 and 0.64, much lower than exercise echocardiogram, which was 0.89 and 0.79 *(57)*. The advent of technetium (Tc)-labeled perfusion agents, along with electrocardiogram gating of images, has significantly enhanced the specificity of SPECT imaging *(63)*. These Tc-labeled agents yield images with higher count density, less scatter, and attenuation than Tl. Taillefer demonstrated that in 115 women undergoing both Tc and Tl SPECT imaging, the sensitivity of Tl and Tc to detect lesions ≥70% was not significantly different: 84 and 80% respectively. However, the specificity was only 59% with Tl and 82% with Tc, increasing to 92% when gated images were added to Tc perfusion imaging *(64)*.

Myocardial perfusion imaging (MPI) also gives important prognostic information. In 3402 women undergoing MPI, the number of abnormal territories was the strongest predictor of mortality during 2.4 years of follow-up after adjustment for exercise variables *(65)*. Boyne et al. *(66)* showed that the combined incidence of death or myocardial infarction was 0.8% per year in patients with normal scans.

4.3. Stress Echocardiography

Exercise echocardiography has similar prognostic value in predicting cardiac events in both men and women. Work load and exercise wall motion score index have the strongest correlation with outcomes such as death or nonfatal myocardial infarction *(67)*.

The available data on stress testing is limited by the test verification bias and small sample sizes of the studies. In an observational study of 3679 consecutive patients undergoing exercise echocardiogram, the sensitivities and specificities were similar in men and women (78 and 44% in men and 79 and 37% in women). After adjusting for test verification bias, the sensitivities drop significantly in both sexes. However, the decrease is higher in women (32% vs 42%), while the specificities remain similar. The positive predictive value is lower in women compared to men (66% vs 84%) which may be a reflection of the lower prevalence of obstructive CAD in women *(68)*.

In a much smaller study of 70 women with intermediate pretest probability of CAD who underwent bicycle exercise protocol and coronary angiograms, the sensitivity of stress echocardiogram to predict angiographic stenosis of >50% was 88% compared with 67% using electrocardiogram alone. The specificity was also higher at 84% vs 51% with only the electrocardiogram. The clinical and hemodynamic significance of a 50% stenosis may not be very important, but the fact that there was intermediate pretest probability may have a role in the higher sensitivity and specificity of this study *(69)*.

Pharmacologic stress testing such as dobutamine stress echocardiography (DSE) can be done in patients who cannot exercise. In low-risk women, DSE, yielded a sensitivity of 50%, increased to 82% for detection of multivessel stenosis when women with inadequate HR response were excluded *(70)*. Meta-analysis of pharmacological stress testing revealed that DSE has the highest combination of sensitivity and specificity, about 80 and 84%, respectively *(71)*. Unfortunately, pharmacologic stress testing does not give the useful functional capacity information obtained from exercise stress testing *(72)*.

4.4. Coronary Calcium Score EBCT

Electron beam computed tomography can offer additional prognostic information. There is a 10-fold higher increase in event rate in patients with calcium scores above the 75th percentile compared to those below the 25th percentile in patients undergoing coronary angiography *(73)*. A prospective study of patients presenting to the emergency room with chest pain revealed that patients with absent coronary artery calcium had an annual event rate of 0.6% over 7-year follow-up *(74)*.

Investigators from the WHI and WHI-Coronary Artery Calcium Study (CACS) found that among patients aged 50–59 years old, those taking estrogen had lower coronary artery calcium scores *(75)*. Alternatively, Becker et al. *(76)* could not demonstrate a difference in the coronary artery calcium score in 277 postmenopausal women on combination estrogen/progestin therapy.

4.5. What Is the Best Noninvasive Diagnostic Test for Women?

Noninvasive testing for detection of CAD in women should be based on the pretest risk of CAD. In patients with low (<25%) or intermediate risk of CAD (25–75%) and a normal baseline electrocardiogram, either exercise treadmill testing or treadmill testing with echocardiography should be considered. Exercise echocardiography or radionuclide studies are preferred for women with abnormal baseline electrocardiogram or those who had revascularization in the past. Women who cannot exercise should undergo pharmacologic stress testing or dobutamine echocardiography, which has the highest combination of sensitivity and specificity. Additionally, high-risk women should have coronary angiography *(77)*.

Cardiovascular disease in women is very unique in that there is greater symptom burden, despite a lower prevalence of obstructive CAD by coronary angiography as compared to men. Even in the presence of angiographically normal coronaries, women were found to have worse in-hospital mortality, based on data from the National Registry of Myocardial Infarction. They found that women presenting with acute myocardial infarction had an overall mortality rate of 16.7% compared to 11.5% in men. This difference was most apparent in younger women *(78)*.

5. VARIED PRESENTATION

5.1. Chest Pain

The Coronary Artery Surgery Study has shown that the prevalence of CAD (stenosis ≥70% or left main stenosis >50%) among men with typical angina was 93%, with probable angina 66%, and 14% in men with nonspecific chest pain. This contrasts with 72, 36, and 6% in women with typical, angina probable angina, and non specific chest pain, respectively, *(79)*. Thus, symptoms of chest pain were less specifically associated with coronary disease in women compared to men.

6. ANGINA WITH "NON-OBSTRUCTIVE CORONARY DISEASE"

Non-obstructive coronary disease at coronary angiography is present more often in women as compared to men. According to the Global Use of Strategies To Open Occluded Arteries in Acute Coronary Syndromes study (GUSTO- IIb), 10.2% of women compared to 6.8% of men presenting with ST-segment elevation myocardial infarction, 9.1% of women compared to 4.2% of men presenting with non-ST-segment elevation myocardial infarction, and 30.5% of women vs 13.9% of men presenting with unstable angina had non-obstructive coronary arteriosclerosis on coronary angiogram *(80)*.

In the Thrombolysis in Myocardial Infarction (TIMI)-IIIA study, patients with non-critical coronary obstruction were more likely to be women and non-white and less likely to have ST-segment deviation on presenting electrocardiogram *(81)*. Some of these women may have pathologically significant atherosclerosis despite the absence of angiographically significant disease due to remodeling of the arterial wall. Among the patients in the TIMI-IIIA with unstable angina and no critical coronary obstruction, 2% had a myocardial infarction or died at 30 days despite absence of angiographically significant CAD *(81)*. Additionally, more than 40% were re-hospitalized more than once and about 30% underwent repeat angiograms for recurrent symptoms.

6.1. Pathology-Endothelial Function

The pathophysiology of chest pain with non-obstructive epicardial CAD is very variable. Some patients have non-cardiac chest pain while others have endothelial dysfunction, variant angina, or an overlap of these conditions. Other explanations include elevation of left ventricular diastolic pressure and microvascular CAD. Endothelial dysfunction is thought to be a precursor of atherosclerosis and has been linked to cardiac events (82). This is associated with increased adhesion of leukocytes, increased thrombogenicity, enhanced expression of matrix metalloprotcinases, and increased inflammation which results in destabilization of an atherosclerotic plaque making it more likely to rupture.

6.2. Evaluation for Endothelial Dysfunction

Intracoronary acetylcholine testing is the gold standard for detecting endothelial dysfunction. In a subgroup of the WISE study, which included 163 women who underwent coronary angiography and endothelial function assessment with intracoronary administration of acetylcholine (Ach), adenosine, and nitroglycerin, there was a significant independent correlation between decreased coronary cross sectional area with Ach, suggesting endothelial dysfunction and CV events such as death, myocardial infarction, heart failure, and stroke. Seventy-five percent of these women had less than 50% angiographic stenosis (83). Noninvasive evaluation with nuclear magnetic resonance spectroscopy has shown that 20% of women who had no angiographically significant stenosis had evidence of abnormal metabolic response to handgrip exercise (84). There was a decrease in phophocreatine:ATP ratio during stress in these women, suggesting microvascular CAD without significant epicardial disease. Three-year follow-up has shown that their event rates are similar to women with obstructive CAD and significantly worse than women with no obstructive CAD and normal spectroscopy (85).

6.3. Treatment

Tricyclic antidepressants, beta-blockers, ACEI, L-arginine, statins, and exercise may relieve symptoms, vascular dysfunction, or both. Blockade of norepinephrine uptake by tricyclic antidepressants like imipramine has shown to decrease the frequency of chest pain by 50% in an unselected group of patients with chest pain and normal coronaries (86). The norepinephrine may enhance the inhibitory action of pain-modulating neurons and act by causing visceral analgesia. It has been shown that on long-term follow-up in women with persistent chest pain with normal coronaries and endothelial dysfunction on initial evaluation, there was subsequent development of obstructive CAD (87). Thus, patients with persistent chest pain and multiple risk factors or evidence of endothelial dysfunction should be reevaluated as well as provided with aggressive treatment of risk factors.

7. HEART FAILURE

Heart failure continues to be the leading principal hospital diagnosis among the Medicare population, costing about $28.8 billion in 2004. In this group, the prevalence of heart failure hospitalizations was highest among African-American women (24.7 per 1000) in 1990 compared to white women (17.8 per 1000). This rate has increased steadily over a decade to 32.4 for African-American women, while it has increased only slightly in white women to 19.5 *(88)*, suggesting an approximately 50% higher prevalence of this disease in black women. Heart failure occurs at an earlier age, with more advanced LV dysfunction at time of initial diagnosis in African-Americans. The rates of heart failure mortality are 40% higher in blacks vs whites and 25% higher in men vs women *(89)*. The overall mortality of blacks was 8.1 per 100 person years and whites was 5.1 per 100 person years in the Studies of Left Ventricular Dysfunction (SOLVD) prevention trial, where blacks also had a higher risk of death from all causes (RR 1.36 95% CI 1.04–1.50 $p = 0.02$) *(90)*.

8. PROGNOSIS

The prognosis of women with heart failure is better than men. According to the Framingham study, the median survival after diagnosis was 1.7 years for men and 3.2 years for women *(89)*. Adams et al. studied the relationship of etiology, gender, and survival in patients with symptomatic heart failure and found that women survived longer than men when heart failure was due to non-ischemic etiology, but this survival benefit was lost in ischemic heart disease. Interestingly, this survival difference depended on etiology of heart failure but not baseline ventricular function *(91)*.

8.1. Etiology

Women admitted for heart failure are in general older and more likely to have history of HTN compared to men, who are more likely to have had previous CAD. Women more frequently have preserved LV function and higher systolic blood pressure at presentation *(92)*. Echocardiographic analysis of 556 participants diagnosed with heart failure in Olmsted County revealed heart failure with preserved ejection fraction in 55% and was more frequent in patients who were older, female, and with no history of myocardial infarction *(93)*.

Hypertension, along with LVH, seems to be the major etiology of heart failure in black patients. Conversely, CAD is the major cause of LV systolic dysfunction in whites *(94)*.

8.2. Management and Response to Different Treatments

Even though women bear about 50% of the burden of heart failure in the United States, their representation in the randomized controlled heart failure trials has been about 20% and it has not changed over the past two decades. The enrollment of non-whites in heart failure trials also follows a similar trend, with only 15% representation, while over 30% of patients with heart failure are non-whites *(95)*. These sex-specific data on treatment effects of heart failure therapies have been limited. A meta-analysis of 12 ACEI and beta-blocker trials has suggested that ACEI were not as beneficial in women as compared to men. Pooled random effects estimates for reduction in mortality yielded 0.82 (95% CI 0.74–0.90) for men and 0.92 (95% CI 0.81–1.04) for women *(96)*. Analysis of the prevention arm of SOLVD suggested ACEI use in prevention of HF progression in women was less beneficial *(96)*. Beta-blockers were shown to have similar efficacy in both men and women in reducing mortality in symptomatic heart failure *(96)*. However, the numbers of women in these studies were small thus leaving unanswered the question whether the difference was a real biologic difference or an effect of inadequate sample size *(96)*.

Pooled analysis of SOLVD prevention and treatment trials showed no difference in mortality benefit from enalapril in black and white patients but there was a 44% reduction in risk of hospitalization for heart failure in whites compared to blacks, suggesting there may be significant effects of race on the benefits of heart failure medications *(97)*. In another study, there was a 5.8% higher absolute risk of all-cause mortality in women compared to men taking digoxin *(98)*. Retrospective analysis of the Digitalis Investigation Group (DIG) trial suggested increased mortality in women with serum digoxin concentrations in the range of 1.2–2 ng/ml but there was a beneficial effect of digoxin on morbidity at serum concentrations from 0.5 to 0.9 ng/ml *(99)*. Progestin may increase serum digoxin levels by inhibiting P-glycoprotein and decreasing the excretion of digoxin. This may contribute to higher serum digoxin levels and thus increased toxicity in women *(98)*.

Brachial artery reactivity studies comparing blacks and whites have shown decreased flow-mediated dilation in blacks *(100,101)*. Data from the Vasodilator Heart Failure Trial (V-HeFT) I and II suggested that an hydralazine/isosorbide dinitrate combination has greater mortality benefits in blacks compared to whites, but the benefit of enalapril was not as pronounced in blacks *(102)*.

The A-HeFT trial addressed this issue further and showed that in African-American patients with NYHA Class III or IV heart failure, the addition of fixed dose of hydralazine plus isosorbide dinitrate to standard neurohormonal inhibition improved survival, hospitalizations, and quality of life

(103). The A-HeFT had 40% women and provides the only data for this ther-apy in women. Subgroup analysis showed the therapy to be highly effective in women *(104)*.

9. CONCLUSION

Cardiovascular disease in minority women is becoming increasingly an area of clinical concern with a need for further research. Among tradi-tional risk factors, obesity and associated metabolic syndromes are dispro-portionate in non-Hispanic black women and Mexican American women. Abdominal obesity, with increases in visceral fat is directly related to inflam-matory markers, dyslipidemia, and associated risk. Hypertension is much more common in African-Americans and increases among postmenopausal women of all races and ethnicities. Similarly, left ventricular hypertrophy is more common in African-American women compared to Caucasian women. Diabetes is more common in certain racial/ethnic minority women with severe consequences. Sedentary lifestyle also contributes to cardiac risk, especially in women. Non-traditional risk factors, including high sensitivity to C-reactive protein, anemia, and retinal artery disease are important emerg-ing areas of clinical research related to cardiovascular disease in women. In the clinical assessment of women, unique consideration should be utilized in performing stress testing, SPECT imaging, stress echocardiography, and coronary calcium storing. Variation in symptoms with coronary heart disease and unique aspects of heart failure in women continue to emerge. Ongoing and future clinical studies must include adequate representation of women, especially underrepresented minorities to further refine clinical approaches in therapies.

REFERENCES

1. Rosamond W, Flega K, Friday G, et al., for the American heart association statistics committee and stroke statistics subcommittee. Heart disease and stroke statistics—2007 Update: A Report from the American Heart Association Statistics Committee and Stroke Statistics Subcommittee. *Circulation* 2007; 115(5):e69–e171.
2. Winkleby MA, Kraemer HC, Ahn DK, et al. Ethnic and socioeconomic differ-ences in cardiovascular disease risk factors: Findings for women from the Third National Health and Nutrition Examination Survey, 1988–1994. *JAMA* 1998; 280(4): 356–362.
3. Howard BV, Lee ET, Cowan LD, et al. Rising tide of cardiovascular disease in American Indians. The Strong Heart Study. *Circulation* 1999; 99(18):2389–2395.
4. Bild DE, Deliano R, Peterson D. Ethnic differences in coronary calcification: the Multi-Ethnic Study of Atherosclerosis (MESA). *Circulation* 2005; 111(10):1313–1320.
5. Thom T, Haase N, Rosamond W, et al. Heart disease and stroke statistics—2006 Update: a report from the American Heart Association Statistics Committee and Stroke Statistics Subcommittee. *Circulation* 2006; 113(6):e85–e151.

6. Mosca L, Ferris A, Fabunmi R, et al. Tracking women's awareness of heart disease: An American Heart Association National Study. *Circulation* 2004; 109(5):573–579.

7. DuBard CA, Garrett J, Gizlice Z. Effect of language on heart attack and stroke awareness among U.S. hispanics. *Am J Prev Med* 2006; 30(3):189–196.

8. Mosca L, Mochari H, Christian A, et al. National study of women's awareness, preventive action, and barriers to cardiovascular health. *Circulation* 2006; 113(4):525–534.

9. Mosca L, Linfante AH, Benjamin EJ. National study of physician awareness and adherence to cardiovascular disease prevention guidelines. *Circulation* 2005; 111(4): 499–510.

10. Hedley AA, Ogden CL, Johnson CL, et al. Prevalence of overweight and obesity among U.S. children, adolescents, and adults, 1999–2002. *JAMA* 2004; 291(23):2847–2850.

11. Wajchenberg BL. Subcutaneous and visceral adipose tissue: their relation to the metabolic syndrome. *Endocr Rev* 2000; 21(6):697–738.

12. Regitz-Zagrosek V, Lehmkuhl E, Weickert MO. Gender differences in the metabolic syndrome and their role for cardiovascular disease. *Clin Res Cardiol* 2006; 95(3): 136–147.

13. Lau DC, Dhillon B, Yan H, et al. Adipokines: molecular links between obesity and atherosclerosis. *Am J Physiol Heart Circ Physiol* 2005; 288(5):H2031–2041.

14. Gupta M, Singh N, Verma S. South Asians and cardiovascular risk: what clinicians should know. *Circulation* 2006; 113(25):e924–e929.

15. Powers DR, Wallin JD. End-Stage renal disease in specific ethnic and racial groups: Risk factors and benefit of antihypertensive therapy. *Arch Intern Med* 1998; 158(7):793–800.

16. Oparil S. Women and hypertension: what did we learn from the women's health initiative? *Cardiol Rev* 2006; 14(6):267–275.

17. Wright JT. Outcomes in hypertensive black and non-black patients treated with chlorthalidone, amlodipine, and lisinopril. *JAMA* 2005; 293(13):1595–1608.

18. Douglas JG, Bakris GL, Epstein M, et al. Management of high blood pressure in African Americans: Consensus Statement of the Hypertension in African Americans Working Group of the International Study on Hypertension in Blacks. *Arch Intern Med* 2003; 163(5):525–541.

19. Drazner MH, Dries DL, Peschock RM, et al. Left ventricular hypertrophy is more prevalent in blacks than whites in the general population: The Dallas Heart Study. *Hypertension* 2005; 46(1).124–129.

20. Levy D, Garrison RJ, Savage DD, et al. Prognostic implications of echocardiographically determined left ventricular mass in the Framingham heart study. *N Engl J Med* 1990; 322(22):1561–1566.

21. Drazner MH, Rame JE, Marino EK, et al. Increased left ventricular mass is a risk factor for the development of a depressed left ventricular ejection fraction within five years: the Cardiovascular Health Study. *J Am Coll Cardiol* 2004; 43(12):2207–2215.

22. Lee WL, Cheung AM, Cape D, et al. Impact of diabetes on coronary artery disease in women and men: a meta-analysis of prospective studies. *Diabetes Care* 2000; 23(7):962–968.

23. Franco OH, Steyerberg EW, Hu FB. Associations of diabetes mellitus with total life expectancy with and without cardiovascular disease. *Arch Intern Med* 2007; 167(11):1145–1151.

24. Steinberg HO, Paradisi G, Cronin J, et al. Type II diabetes abrogates sex differences in endothelial function in premenopausal women. *Circulation* 2000; 101(17): 2040–2046.

25. Koh KK, Kang MH, Jin DK, et al. Vascular effects of estrogen in type II diabetic postmenopausal women. *JACC* 2001; 38(5):1409–1415.

26. Wexler DJ, Grant RW, Meigs JB, et al. Sex disparities in treatment of cardiac risk factors in patients with type II diabetes. *Diabet Care* 2005; 28(3):514–520.

27. Centers for Disease Control and Prevention. Smoking and tobacco use. (Accessed September 2007 at http://www.cdc.gov/tobacco)

28. Willett WC, Green A, Stampfer MJ, et al. Relative and absolute excess risks of coronary heart disease among women who smoke cigarettes. *NEJM* 1987; 317(21): 1303–1309.

29. Kawachi I, Colditz GA, Stampfer MJ, et al. Smoking cessation and time course of decreased risks of coronary heart disease in middle-aged women. *Arch Intern Med* 1994; 154(2):169–175.

30. Kaur S, Cohen A, Color R, et al. The impact of environmental tobacco smoke on women's risk of dying from heart disease: a Meta-Analysis. *J Womens Health (Larchmt)* 2004; 13(8):888–897.

31. Centers for Disease Control and Prevention. early release of selected estimates based on data from the 2007 National health interview survey. (Accessed September 14, 2008 at http://www.cdc.gov/nchs/data/nhis/earlyrelease/200709˙07.pdf)

32. Mosca L, Manson JE, Sutherland SE, et al. Cardiovascular disease in women: a statement for healthcare professionals from the American heart association writing group. *Circulation* 1997; 96(7):2468–2482.

33. Lemaitre RN, Heckbert SR, Psaty BM, et al. Leisure-time physical activity and the risk of nonfatal myocardial infarction in postmenopausal women. *Arch Intern Med* 1995; 155(21):2302–2308.

34. Krummel DA, Koffman DM, Bronner Y, et al. Cardiovascular health interventions in women: what works? *J Womens Health Gend Based Med* 2001; 10(2):117–136.

35. Ridker PM, Buring JE, Shih J, et al. Prospective study of C-reactive protein and the risk of future cardiovascular events among apparently health women. *Circulation* 1998; 98(8):731–733.

36. Ridker PM, Rifai N, Rose L, et al. Comparison of C-reactive protein and low-density lipoprotein cholesterol levels in the prediction of first cardiovascular events. *N Engl J Med* 2002; 347(20):1557–1565.

37. Mora S, Ridker PM. Justification for the use of statin in primary prevention: an intervention trial evaluating rosuvastatin (JUPITER)—can C-reactive protein be used to target statin therapy in primary prevention? *Am J Cardiol* 2006; 97(2A):33A–41A.

38. Pai JK, Pischon T, Ma J, et al. Inflammatory markers and the risk of coronary heart disease in men and women. *N Engl J Med* 2004; 351(25):2599–2610.

39. Vlagopoulos PT, Tighiouart H, Weiner DE, et al. Anemia as a risk factor for cardiovascular disease and all-cause mortality in diabetes: the impact of chronic kidney disease. *J Am Soc Nephrol* 2005; 16(11):3403–3410.

40. Muntner P, He J, Astor BC, et al. Traditional and nontraditional risk factors predict coronary heart disease in chronic kidney disease: results from the atherosclerosis risk in communities study. *J Am Soc Nephrol* 2005; 16(2):529–538.

41. Arant CB, Wessel TR, Olson MB, et al., for the National Heart, Lung, and Blood Institute Women's Ischemia Syndrome Evaluation Study. Hemoglobin level is an independent predictor for adverse cardiovascular outcomes in women undergoing evaluation for chest pain: results from the National Heart, Lung, and Blood Institute Women's Ischemia Syndrome Evaluation Study. *J Am Coll Cardiol* 2004; 43(11): 2009–2014.

42. Tedeschi-Reiner E, Strozzi M, Skoric B, et al. Relation of atherosclerotic changes in retinal arteries to the extent of coronary artery disease. *Am J Cardiol* 2005; 96(8): 1107–1109.

43. Bressler NM. Retinal arteriolar narrowing and risk of coronary heart disease. *Arch Ophthalmol* 2003; 121(1):113–114.

44. Wong TY, Klein R, Sharrett AR, et al. Retinal arteriolar narrowing and risk of coronary heart disease in men and women. The Atherosclerosis Risk in Communities Study. *JAMA* 2002; 287(9):1153–1159.

45. Palaniappan L, Anthony MN, Mahesh C, et al. Cardiovascular risk factors in ethnic minority women aged < or = 30 Years. *Am J Cardiol* 2002; 89(5):524–529.

46. Berglund L, Ramakrishnan R. Lipoprotein(a): an elusive cardiovascular risk factor. *Arterioscler Thromb Vasc Biol* 2004; 24(12):2219–2226.

47. de Gaetano G; Collaborative Group of the Primary Prevention Project. Low-dose aspirin and Vitamin E in people at cardiovascular risk: a randomised trial in general practice. Collaborative Group of the Primary Prevention Project. *Lancet* 2001; 357(9250):89–95.

48. Lee IM, Cook NR, Gaziano JM, et al. Vitamin E in the primary prevention of cardiovascular disease and cancer: the women's health study: a randomized controlled trial. *JAMA* 2005; 294(1):56–65.

49. Ridker PM, Cook NR, Lee IM, et al. A randomized trial of low-dose aspirin in the primary prevention of cardiovascular disease in women. *N Engl J Med* 2005; 352(13):1293–1304.

50. Berger JS, Roncaglioni MC, Avanzini F, et al. Aspirin for the primary prevention of cardiovascular events in women and men: a sex-specific meta-analysis of randomized controlled trials. *JAMA* 2006; 295(3):306–313.

51. The Writing Group for the PEPI Trial. Effects of estrogen or estrogen/progestin regimens on heart disease risk factors in postmenopausal women. The Postmenopausal Estrogen/Progestin Interventions (PEPI) Trial. The Writing Group for the PEPI Trial. *JAMA* 1995; 273(3):199–208.

52. Manson JE, Hsia J, Johnson KC, et al. Estrogen plus progestin and the risk of coronary heart disease. *N Engl J Med* 2003; 349(6):523–534.

53. Hulley S, Grady D, Bush T, et al. Randomized trial of estrogen plus progestin for secondary prevention of coronary heart disease in postmenopausal women. Heart and Estrogen/progestin Replacement Study (HERS) Research Group. *JAMA* 1998; 280(7):605–613.

54. Ouyang P, Michos ED, Karas RH. Hormone replacement therapy and the cardiovascular system lessons learned and unanswered questions. *J Am Coll Cardiol* 2006; 47(9):1741–1753.

55. Rossouw JE, Prentice RL, Manson JE, et al. Postmenopausal hormone therapy and risk of cardiovascular disease by age and years since menopause. *JAMA* 2007; 297(13):1465–1477.

56. Shaw LJ, Bairey Merz CN, Pepine CJ, et al. the WISE Investigators. Insights from the NHLBI-Sponsored Women's Ischemia Syndrome Evaluation (WISE) Study: Part I: gender differences in traditional and novel risk factors, symptom evaluation, and gender-optimized diagnostic strategies. *J Am Coll Cardiol* 2006; 47(3 Suppl.): S4–S20.

57. Kwok Y, Kim C, Grady D, et al. Meta-analysis of exercise testing to detect coronary artery disease in women. *Am J Cardiol* 1999; 83(5):660–666.

58. Lloyd GW, Patel NR, McGing E, et al. Does angina vary with the menstrual cycle in women with premenopausal coronary artery disease? *Heart* 2000; 84(2): 189–192.

59. Shaw LJ, Olson MB, Kip K, et al. The value of estimated functional capacity in estimating outcome: results from the NHLBI-Sponsored Women's Ischemia Syndrome Evaluation (WISE) Study. *J Am Coll Cardiol* 2006; 47(3 Suppl.):S36–S43.

60. Mora S, Redberg RF, Cui Y, et al. Ability of exercise testing to predict cardiovascular and all-cause death in asymptomatic women: a 20-year follow-up of the lipid research clinics prevalence study. *JAMA* 2003; 290(12):1600–1607.

61. Pancholy SB, Fattah AA, Kamal AM, et al. Independent and incremental prognostic value of exercise thallium single-photon emission computed tomographic imaging in women. *J Nucl Cardiol* 1995; 2:110–116.

62. Hansen CL, Crabbe D, Rubin S. Lower diagnostic accuracy of Thallium-201 SPECT myocardial perfusion imaging in women: an effect of small chamber size. *J Am Coll Cardiol* 1996; 28(5):1214–1219.

63. Beller GA, Zaret BL. Contributions of nuclear cardiology to diagnosis and prognosis of patients with coronary artery disease. *Circulation* 2000; 101(12):1465–1478.

64. Taillefer R, DePuey EG, Udelson JE, et al. Comparative diagnostic accuracy of TI-201 and Tc-99m Sestamibi SPECT imaging (perfusion and ECG-gated SPECT) in detecting coronary artery disease in women. *J Am Coll Cardiol* 1997; 29(1): 69–77.

65. Marwick TH, Shaw LJ, Lauer MS, et al. The noninvasive prediction of cardiac mortality in men and women with known or suspected coronary artery disease. Economics of Noninvasive Diagnosis (END) Study Group. *Am J Med* 1999; 106(2)172–178.

66. Boyne TS, Koplan BA, Parsons WJ, et al. Predicting adverse outcome with exercise SPECT Technetium-99m Sestamibi imaging in patients with suspected or known coronary artery disease. *Am J Cardiol* 1997; 79(3):270–274.

67. Arruda-Olson AM, Juracan EM, Mahoney DW, et al. Prognostic value of exercise echocardiography in 5798 patients: is there a gender difference? *J Am Coll Cardiol* 2002; 39(4):625–631.

68. Roger VL, Pellikka PA, Bell MR, et al. Sex and test verification bias. Impact on the diagnostic value of exercise echocardiography. *Circulation* 1997; 95(2):405–410.

69. Williams MJ, Marwick TH, O'Gorman D, et al. Comparison of exercise echocardiography with an exercise score to diagnose coronary artery disease in women. *Am J Cardiol* 1994; 74(5):435–438.

70. Ho YL, Wu CC, Huang PJ, et al. Assessment of coronary artery disease in women by dobutamine stress echocardiography: comparison with stress Shallium-201 single-photon emission computed tomography and exercise electrocardiography. *Am Heart J* 1998; 135(4):655–662.

71. Kim C, Kwok YS, Heagerty P, et al. Pharmacologic stress testing for coronary disease diagnosis: a meta-analysis. *Am Heart J* 2001; 142(6):934–944.

72. Tong AT, Douglas PS. Stress echocardiography in women. *Cardiol Clin* 1999; 17(3):573–582.

73. Detrano R, Hsiai T, Wang, S, et al. Prognostic value of coronary calcification and angiographic stress stenoses in patients undergoing coronary angiography. *J Am Coll Cardiol* 1996; 27(2):285–290.

74. Georgiou D, Budoff MJ, Kaufer E, et al. Screening patients with chest pain in the emergency department using electron beam tomography: a follow-up study. *J Am Coll Cardiol* 2001; 38(1):105–110.

75. Manson JE, Allison MA, Rossouw JE, et al., for the WHI and WHI-CACS Investigators. Estrogen therapy and coronary-artery calcification. *N Engl J Med* 2007; 356(25):2591–2602.

76. Becker A, Leber A, von Ziegler F, et al. Comparison of progression of coronary calcium in postmenopausal women on versus not on Estrogen/progestin therapy. *Am J Cardiol* 2007; 99(3):374–378.

77. Nasir K, Redberg RF, Budof MJ, et al. Utility of stress testing and coronary calcification measurement for detection of coronary artery disease in women. *Arch Intern Med* 2004; 164(15):1610–1620.

78. Vaccarino V, Parsons L, Every NR, et al. Sex-based differences in early mortality after myocardial infarction. National Registry of Myocardial Infarction 2 Participants. *N Engl J Med* 1999; 341(4):217–225.
79. Chaitman BR, Bourassa MG, Davis K, et al. Angiographic prevalence high-risk coronary artery disease in patient subsets (CASS). *Circulation* 1981; 64(2):360–367.
80. Hochman JS, Tamis JE, Thompson TD, et al. Sex, clinical presentation, and outcome in patients with acute coronary syndromes. global use of strategies to open occluded coronary arteries in acute coronary syndromes IIb investigators. *N Engl J Med* 1999; 341(4):226–232.
81. Diver DJ, Bier JD, Ferreira PE, et al. Clinical and arteriographic characterization of patients with unstable angina without critical coronary arterial narrowing (from the TIMI-IIIA Trial). *Am J Cardiol* 1994; 74(6):531–537.
82. Widlansky ME, Gokce N, Keaney JF, Jr, et al. The clinical implications of endothelial dysfunction. *J Am Coll Cardiol* 2003; 42(7):1149–1160.
83. von Mering GO, Arant CB, Wessel TR, et al. Abnormal coronary vasomotion as a prognostic indicator of cardiovascular events in women: results from the National Heart, Lung, and Blood Institute-Sponsored Women's Ischemia Syndrome Evaluation (WISE). *Circulation* 2004; 109(6):722–725.
84. Buchthal SD, den Hollander JA, Merz CN, et al. Abnormal myocardial phosphorus-31 nuclear magnetic resonance spectroscopy in women with chest pain but normal coronary angiograms. *N Engl J Med* 2000; 342(12):829–835.
85. Johnson BD, Shaw LJ, Buchthal SD, et al. Prognosis in women with Myocardial ischemia in the absence of obstructive coronary disease: results from the National Institutes of Health-National Heart, Lung, and Blood Institute-Sponsored Women's Ischemia Syndrome Evaluation (WISE). *Circulation* 2004; 109(24):2993–2999.
86. Bugiardini R, Bairey Merz CN. Angina with "Normal" coronary arteries: a changing philosophy. *JAMA* 2005; 293(4):477–484.
87. Bugiardini R, Manfrini O, Pizzi C, et al. Endothelial function predicts future development of coronary artery disease: a study of women with chest pain and normal coronary angiograms. *Circulation* 2004; 109(21):2518–2523.
88. Brown DW, Haldeman GA, Croft JB, et al. Racial or ethnic differences in hospitalization for heart failure among elderly adults: Medicare, 1990 to 2000. *Am Heart J* 2005; 150(3):448–454.
89. Wilson PW. An epidemiologic perspective of systemic hypertension, ischemic heart disease, and heart failure. *Am J Cardiol* 1997; 80(9B):3J–8J.
90. Dries DL, Exner DV, Gersh BJ, et al. Racial differences in the outcome of left ventricular dysfunction. *N Engl J Med* 1999; 340(8):609–616.
91. Adams KF, Jr, Dunlap SH, Sueta CA, et al. Relation between gender, etiology, and survival in patients with symptomatic heart failure. *J Am Coll Cardiol* 1996; 28(7): 1781–1788.
92. Vaccarino V, Chen VT, Wang Y, et al. Sex differences in the clinical care and outcomes of congestive heart failure in the elderly. *Am Heart J* 1999; 138(5 Pt 1):835–842.
93. Bursi F, Weston SA, Redfield MM, et al. Systolic and diastolic heart failure in the community. *JAMA* 2006; 296(18):2209–2216.
94. Yancy CW. Heart failure in African Americans: pathophysiology and treatment. *J Card Fail* 2003; 9(5 Suppl. Nitric Oxide):S210–S215.
95. Heiat A, Gross CP, Krumholz HM. Representation of the elderly, women, and minorities in heart failure clinical trials. *Arch Intern Med* 2002; 162(15):1682–1688.
96. Shekelle PG, Rich MW, Morton SC, et al. Efficacy of angiotensin-converting enzyme inhibitors and beta-blockers in the management of left ventricular systolic dysfunction according to race, gender, and diabetic status: a meta-analysis of major clinical trials. *J Am Coll Cardiol* 2003; 41(9):1529–1538.

97. Exner DV, Dries DL, Domanski MJ, et al. Lesser response to angiotensin-converting-enzyme inhibitor therapy in black as compared to white patients with left ventricular dysfunction. *N Engl J Med* 2001; 344(18):1351–1357.
98. Rathore SS, Wang Y, Krumholz HM. Sex-based differences in the effect of digoxin for the treatment of heart failure. *N Engl J Med* 2002; 347(18):1403–1411.
99. Adams KF, Jr, Patterson JH, Gattis WA, et al. Relationship of serum digoxin concentration to mortality and morbidity in women in the digitalis investigation group trial: a retrospective analysis. *J Am Coll Cardiol* 2005; 46(3):497–504.
100. Campia U, Choucair WK, Bryant MB, et al. Reduced endothelium-dependent and independent dilation of conductance arteries in African Americans. *J Am Coll Cardiol* 2002; 40(4):754–760.
101. Cardillo C, Kilcoyne CM, Cannon RO 3rd, et al. Attenuation of cyclic nucleotide-mediated smooth muscle relaxation in blacks as a cause of racial differences in vasodilator function. *Circulation* 1999; 99(1):90–95.
102. Carson P, Ziesche S, Johnson G, et al. Racial differences in response to therapy for heart failure: analysis of the vasodilator-heart failure trials. Vasodilator-Heart Failure Trial Study Group. *J Card Fail* 1999; 5(3):178–187.
103. Taylor A, Ziesche S, Yancy C, et al., for the African-American Heart Failure Trial Investigators. Combination of isosorbide dinitrate and hydralazine in blacks with heart failure. *N Engl J Med* 2004; 351(20):2049–2057.
104. Taylor AL, Lindenfeld J, Ziesche S, et al., for the A-HeFT Investigators. Outcomes by gender in the African-American Heart Failure Trial. *JACC* 2006; 48(11):2263–2267.

SUBJECT INDEX

321